THE PRINCIPLES AND PRACTICAL APPLICATION
OF ACUPUNCTURE POINT COMBINATIONS

of related interest

The Living Needle
Modern Acupuncture Technique
Justin Phillips
ISBN 978 1 84819 381 9
eISBN 978 0 85701 339 2

The Fundamentals of Acupuncture
Nigel Ching
Foreword by Charles Buck
ISBN 978 1 84819 313 0
eISBN 978 0 85701 266 1

Developing Internal Energy for Effective Acupuncture Practice
Zhan Zhuang, Yi Qi Gong and the Art of Painless Needle Insertion
Ioannis Solos
ISBN 978 1 84819 183 9
eISBN 978 0 85701 144 2

Intuitive Acupuncture
John Hamwee
ISBN 978 1 84819 273 7
eISBN 978 0 85701 220 3

The Spark in the Machine
How the Science of Acupuncture Explains the Mysteries of Western Medicine
Dr. Daniel Keown MBChB MCEM LicAc
ISBN 978 1 84819 196 9
eISBN 978 0 85701 154 1

THE PRINCIPLES AND PRACTICAL APPLICATION OF ACUPUNCTURE POINT COMBINATIONS

David Hartmann

Foreword by John McDonald

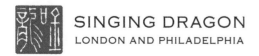

SINGING DRAGON
LONDON AND PHILADELPHIA

First published in 2020
by Singing Dragon
an imprint of Jessica Kingsley Publishers
73 Collier Street
London N1 9BE, UK
and
400 Market Street, Suite 400
Philadelphia, PA 19106, USA

www.singingdragon.com

Library of Congress Cataloging in Publication Data
Names: Hartmann, David, author.
Title: The principles and practical application of acupuncture point
    combinations / David Hartmann.
Description: London ; Philadelphia : Jessica Kingsley Publishers, 2020. |
    Includes bibliographical references and index.
Identifiers: LCCN 2018059823 | ISBN 9781848193956
Subjects: | MESH: Acupuncture Points
Classification: LCC RM184.5 | NLM WB 369.5.M5 | DDC 615.8/92--
dc23 LC record available at https://lccn.loc.gov/2018059823

British Library Cataloguing in Publication Data
A CIP catalogue record for this book is available from the British Library

ISBN 978 1 84819 395 6
eISBN 978 0 85701 352 1

Printed and bound by CPI Group (UK) Ltd, Croydon, CR0 4YY

Contents

Foreword

In the education and training of acupuncturists, it has been my experience as a teacher over more than four decades that it is much more difficult to teach process than content. There are two vital process steps with which I have seen many students struggle. The first is transforming a list of signs and symptoms and clinical observations into a Traditional Chinese Medicine (TCM) pattern differentiation (or other diagnostic conclusion). The second is constructing the most appropriate acupuncture point combination to address the specific health needs of the presenting patient.

This new book by David Hartmann is a very valuable contribution to assist not only students but even veteran practitioners with the thinking processes which underpin creating optimal acupuncture point combinations.

In the words of the author, do you want to be a cook following a recipe or do you want to be a chef creating unique dishes? Of course, most chefs reach their level of culinary expertise by first familiarizing themselves with the best recipes from the past, much as acupuncturists begin with tried-and-true acupuncture point combinations from the historical literature of the last two millennia. This historical acupuncture literature is an extremely valuable but often under-valued resource. To put our Chinese medicine history into context, very few pharmaceuticals in current use have a recorded history of use extending back more than 50 years, whereas we have access to the treatment recommendations of hundreds of famous doctors from competing schools of thought, with their commentaries on each other's treatment approaches, spanning more than 2000 years.

To make the best use of historical literature, however, we must learn to understand the thinking behind each acupuncture formula, so that we can distill the principles of acupuncture point combination. The author has outlined many different approaches to acupuncture point combination, including Zàng Fǔ pattern-based approaches, Wǔ Xíng (Five Element) approaches, Six Division (Channel) combinations and many of the traditional point combination principles (left and right, above and below, front and back, four limbs, chain of points along a channel, etc.). Each point combination method is illustrated with a clinical example, which is helpful in an area which can easily become confusing. Some of these point combinations are common, but a lot of them are more obscure, and rarely taught in TCM institutions. The writing style is more conversational than academic, but this is quite appropriate for making this information easily accessible for the reader. In fact, this conversational tone assists the author in the challenging task of bringing some of the historical point combinations to the reader in a fresh and uncomplicated manner.

This is not a book to be read through once and then put on the library shelf. It is a book to come back to many times, and each time it is likely that the reader will come away with some fresh ideas about how to combine points.

This book embodies the true definition of 'education', from the Latin *educare*, to lead out. This is a book that does not tell you what to think, but how to think about acupuncture point combination.

David's book fills an important gap in the acupuncture literature. The process of critically collating, organizing and sharing specific information from historical acupuncture literature is a vital task for a living, growing medicine with deep roots. David Hartmann shares my twin passions for history and research, both of which are fundamental to the future development of acupuncture.

John McDonald, PhD

Acknowledgements

First and foremost, I would like to thank my amazing family – in particular my wife, Amanda, and my kids, Abby, Olivia and Jessie. I would also like to thank my mum. You are all so special to me in ways too numerous to count and mention here. I love you all dearly and I thank you for your patience and understanding while I was writing this book.

Second, I would like to thank John McDonald for being, well, John McDonald. Your foreword was amazing and humbling, and I thank you for taking the time to read my original transcripts. Ever since I started studying Chinese medicine in 1993, you have been there for me, and I can't possibly thank you enough for being that person.

I also have to thank two people that got this project off the ground to begin with: Georgina Black and Claire Wilson. Georgina has always encouraged me to write and teach, and she found me the contact details for Claire Wilson, senior commissioning editor at Singing Dragon. By an awesome twist of fate, Claire was working at Elsevier when my *Acupoint Dictionary* was published in 2009, so she had a base level to work off for my writing. Thank you both for everything you have done to date, and for the future, which I know will be bright and beautiful.

I have to thank Amie Whittington, Joshua Brookes, Kathleen Crow, Chris Fehres and Megan Davern for proofreading the different chapters in this book. I can say, with complete honesty, that I wouldn't have finished the book on time without you all. Further, you spotted my spelling errors, punctuation issues and errors in past tense/present tense – one of the banes of my writing life. Ha!

When I was mulling this project around in my brain, I had a few people who allowed me to use them as a sounding board – those people were Megan Davern, Murray Barton, Joshua Brookes, Amie Whittington, Chris Fehres, my mother, Toni Cross, and my lovely wife, Amanda. Without your silence, and then suggestions, this book wouldn't have been half as good. Thank you all so much for that.

Thank you to Amie Whittington and Joshua Brookes for your help with referencing. This was always going to be a huge challenge, but I really wanted to use a wide range of different sources. I couldn't have managed it all on my own.

Big thanks must go to Amie Whittington, my daughters, Abby and Olivia, and my mum, Toni Cross, for constructing the appendices, and my wife, Amanda, for helping me with the images. I appreciate that the images are a little raw, but I think it really adds to the flavor and feel of the book.

Thanks also to Patrick Wang, Li Li, Jefferson Wang and Cathy Wang for helping me with the traditional Chinese characters and the Pīn Yīn, as well as directing me to some awesome websites that helped me navigate this perilous project. I really wanted this book to be available to as many people across the planet as possible, so I felt it very important to provide the reader with a range of different tools for learning. I hope that I have done it justice. Any errors in Pīn Yīn or traditional Chinese characters are mine alone.

I also need to thank Tania Durham and Amie Whittington for their assistance with computers. Although I can type quite fast, I have minimal knowledge about computers and what they can do. I think my favorite was using 'Control F' – my goodness, the hours that saved me.

I know I will have missed some people out and for that I am sorry. Please know, anyone who has been in my life, that I value you dearly and thank you for being who you are.

Disclaimer

The calligraphy of the traditional Chinese characters used for the front cover was something that my daughters Abby and Olivia helped me with. Apart from the stress of doing a good job, the three of us had quite a bit of fun. Although I appreciate the effort we made was far from perfect, I can assure you we tried our best.

As I stated in my acknowledgements, there may be times where my Pīn Yīn (along with the tone lines) and traditional Chinese characters are wrong. I have tried to avoid that happening. If it has occurred, I apologize.

After a lengthy process, I decided on using the traditional Chinese characters rather than the simplified because I wanted to honor Chinese traditions. I want to see the traditional Chinese characters survive into the future, in the same way that I want to see the Aboriginal culture in Australia stay true to its origins of language. Too many languages are being lost around the world.

Finally, when specific authors and quotations are found in the text, I have referenced there; I chose the endnote referencing style for everything else, because I didn't want the flow of my paragraphs to be disrupted by continual written referencing. By simply having a number, the reader can finish the paragraph and then flip to the end of the chapter to check the reference (or additional comments) if they so wish.

Abbreviations and the Appendices

As with any Chinese medicine book, it's very hard to decide what terms should be in English, which terms should be Pīn Yīn and which should be abbreviated. For the most part I have used English terms, referring to the WHO (2007) book *WHO International Standard Terminologies on Traditional Medicine in the Western Pacific Region.*

For the acupuncture points, I have also used the recommended abbreviations from the WHO book – for example, TE for Triple Energizer or Sān Jiāo. Therefore, you will see an acupuncture point written as TE 5; you won't see it written as Triple Energizer 5 or Sān Jiāo 5, or Wài Guān, or 外關.

If you refer to Appendix 2 or 3, you will see each point written in its entirety, including the abbreviation, full English title, Pīn Yīn and the traditional Chinese character.

When considering the use of other key terms, there were times when I thought that the best term I could use was actually the Pīn Yīn term – for example, Shén, as opposed to spirit or mind.

Every single term used, whether in English, Pīn Yīn or its abbreviated self, has been included in Appendices 1–3:

- Appendix 1: Key Terms – English, Pīn Yīn and Traditional Chinese Characters

- Appendix 2: Acupuncture Point Terms – English, Pīn Yīn and Traditional Chinese Characters

- Appendix 3: Acupuncture Point Terms – Pīn Yīn, English and Traditional Chinese Characters

There are two further appendices:

- Appendix 4: Cautions and Contraindications When Using Acupuncture

- Appendix 5: Special Point Category Tables

Preface

The Master said, 'Learn as if you were following someone whom you could not catch up, as though it were someone you were frightened of losing.'

Confucius/Kǒng Zǐ/孔子 (551–479 BCE)[1]

My pathway into a career in Chinese medicine wasn't straightforward. My original plan was to study physiotherapy but this required quite a high mark in the Australian higher school certificate and I didn't quite get the marks I needed in 1991 (my final year of schooling). Therefore, I had a fallback plan, and this was to leave home, which was in a small coastal town called Bonny Hills in New South Wales, Australia, and move up to the Whitsundays (North Queensland) where I would work in the hospitality industry on one of the dozens of island resorts.

It soon became apparent that if I wanted to make a career out of hospitality, then I needed to study first. I found a course in Sydney and moved there for six months. It didn't work out, so I moved back home for a while and helped a friend of the family build a mud-brick house.

By early 1993 I hadn't really achieved much and so I knew I had to leave my small town for a bigger city. Sydney had burnt me, so I tried Brisbane, Queensland. One of Mum's friends had a daughter looking for a flatmate and I jumped at the chance. That arrangement didn't last long and I ended up in shared accommodation with a bunch of guys. It was during this house move that Mum came and helped me. On her trip back to Bonny Hills (a six-and-a half-hour drive) the front windscreen of her car shattered just outside Coffs Harbour (4 hours). This was quite an impressive feat considering her car was fitted with a shatterproof windscreen.

She found a mechanic and, while she waited for the car to be repaired, went and got a cup of tea from a café nearby. Looking for something to read, she came across a pamphlet for a natural medicine institution called Australian College of Natural Medicine (now called Endeavour College of Natural Health) which was located in Brisbane. Mum had an epiphany, and when her windscreen was repaired she didn't drive home – she drove back to Brisbane.

We booked an interview with the college and it just seemed perfect. I chose acupuncture rather than one of the other natural medicines because I had received treatment with it in the past and had marveled at the results. There was just one problem – neither Mum nor I had any money and the semester fees had to be paid upfront. We tried a few banks for personal loans but we found out you can't borrow money if you don't have money to begin with. Dad was also unable to help, so I tried my dad's dad, Grandpa.

Grandpa had seven kids and 21 grandkids, so I wasn't hopeful, but I have always been of the view that you don't know if you don't try. So I tried and Grandpa loaned me money.

Meanwhile, I found a casual job, in hospitality, and started the course, and the most amazing thing happened. I loved it! I loved acupuncture and I got really high grades, too. The old saying that you do well at something you love couldn't have been more accurate.

I was a sponge and took it all in. When I graduated, I went back through all my textbooks and handwritten notes and pulled out all the clinically relevant content, which eventually became my first published textbook titled *Acupoint Dictionary*.

I also put any Chinese medicine theme that was barely discussed throughout the course into a different folder. These obscure medical ideas intrigued me and this folder allowed me the opportunity to work through each theme one at a time. Some of these included the Eight Extraordinary Vessels, Wǔ Xíng/Five Elements, the Shāng Hán Lùn/Treatise on Cold Injury and Acupuncture Point Combinations – how/why did the points work together in an acupuncture treatment?

Over time I have been compelled to know the how and the why. I knew the answers could be found in books and so I hit the books hard. Gradually, I started to learn how each acupuncture point on the body worked, and then why the different combinations had been chosen. Even so, it's still incredibly difficult to find detailed discussion about how/why the acupuncture point combinations work.

I'm not sure what it's like in other countries but in Australia, and specifically where I studied, students are taught how to diagnose patients using the Zàng Fǔ patterns. This results in a diagnosis for your patient, which then has a list of points used to treat that pattern of disharmony.

When I studied back in the mid-1990s, we weren't told how every single one of the points worked together (in combination) to achieve balance and harmony for our patients; we were just told that those were the best points! Some of the point combinations were explained but not all of them. For example, LR 3 and LI 4 were discussed as a combination, as were SP 6 and ST 36, and plenty of others. What was missing was how the *entire* point combination worked as a collective.

Even in the present day, the college still doesn't explain how all of the points work together in combinations. But that's not a slight on the college, because the course is so jam-packed full of incredible content that we can't, as lecturers, find the time to include this in the classes/clinics.

In the end, this dilemma has prompted me to write this book so that you, the reader, have a place to go that teaches you how to combine acupuncture points and, in so doing, create better treatment outcomes for your patients.

Before I sign off, I wanted to tell you that the acupuncture point combinations that fill this book are from four different sources:

- classical texts

- modern classics

- my own clinical experience

- a point combination from a classic text that is given a modern twist.

Regardless of the source, the point combinations are almost always explained, and will often include a step-by-step process so that you can see how the combination was constructed. This should then help you do the same thing in your own clinic.

I also hope you get three things out of reading this book:

- you learn something new

- you are reminded of something you had forgotten

- you learn how to construct your own acupuncture point combinations.

If I can do that, then I have achieved what I set out to do.

I really do hope that you enjoy this book on acupuncture point combinations. It has been a labor of love and I would be humbled and honored if you ended up loving it too.

Love and light to you all

David Hartmann

Note

1 Liang 1996, p.149. Confucius or Kǒng Zǐ (551–479 BCE) has become one of the most famous philosophers of all time, Eastern or Western. He became so popular in Europe in the Middle Ages that Western society latinized his name so they could pronounce it better. His popularity came about because he never proclaimed himself to be a god, and nothing that he said went directly against Christian beliefs in Western countries, where Christianity was still the ruling power of thought. He is, in my view, one of the most remarkable men to have ever lived.

Part 1

The Foundations of Acupuncture Point Combinations

I have a certain medicine –
I keep with me at all times,
I call it the wish-fulfilling jewel

Li Zhongzi (late 1500s to early 1600s CE)[1]

Welcome to Part 1 of *The Principles and Practical Application of Acupuncture Point Combinations*. In Chapters 1 and 2 I will be laying the groundwork for acupuncture point combinations. Chapter 1 outlines my treatment approach. I feel this is important because it gives you a sense of who I am as a therapist. Chapter 2 guides you through a better understanding of point combinations.

Note
1   Bertschinger 2013, p.35.

The physician is only nature's assistant.

Galen (129–216 CE)[1]

It is more important to know what sort of person has a disease than to know what sort of disease a person has.

Hippocrates (460–375 BCE)[2]

1

How I Treat Patients

I have a number of different treatment strategies that need some discussion. This will give you a better understanding of how/why my treatments are structured the way they are.

1. Potential new patient

Typically, I get new patients via phone calls, walk-ins or from friends' gatherings. The first thing I need to do is to convince the person that acupuncture can help them with their complaint. Sometimes this isn't hard because the person has had acupuncture before or because they have been referred to me by an existing patient.

Sometimes, however, it's difficult to convince them about the benefits of acupuncture. They could be worried about the needles hurting. They might be concerned about the cost of the treatment. They might even be convinced (by whom, I have no idea) that Chinese medicine only requires one treatment and their complaint will be healed.

As the 6th essay in *The Spiritual Pivot* (Líng Shū/靈樞)[3] guides us, 'For a disease of nine days, three acupuncture treatments. For a disease of a month, ten acupuncture treatments. More or less, near or far, treat in accord with the dimensions of the disease' (Wu 1993, p.32).

I'm not sure what your experience has been in other countries, but I have found that in Australia these are the typical concerns that potential new patients have when deciding whether to try acupuncture. But I don't shy away from these questions.

For starters, we know that acupuncture doesn't hurt very much, and I often say that an acupuncture needle is thinner than a strand of hair. I also mention that about one in every ten needles might bite a little – like a mosquito bite – but that the sensation goes away almost immediately.

As for cost, the Chinese medicine community in Australia charges very little compared with other medicines. If they need further explanation, then I might discuss the call-out costs of plumbers and electricians. Or I might mention the costs of seeing a naturopath initially and then the ongoing appointment/supplement costs. I may even discuss the ongoing costs of visiting a medical doctor (MD) or a general practitioner (GP).

The number of treatments that a new patient might need is not that simple to answer – it really is educated guesswork on our part. We can't be 100% certain that, for example, five weekly treatments will effectively treat a chronic cough they have had for six years. There are so many factors, known and unknown, which will determine whether five treatments are the magic number for that patient.

But we can draw on our experience in order to make our estimate more accurate. I never tell my patient they could be completely healed after one treatment. In fact, I tend to aim on the higher side when it comes to predicting the number of treatments they will need. I'd rather they got better earlier than my estimate rather than still only being 50% improved when we reach that number.

I don't want to shy away from the sometimes brutal reality of their complaint. If a potential patient has had a problem for more than 20 years, then it's just not ethical for me to say they could be better in a couple of months. I'd much prefer to explain the chronic nature of their complaint and advise a series of treatments across several treatment blocks. I would focus on their newer signs and symptoms, and explain that these should improve faster than the chronic ones. I would also talk to them about targeting these small victories throughout the treatment blocks because each of these improvements gets them closer to the *big heal*. I like metaphors, and so this is where I get them to visualize us both climbing a mountain: the healing of their body is the climb up, but also the descent down the other side.

The climb up is the hardest bit and is the bit we have to do first. The climb is where we focus on the little improvements – these are generally the more recent complaints that a patient has. The newer/acute disorders are almost always easier to treat than the old/chronic ones.

The same applies when we climb a mountain. We focus on the enjoyable little experiences along the way – the gorgeous flowers on the hillside, the subtle breeze gently rubbing the side of our face, the brief rest and snack under a shaded rocky outcrop, a pause to turn back and stare at the stunning view, even the feeling that we are achieving something of critical importance as we get closer to the top of the climb, the knowing in the back of our minds that it's going to be so much easier on the way back down.

As we climb the metaphorical mountain together, we tough it out together. We celebrate improvements in our patient's complaints. We know that as each of these complaints clears away, we are getting closer to the big heal – the top of the mountain. All these toxic little complaints should be celebrated as they disappear.

Assuming I do a good job, then we get to the top of the mountain and the patient has the big heal. This is often accompanied by a healing crisis (where the patient feels as if we went backwards rather than forwards), but this is rarely a bad thing – well, as long as the patient knows it could occur (and they always do with me).

Similarly, on our trek up the mountain, when we finally reach the top and our exhaustion is mixed in with our euphoria, it can all be a little much and we find ourselves slumping to the ground. This is the healing crisis, but the good news is that it rarely lasts long, and before you know it, you are standing back up and taking in the splendour of the view, and you are fortified for the trip back down.

My experience has advised me that the healing crisis is the body reaching the point where health *could* take over from disease. I say 'could' rather than 'will' or 'should' because this is often where a patient decides they have improved enough and stop coming for treatment. The problem here is that the patient is not completely healed and still needs additional treatments. If they stay the course, then the rest of the treatments are easier than the previous ones, in the same way that the trip back down the mountain is far easier than the climb. Their body should be healed and stronger than it's been in years. Strong enough to fight to stay healthy.

Regardless of whether my patients have healed quickly or slowly, from acute complaints or chronic disorders, I always encourage regular appointments into the future. These are what I call 'top-ups'. Prevention is better than cure, after all.

Most of all, I make sure that my patients understand that Chinese medicine helps their body heal itself, and to heal itself much faster than it likely could have managed on its own.

2. How I choose my points

In part this is done via my Chinese medicine diagnosis; it is also done via the patient's Qì telling me (discussed shortly); and part of this is done via point combinations.

My point combinations are designed to tonify together, sedate together, move stagnations together; no matter what the diagnosis is, I can construct a treatment that has the points working together for optimal benefit.

I don't usually lift and thrust a needle to tonify or sedate; I don't typically twirl or shake the needle a certain way to tonify or sedate. It's the sum of the parts that will tonify together, sedate together and/or move stagnations together. It's the combination of points performing a function together that I am interested in. This will be discussed in a lot more detail throughout the book – in fact, that is what this book is all about!

I can even construct a treatment where some points tonify and some points sedate.

One of my favorite point combinations is when I am treating a patient with a common cold resulting from an External Pathogenic Factor invasion. In that instance I have combinations of points that can tonify Wèi Qì, some that can clear the External Pathogenic Factor, and some that can do both.

3. Number of needles

The typical number of needles I use ranges from eight to 16. My view is that either side of those numbers is either not enough or too much. This view is based on my 20-plus years of experience as well as extensive research and reading.

I don't have a problem with other acupuncturists needling outside of those numbers. In fact, the acupuncturist that I currently frequent uses between 30 and 40 needles.

The other reason I have a range of 8–16 needles is for the point combinations to be most effective. I will discuss this concept shortly, but the sum of the parts is more important than individual point function. I find that if I do fewer than eight needles, I haven't been able to get a good enough combination of points, which may negatively impact on the success of the treatment.

On the other hand, if I go beyond 16 needles, I feel that I'm moving beyond my preferred targeted approach. The combinations of points can therefore become diluted, and the purpose of the treatment may even get lost within the vast function list of each point used.

I want to target my treatments – I don't want to put stacks of needles in and hope that some of them will have an effect – and that is why my preference is to use 8–16 needles. This range allows me to give each point a job to do and a point partner/s to help.

Lastly, the number of needles used is almost always an odd number. This is because my favorite channel, the Rèn Mài, is unilateral and often one or three needles are included in the treatment.

4. Bilateral needling

I almost always do bilateral needling. I am of the view that if there are two of the same point, then I should needle both. It's like a double-shot benefit – as in, two LI 4 points are far better than one.

I have experimented with this in the past and done unilateral needling. I found my treatments to be less effective as a result. I have also observed that my point combinations typically rely on bilateral needling for a more rounded effect.

5. Deliberate/sensible scattering

The deliberate, sensible – and planned – scattering of needles is very important to me, and for each treatment I look to cover some/all the areas of the head/face, trunk (front or back), arms/hands and legs/feet. Over the years I have found that this ensures the best chance of breaking through any stagnations. If I stack my needles in one area, then I line myself up for failure.[4]

None of us can be 100% sure that we know where blockages are located. Therefore, I take that out of the equation and deliberately 'scatter shot' my points. These are across a wide area of the body, using a range of different channels that travel in different directions. The points and channels chosen are deliberate and combine well with one another. It's not random stabbing of points. As you work your way through this book, you will learn how to do this too.

6. Patient positioning

Once I have decided on the diagnosis, and written up a sticky label for my patient's forehead (see Chapter 2), I must then decide on whether my patient will lie prone or supine (face down or face up). I don't flip my patient midway through a treatment. I don't like it when practitioners have done that to me in the past. Also, my patients have commented to me that they lose that sense of relaxation right at the point where they were starting to relax, and they don't get that relaxed feeling back after they have been flipped. They comment that their brain starts going a million miles an hour and they get restless. A restless brain isn't conducive to good treatment results.

7. Points on paper

The points I start with on paper almost always end up slightly different by the time all the needles have been inserted. As therapists, I feel we need to be conduits of energy, or Qì, if you like. That's the patient's Qì and Universal Qì (discussed further in Sections 12 and 13 below). This Qì tells us a lot, and in regard to treatment, it tells us which points need special attention and which don't.

I don't get a full sense of that when I am sitting across a table from someone. I get a bit, but I get the rest once I start touching their aura and their body. If you are sensitive to this Qì, you can pick up a lot on what the person really needs. This sensitivity bypasses the patient's (and my) rational brain. With the rational brain out of the way, we can get to the deeper layer of healing energy – one that neither the patient nor I have any real idea about. In my view this is the area where the best healing occurs.

8. In what order do I needle my points?

For the most part I don't needle points in a particular order. As I said earlier, I consider the sum of the parts to be more important than the individual points. I know that once all my needles are in, the treatment will start its healing journey; and it's the collective that will achieve that.

There are exceptions to this rule and I will give a few examples here.

Patient stress and anxiety

If my patient is incredibly stressed and anxious (for whatever reason), then I like to 'open the Four Gates' before I do anything else (see Chapter 6). These are LI 4 and LR 3 needled bilaterally. As some of you know, this is a great point combination to calm the patient down.[5]

Another great treatment for calming a patient is GV 20 and M-HN-3 (Yìn Táng) or GV 20 and HT 7.[6] I may choose one of those combinations before needling any others.

The Eight Extraordinary Vessels

I also put the points in a certain order when I open the Eight Extraordinary Vessels. In that instance I will always start with the opening point, use the coupled point next and then put at least one point in the vessel I am opening (see Chapter 12).

For example, if I wanted to open the Chōng Mài, I would first needle SP 4 bilaterally; then I would needle PC 6 bilaterally; then I would put a point in the Chōng Mài, such as KI 14 bilaterally. This makes it completely clear what I am trying to achieve with my treatment because SP 4, PC 6 and KI 14 perform multiple functions in the body, and the last thing I want is for the points to be confused about why they are being used. Yes, that can really happen – but more on that later!

I'm not saying that the body wouldn't work it out, but in this situation I want the treatment to start working as quickly as possible. There will be a more thorough explanation of these scenarios later in the book.

So, because I don't have to needle points in a particular order, I tend to choose the sequence of my needling in other ways. Therefore, the points that are likely to hurt the most are needled last. I want to limit the stressful experience that a lot of people feel when they know needles are about to penetrate their skin. I have found that the best way to do this is to keep the nasty points till the end.

I have experimented with this over the years by either doing the nasty points first or trying to hide them in the middle of the treatment. I even went through a phase where I left them out altogether and chose other, less effective, points to limit the pain potential for my patients (obviously, this wasn't the most sensible decision I have made in my Chinese medicine career, but we learn from our mistakes just as much as we learn from our successes).

I also tend to leave the points on the feet until the end of the treatment. This is partly because they can be a bit nasty, but mostly it's for reasons of hygiene. After I touch the feet, I need to wash my hands before I touch the patient's body again. It can get a little stop-start if I am having to wash my hands multiple times in a treatment. So, if I leave all my feet points until the end, I only have to wash my hands after all the needles have been inserted.

9. How do I needle?

Over the past 20-plus years of treating patients I have tried a range of different techniques. Some have been very traditional Chinese and some have been more Japanese-style. My needle types have ranged from 0.35 by 40mm down to 0.12 by 15mm. My stimulation methods have ranged from strong stimulation to obtain Dé Qì down to barely inserting the needle at all.

In the end, I have come to a middle ground. I now almost always use 0.18 by 15mm, 0.20 by 30mm or 0.25 by 40mm needles. Sometimes I need to use longer ones and they may end up 0.30 thick by 75mm long, but for the most part the needles mentioned above are the ones I use.

These needles are chosen based on how far I need to insert them. I use a guide tube and tap the needle into the skin. I then push the needle in further and leave it at a certain depth in the body. I don't generally do any further lifting and thrusting to acquire Dé Qì. My needle tip will be activating the Dé Qì because I have needled into the pocket of Qì. This principle applies no matter what angle I insert the needle. A few examples are given here.

Needling LU 7

For LU 7, I use a 0.20 by 30mm needle and I angle it transverse along the channel. Needling with the flow of Qì or against it doesn't bother me too much but is sometimes a consideration.[7] I start the needle tip just proximal or distal to the point and then needle about 0.5 cùn transverse.

Needling SP 6

For SP 6, I use a 0.20 by 40mm needle and I angle it perpendicular, 0.5 cùn to 1 cùn deep.

Needling BL 15

For BL 15, I use a 0.20 by 30mm needle and I angle it oblique 0.5 cùn towards the spine, away from the spine, up the channel or down the channel.

I haven't found any negatives with needling this way. I haven't seen any lessening of benefit from treatment. In fact, my patients are delighted because acupuncture doesn't hurt them and more of them continue to attend therapy as a result.

10. Write the needle number down

I write the number of needles used in the treatment on the patient file and circle it. Then, when I remove the needles, I count them to ensure I don't forget any that might be hidden away. I put needles straight into the sharps container as I remove them.

This was something I started to do consistently when I had a couple of near misses with hidden needles. But it's something I have been doing for a long time now. I think it probably became a habit pretty soon after I graduated.

11. Patient explanation

If the patient is interested, I will explain what I am doing before, during and after the treatment. The mind is a powerful tool and can be used to aid us in healing. As I'm explaining the treatment, I want my patient to start visualizing this in their mind. I'm convinced that this actually helps the patient's healing.

I realize that this feeds into the whole placebo argument, so I won't go into any more detail, but I do consider it an important part of my treatment.

12. Universal Qì

I use Universal Qì in every single treatment. Apart from what I stated above, Universal Qì is also important in other ways. One of those is to ensure that you don't use your own Qì when treating patients. You must always ensure that you keep some of your own personal Qì supply each day or you will burn out. I'm not suggesting that we don't give of ourselves in our desire to help the injured and sick, but we must do that with Universal Qì as our partner.

Some of you will have different ways to keep yourself strong and healthy throughout a busy clinic day. Perhaps you do some energy exercises such as Tài Jí Quán[8] or Qì Gōng.

I really like to make sure I have at least three breaks in a busy day. They don't have to be long – but they need to be there so I can recharge and be ready for my next influx of patients.

13. Accessing Universal Qì

How do I access and use Universal Qì? First of all, I recognize that it's everywhere and that I can gain access to it immediately because I am in it; because my patient is also in it, we can both use this Universal Qì to our benefit. Second, when I want to target a specific area, I place my hands over the zone (either just above or on the skin), close my eyes and visualize white puffy clouds. I breathe in and draw the white puffy clouds into myself; then, as I breathe out, I send the white puffy clouds out through my hands and into the patient. I repeat this 3–5 times.

Sometimes when I am doing this, the color and image change. I could get an image of red fire, blue waterfalls and purple sunsets, for example. When this happens, I go with it and stay with the new color and image. One of two things tend to occur during this – either the patient describes the area getting hot, cold or incredibly energetic, or when I ask them what their favorite color is, it turns out to be the color that I've been sending into their body. This color appears to be their Universal Qì color of choice.

14. Needle retention time

I like to give my patients about 30 minutes with the needles in. That means that the 30-minute period starts once all the needles have been inserted. This isn't a conscious choice because I want to tonify, sedate or disperse; I do it because experience has shown that a patient has generally been able to relax in that time and that they are just about to get to the point where the brain starts to kick in again and they want to get up. My mum will regularly yell out 'I'm cooked, David!' around that 30-minute mark of treatment.

15. Expecting results

I expect results! I go into every treatment with the belief that my patient will improve. I have to believe this, because to do otherwise could compromise our treatment goals. Positivity and real belief in my medicine is crucial to good results. And if I can get my patients expecting results too, then we are even more likely to achieve our goals.

I never tell my patients that they will be cured or fixed as a result of my treatments. I don't tell them that I can definitely help them to get better. My patients choose me and choose acupuncture because I explain what we will be trying to achieve in their healing. I talk about past patient successes with them if they ask me about whether I have treated their particular complaint before. If I have never treated their particular complaint, but I know about the research associated with their complaint, then I can talk to them about the research successes.

If I don't think I can help someone, then I won't start treating them. If I know of someone in my field who is far more experienced at treating the person's complaint, then I will refer them on. If they have been referred to me, then they specifically want to be treated by me; therefore, if I know I can treat their complaint, I will take them on as a patient.

16. Favorite channel

Do I have a favorite channel? Definitely! It's the Rèn Mài. I can achieve so much with this channel. Every single organ can be treated using the Rèn Mài. Apart from the obvious reason that the channel travels past every organ, the other reason is because the Rèn Mài activates the Sān Jiāo.

According to the 66th difficulty (Flaws 2004, p.121) of *The Classic of Difficulties* (*Canon of the Yellow Emperor's Eighty-One Difficult Issues*/Huáng Dì Bā Shí Yī Nán Jīng/黃帝八十一難經): 'The triple burner [Sān Jiāo] is the special messenger of this original qi, governing the free flow and movement of the three qi through the five viscera and six bowels.'[9] By activating the Sān Jiāo, you can use the Rèn Mài to treat every single organ in the body.

It's a sensational channel to use when you want to link up combinations of points (see Chapter 12). The Rèn Mài can also be used to treat organs in different parts of the Sān Jiāo.

For example, if the patient has disharmony between their Lung and Kidney organs, leading to asthma and wheezing, then I can use the Rèn Mài to reconnect the Lung/Kidney organ imbalance. This might include CV 4, CV 6, CV 17 and CV 22, along with points on different channels and in other areas of the body.

I also like the Rèn Mài because I have direct and *local* access to each organ. This allows me to use local points and distal points in my treatment for organ-based problems. So, using the example above, I could include KI 4 and LU 9 for a patient with asthma and wheezing as a result of a Lung/Kidney organ imbalance along with CV 4, CV 6, CV 17 and CV 22.

17. Favorite points

Do I have favorite points? Of course! I'm sure most of you have, too. A lot of these points are included in this book. Table 1.1 outlines my 100 favorite points. There are plenty of other points not in the list that I use on a regular basis, but I had to be ruthless when narrowing my list down to only 100.

My favorite points are the ones I use most often in clinic and so they are, to some degree, based on the patient's presenting complaints. Currently, the two most common categories of complaints that my patients present with are Shén disorders and musculoskeletal complaints.

Table 1.1 Favorite 100 acupuncture points

Channels	Points	
Lung channel	LU 5 LU 7	LU 9
Heart channel	HT 6	HT 7
Pericardium channel	PC 6	
Large Intestine channel	LI 4 LI 10	LI 11 LI 20
Small Intestine channel	SI 3 SI 7	SI 14
Sān Jiāo channel	TE 4 TE 5	TE 6 TE 17
Spleen channel	SP 3 SP 4 SP 6	SP 9 SP 10 SP 21
Liver channel	LR 2 LR 3	LR 13 LR 14
Kidney channel	KI 1 KI 3 KI 6 KI 7 KI 22	KI 23 KI 24 KI 25 KI 26 KI 27
Stomach channel	ST 8 ST 21 ST 25 ST 34	ST 36 ST 40 ST 44
Gall Bladder channel	GB 20 GB 21 GB 24 GB 25 GB 29	GB 30 GB 34 GB 37 GB 40 GB 41

Urinary Bladder channel	BL 2	BL 24
	BL 10	BL 25
	BL 12	BL 26
	BL 13	BL 40
	BL 14	BL 42
	BL 15	BL 43
	BL 17	BL 44
	BL 18	BL 47
	BL 19	BL 49
	BL 20	BL 52
	BL 21	BL 57
	BL 22	BL 60
	BL 23	BL 62
Rèn Mài	CV 4	CV 14
	CV 6	CV 15
	CV 9	CV 17
	CV 12	CV 21
Dū Mài	GV 4	GV 20
	GV 14	GV 23
	GV 16	GV 24
Extra points	M-BW-35 (Huá Tuó Jiā Jǐ)	M-HN-30 (Bǎi Láo)
	M-HN-3 (Yìn Táng)	MN-LE-16 (Xī Yǎn)
	M-HN-14 (Bí Tōng)	M-UE-48 (Jiān Qián)

I have shown this table to my students over the years, and the points have varied from year to year as I change some of my choices around a bit. What typically happens when I list my top 100 is that my students then tell me to narrow the 100 down to a top ten, a top five, and then to my absolute favorite point. Tables 1.2, 1.3 and 1.4 list my current favorites.

Table 1.2 Favorite ten acupuncture points

Channels	Points
Heart channel	HT 7
Large Intestine channel	LI 4
Spleen channel	SP 6
Liver channel	LR 3
Kidney channel	KI 3
Stomach channel	ST 36
Gall Bladder channel	GB 20
Rèn Mài	CV 17
Dū Mài	GV 20
Extra points	M-HN-3 (Yìn Táng)

Table 1.3 Favorite five acupuncture points

Channels	Points
Heart channel	HT 7
Large Intestine channel	LI 4
Spleen channel	SP 6
Stomach channel	ST 36
Dū Mài	GV 20

Table 1.4 Favorite acupuncture point

Channels	Points
Dū Mài	GV 20

My top ten and top five points are chosen because of the wide range of disorders/complaints that they can treat. I know I can rely on them to do their job when I use them.

My favorite point is chosen because it's my favorite point to have done on me. The feeling that comes over me when GV 20 is needled is one of pure bliss. Therefore, I want as many patients as possible to get that same feeling from my treatments. For a variety of reasons, not everyone likes to receive GV 20, so I don't use it on them.

18. Follow-up phone call

It has become common practice for me to call, text or email my patients one or two days after their treatment. This does two things:

- First, it shows I care for my patients even when they are not in my clinic.

- Second, it often guides when the next appointment should be. I'm not a fan of booking patients in every week and sticking to the schedule rigidly. This is because patients' signs and symptoms change at different speeds and on different days. As they change, this should dictate when they need their next appointment.

So I set out a treatment plan for my patients. This might very well be one treatment a week for six weeks, but my patients know that this could change somewhat based on how they respond to their treatment. They may end up coming in again three days later and then it might be ten days before the next appointment.

My purpose is to stick to the framework of treating my patient and not the disease. So as my patient changes, I must change too.

Notes

1   There is some dispute about the actual years of birth and death for Galen. Most sources I reviewed suggested 129 CE as his year of birth and 216 CE as his year of death. That aside, Galen is considered by many to be the father of Western medicine. The quotation was taken from www.azquotes.com/quote/1306272.

2   Definitely one of the more remarkable quotations I have come across. Very Chinese medicine sounding, which is interesting considering it came from Western culture. Hippocrates (460–375 BCE) laid the groundwork for Greek medicine, and the Hippocratic Oath is still taken by medical graduates in some countries, which is amazing considering Hippocrates was alive 2500 years ago. The quotation was taken from www.brainyquote.com/authors/hippocrates.

3   *The Spiritual Pivot* (Líng Shū) was written somewhere between 200 and 0 BCE.

4   Maciocia 2015, pp.1191–1192.

5   Ross 1995, p.249.

6   Flaws and Wolfe 2008, p.87.

7   Phillips 2017, pp.55–70. Typically, if you needle with the flow of the channel, you will tonify; if you needle against the flow, you will sedate. There are, of course, alternative views on this.

8   Tài Jí Quán is probably better known as Tai Chi, due to the popular use of the Wade-Giles romanization of the Chinese Mandarin language. This style is no longer in vogue and the Chinese have developed their own Pīn Yīn, which means that Tai Chi is now written as Tài Jí or Tài Jí Quán.

9   The viscera refer to the Yīn organs and the bowels refer to the Yáng organs. The Yīn organ missing is the Pericardium, which was considered to be part of the Heart at that stage in Chinese medicine history.

Qi Bo said, 'In the beginning, wizards originally knew the hundred diseases and what would overcome them. The ancients knew of the body's diseases, that which followed and that which gave birth to them, so that they could use incantations to finish them.'

58th essay – *Spiritual Pivot*/Líng Shū/靈樞[1]

2

Understanding Acupuncture Point Combinations

Before we jump head first into this book, we need to spend a little time making sure that you understand what acupuncture point combinations actually are. This will require some discussion on a variety of topics including why combining points matters and how acupuncture point combinations work.

I also want to ensure that you are familiar with the terminology that will be used throughout the book. Lastly, I wanted to discuss the phrases 'treat the person, not the disease' and 'prevention is better than cure'.

If we become familiar with constructing our own acupuncture point combinations, we can become more like the wizard practitioners of antiquity.

1. Why it matters

There are a number of reasons why accurate combining of acupuncture points matters in a treatment. You no doubt see the treatment combinations in most Chinese medicine books you read. These could be standardized treatment protocols for a variety of diagnostic methods including the Zàng Fǔ patterns, Wǔ Xíng and the Shāng Hán Lùn, to name just a few.

Although these treatment protocols are unique for each diagnostic method, they are still acupuncture point combinations, and they are good ones which have likely been documented over hundreds, even thousands, of years of use. This book isn't designed to make you move away from these learned diagnostic methods; rather, it aims to teach you ways you can edit these treatment protocols where necessary. Because, let's face it, not all of our patients can be diagnosed using only one label.

Let me use a quick example here, with a much more in-depth example in Section 11 below.

I sometimes diagnose my patients with the Zàng Fǔ patterns of Liver Yáng Rising with Kidney Yīn Xū. In this instance, you essentially have three different patterns occurring at once. There is a chronic Liver Xuè Xū or Liver Yīn Xū, along with an acute Liver Heat, and also a chronic Kidney Yīn Xū. In this instance, I often show my students how this might look using what I call 'Zàng Fǔ Pattern Manhattans'. It gives the students a visual cue to make sense of the diagnosis. See Diagrams 2.1–2.4.

This diagnosis is complicated and, according to McDonald and Penner (1994, pp.142–147, 166–168), it requires the practitioner to consider roughly 16 different points and, if needled bilaterally, 30 needles inserted into the patient (see Table 2.1).

Table 2.1 Liver Yáng Rising with Kidney Yīn Xū treatment[2]

Points	Liver Xuè Xū	Liver Yīn Xū	Liver Heat	Kidney Yīn Xū
BL 17	✓			
BL 18	✓	✓		
BL 20	✓			
BL 23		✓		✓
KI 1				✓
KI 3		✓		✓
KI 6				✓
GB 20			✓	
GB 34			✓	
GB 43			✓	
LR 2			✓	
LR 3	✓	✓	✓	
SP 6	✓			✓
CV 4	✓			✓
ST 36	✓			
GV 20			✓	

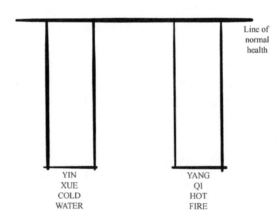

Line of normal health

YIN   YANG
XUE   QI
COLD   HOT
WATER FIRE

Diagram 2.1 Normal Zàng Fǔ Manhattan

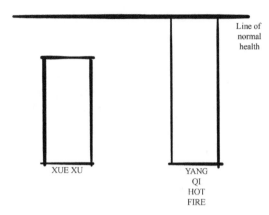

Diagram 2.2 Xuè Xū Manhattan

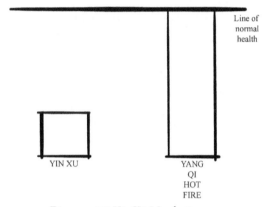

Diagram 2.3 Yīn Xū Manhattan

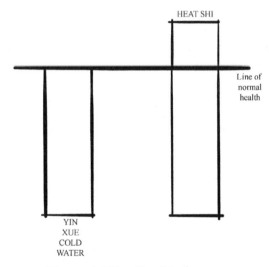

Diagram 2.4 Liver Heat Manhattan

Because I like to use between eight and 16 needles, then I clearly have too many. This scenario and many others are what this book is all about. I will teach you how to take this complicated and excessive number of points and narrow it down to an acceptable number, while keeping the integrity of the treatment.

So, to keep it simple for this example (with explanations later), I will only choose the points above that appeared more than once. This leaves us with BL 18, BL 23, KI 3, LR 3, SP 6 and CV 4. That would be 11 needles bilaterally now, instead of 30. Plus, it sits within my preferred range of 8–16 needles.

But do those points combine well together? In this instance, they do, and you will learn how they do as you read through the book.

I also need to see if they are scattered throughout the body in a sensible manner. For the points listed above, I have two on the trunk and three on the legs. Although that's not a perfect scenario, I am happy enough to stick with these points for this brief example. In reality, I would probably be looking for a point on the arms/hands and/or the head/face to get a more global body approach.

Now I need to check that I'm not having to flip my patient mid-treatment, which I don't like doing. I can get to every point with my patient face down and with a bolster under their ankles (to access LR 3), except for CV 4.

I now have one last decision to make: I can leave that point out and needle ten points bilaterally or I can add in a point that wasn't in Table 2.1. That point is BL 26, which is CV 4 on the back of the body,[3] and that is something I would almost definitely do, which gives me 12 needled points.

This process all happens in my head in a matter of minutes and is something that you will become adept at as you work your way through this book. Why? Because it matters! It really does matter that you become proficient at working out how to construct a treatment. It's simply not good enough to rely solely on your diagnostic method of choice because patients should never be labeled as one disorder/disease/diagnosis. If we do that, we become just like Western medical practitioners and we start treating the disease and not the person.

Furthermore, it's not particularly common for patients to fit perfectly into one diagnosis anyway, so as soon as that happens, you are forced to think about your point choices and how you will change them. The problem is that you probably weren't taught how to adjust your treatment – you were likely told what to do by your well-meaning lecturers and clinic supervisors.

This book will show you how accurate acupuncture point combinations can enhance your treatment benefits.

2. The dynamic movement of Vital Substances

As you probably recall in your studies, the Vital Substances are Qì, Xuè, Jīn Yè and Jīng.[4]

The Qì moves the Xuè, Qì moves Jīn Yè, and Qì moves Jīng.[5] Xuè, Jīn Yè and Jīng are also just a different form of Qì.[6]

These Vital Substances are what we access when we treat patients with acupuncture; they move at different speeds, are in different locations and move at differing depths. Therefore, this requires us to think about which of these substances we want to activate when we construct treatments.

For example, a portion of the Jīn Yè is heavy, and gravity drops it to the lower parts of the body, including the feet, ankles, legs, hips/thighs and abdomen. This means we need to choose a point combination that will work against gravity and force the Jīn Yè to move back up the body. Sensibly, this means that you would choose points that are predominantly on the legs and located on channels that moved Qì up the body. Further, you can also select points on the abdomen to drag the Jīn Yè back up into the trunk for redistribution through the organs involved in Jīn Yè transformation and transportation. But you can also choose points that move Qì down the legs, which can create momentum by forcing the Jīn Yè to move; even though this pushes the Jīn Yè in the opposite direction to the way you want it to go, the momentum you generate provides additional thrust and lift back up the legs.

I explain it to my students (and sometimes my patients) as being like the famous Apollo 13 space voyage in 1970. The spacecraft was critically damaged and needed to return to Earth immediately. Instead of turning the spaceship around (which would have used up too much fuel as well as slowed them down), the commander of the ship flew a further distance to slingshot around the moon in order to generate extra speed and use less fuel by using Earth's gravity for the return journey.

This is exactly what happens when you choose acupuncture points that move Qì down the body; they slingshot the Qì, Xuè, Jīn Yè and Jīng back up the body. The key difference between Apollo 13 and acupuncture is that (in this example) we work *against* gravity.

Acupuncture point combinations can be used to flush the extremities or to nourish the organs. They can be used to sedate excesses or tonify deficiencies. We can bash through stagnations of any type and can expel External Pathogenic Factors. All of this is done through the dynamic flow of Vital Substances.

3. Stagnations, stasis, accumulations

Acupuncture point combinations can be used to bash through stagnations, stasis or accumulations. I teach my students that these terms are often specific to particular Vital Substances. For Qì, I use stagnation, as in Qì Stagnation; for Xuè, I use stasis, as in Xuè Stasis; for Jīn Yè, I use accumulation, as in Phlegm (Damp Heat) Accumulation or Damp Accumulation.

Qì Stagnation is usually the easiest to shift because Qì is the most ethereal Vital Substance. Xuè Stasis is usually the next easiest to shift, leaving Damp or Phlegm (Jīn Yè) the hardest to shift. Phlegm is often the most difficult to move because it has become a sticky, glugging, toxic, inflamed mess. This stickiness adheres to its surroundings and makes it very difficult to shift.[7]

Regardless of which stagnation exists, there are relevant point combinations that can be used to bash through them.

Finally, a patient has the best chance of continued health when they have free flow of their Vital Substances. The minute one, or several, of these substances become stuck, toxins can start to accumulate. This toxicity is where disease starts, so if we can keep the substances in free flow, we give ourselves the best chance of staying healthy.

4. Stacking acupuncture points in one area

I discussed my views on this in Chapter 1. I just don't like putting all my needles in the one area. This isn't just my view either: a lot of authors prefer to have points in multiple areas of the body.[8]

None of us can know for certain where all the stagnations are in the body. If we stack needles in one area, then we might find that the flow of Vital Substances increases but only up/down to where the stagnation lies – and that's where it stops – whereas if I had placed needles more deliberately throughout the body, I can be holistic, particularly if I use a range of different channels that travel in different directions.

The points and channels chosen are deliberate and combine well with one another. It's not random stabbing of points. I look to cover some/all the areas of the head/face, trunk (front or back), arms/hands and legs/feet. Over the years I have found that this ensures the best chance of breaking through any stagnations.

The deliberate, but planned, scattering of needles is very important to me and I apply it to every treatment. As you work your way through this book you will learn how to do this too.

5. How do acupuncture point combinations work?

'They just do, okay!'

I'm sorry but that statement just doesn't fly with me. I don't care how many people have said this to me over the years; I haven't been swayed from my mission to know the how and the why – and because I've never been someone that keeps what I have learned to myself, this book is the end result.

What is the benefit for you, the reader? Perhaps I can use an analogy to get my point across more effectively. I have a few friends who are chefs. When we get together and have a few drinks, I often tease them by calling them cooks rather than chefs. They don't like being called cooks, because to them a cook can be anybody in a kitchen who follows a recipe. They are chefs because they design their own meals.

The same applies to us as acupuncturists. You can be an acupuncturist who follows learned diagnostic treatment protocols (like a cook following a recipe) or you can be an acupuncturist who constructs a treatment specific to your patient that is perfect for them at that exact moment in time (like a chef designing a meal).

Who would you rather be? Personally, both options are more than adequate for excellent treatment results. But wouldn't you like to know how to design your own treatment?

This book will teach you how to create a treatment masterpiece that has the potential to surpass a standard one.

To answer the question, though, there are three main reasons that point combinations work.

They make a particular acupuncture point work stronger, better or faster

Every single acupuncture point in the body has a list of actions and indications (Chinese- and Western-based) that they can treat. Some points only treat a few disorders, whereas some treat a wide range of signs and symptoms. For example, M-UE-24 (Luò Zhěn) really only treats stiffness in the neck and local metacarpophalangeal problems.[9] ST 36, on the other hand, treats pretty much everything.[10]

If we use M-UE-24 (Luò Zhěn) as our case in point (no pun intended), then we can make it work stronger, better and faster for neck stiffness if we combine it with other points that have a similar effect. This might include, but won't be limited to, local points such as GB 20, M-HN-30 (Bǎi Láo) and BL 10, plus some other distal points such as LU 7 and SI 3.[11]

Let's use another example. We all know that LI 4 is great for pain relief – in particular, headaches. Targeting frontal headaches specifically can be enhanced when we combine LI 4 with ST 8, ST 44, GB 14, GB 20 and M-HN-3 (Yìn Táng).[12] This is because the point combination enhances the power of LI 4, and the power of the other points in the combination is boosted by LI 4.

Sensational point combinations occur when each point in the combination enhances the power of the other points.

They enhance one particular function of an acupuncture point and cancel/reduce its other functions

As I stated above, some points treat a wide range of actions and indications. That being the case, we sometimes need to give the point direction – tell it what to target, in other words.

If we use SP 6 as our point example, I have listed the more common actions and indications in Table 2.2 according to a number of my Chinese medicine peers. The actions and indications listed aren't the entire list from each of these authors.

Table 2.2 SP 6 functions

SP 6	Deadman, Al-Khafaji and Baker 2007, pp.189–192	Maciocia 2015, pp.1000–1001	McDonald 1986, pp.28–29
Actions	Tonifies Spleen Tonifies Stomach Resolves Dampness Harmonizes Liver Tonifies Kidneys Regulates menstruation Induces labor Harmonizes Lower Jiāo Regulates urination Benefits genitals Calms the Shén Invigorates Xuè Activates channel Alleviates pain	Strengthens Spleen Resolves Dampness Promotes Liver Qì Tonifies Kidneys Regulates menses Benefits urination Calms the Shén Moves Xuè Stops pain Nourishes Xuè and Yīn Cools Xuè Regulates uterus Stops bleeding	Strengthens Spleen Promotes Stomach Transforms Damp Spreads Liver Qì Benefits Kidneys Regulates menstruation Induces labor Invigorates Qì and Xuè circulation Activates channel Lowers temperature
Indications	Heavy body Borborygmus Edema Diarrhea No desire to eat or drink Irregular menstruation Infertility Impotence Difficult urination Palpitations Insomnia Dizziness Hypertension Leg pain	Feeling heavy Edema Loose stools Poor appetite Irregular menses Infertility Impotence Difficult urination Palpitations Insomnia Dizziness Low abdominal pain	Borborygmus Edema Diarrhea Menstrual disorders Infertility in women Seminal emission Impotence Urinary incontinence Insomnia Leg/foot paralysis Vaginal discharge Uterine prolapse

As you can see, there is a substantial number of actions and indications, many of which all of the authors agree on. So, when I needle SP 6, I know that the point could affect any/all of the actions and indications listed above (as well as the ones I haven't included in the table).

That's why enhancing one particular function of a point and cancelling/reducing its other functions is an important consideration when constructing acupuncture point combinations. I will stick with SP 6 for some examples.

SP 6 can tonify Xuè and Yīn when used in conjunction with HT 6 and KI 6.[13] I call this combination the 'three Yīn sixes'. There are three points in total; they are all on Yīn channels; they are all the sixth point on their channel – hence, the three Yīn sixes. This combination will be discussed in more detail in Chapter 6.

Alternatively, SP 6 can also resolve/transform Dampness when used in conjunction with SP 9 and CV 9.[14]

This same scenario applies for all the other actions and indications – not just for SP 6 but for every point on the body.

It is worth noting that the combination examples just discussed won't exclusively treat that one action. The combination of points will still likely have a positive effect on some of the other actions and indications for each of the points used in the combination. This will be discussed in more detail later.

Each acupuncture point in the combination works on different aspects of the patient's illness

This is a particularly good combination because it allows for multiple patient signs and symptoms to be accessed in the same treatment.

For example, if a patient presents with Damp Heat, you can use LI 11 and TE 5 for clearing the Heat[15] and then use SP 3 and ST 36 for moving the Damp.[16]

Another example is a patient with Kidney Yáng Xū and Cold Damp arthritis in the right knee. In this instance, you could use KI 3, KI 7, BL 23 and GV 4 for the Kidney Yáng Xū;[17] then SP 9, SP 10, ST 34, ST 35 and ST 36 for the right knee arthritis.[18]

You just need to be careful that you don't try to achieve too much in the treatment.

I believe that every treatment has a limit as to what it can accomplish. I doubt that anybody really knows what that limit is – it will just occur in the body and we may/may not find out later.

I have discovered over the years that you can do too much for your patient. I'm sure it's done with good intentions, but we should avoid overdosing the patient with acupuncture. One of the most common side effects of overdosing the patient is that they get a worsening of symptoms,[19] which typically come on almost immediately, or there may be a delay and the symptoms worsen about 24–48 hours after the acupuncture treatment. As you can appreciate, this is rarely a good thing, and the patient will generally associate this worsening as being the direct result of the acupuncture treatment.

If I am ever unsure as to whether a patient *may* get a healing crisis (of sorts), I always err on the side of caution and advise them of this possibility. I also inform them that it's not a bad thing; in fact, it's a good outcome because the body is trying to heal itself and the toxic overload is leading to the perceived worsening of symptoms.

I tell them that if this does occur, they should call me and we will plan our next attack moving forward. Sometimes that will be another acupuncture treatment almost immediately. Sometimes I might suggest a day at home to rest, or even some other option, dependent on how they have reacted to the previous treatment.

Another possible outcome is that the body doesn't really show any noticeable improvement in any of the wide array of signs and symptoms you were trying to treat. You have possibly spread yourself too thin in your endeavor to help the patient heal everything they have wrong with them.

You should focus on only a few actions and indications and construct the best possible point combination for those few things.[20] The treatment will then be specific and will also remain undiluted.

Which brings us to the debate about what you treat first. Do you treat the root? The manifestation(s)? Or try to treat both at the same time?[21] Typically, I treat what the patient wants me to treat, which is almost always the manifestation(s), but I will try to include a few points for the underlying root.

Always remember that acupuncture is an incredibly powerful medicine, and if you are ever in doubt as to whether you might be trying to do too much in a treatment, well, just reassess and consider dropping a few of the points.

6. Local, adjacent, distal

Even if we know where some of the stagnation is located, I still abide by the policy of local, adjacent and distal needle insertion.

As you may already know, local points are directly over the problem area, adjacent points are close by, and distal points are at some distance away from the problem area. By using local, adjacent and distal points, you can get incredibly good results because you aren't stacking one area of the body.[22]

I appreciate that some authors have alternative views on needling local points, but unless the patient won't let you, or you know from experience that certain conditions are not conducive, then I will use some local points.

If I can't use local points, then I will use adjacent and distal points. Allow me to use an analogy of a donut and a cricket ball/baseball, via a short case study, to further emphasize my love of local, adjacent and distal needle insertion.

CASE STUDY 2.1 A 26-YEAR-OLD MALE WITH A TORN LEFT CALF/GASTROCNEMIUS MUSCLE

My patient tore his left calf muscle two days prior and the only treatment he has had is regular ice application. Upon palpation I can feel significant tension, along with patient discomfort in the region just lateral to the Urinary Bladder channel points of BL 56, BL 57 and BL 58.

My plan is to do roughly four local Ā Shì points; adjacent points including BL 56, BL 57, BL 58 and GB 35; and distal points including BL 36, BL 40, BL 60, GB 29, GB 34, LR 3, KI 3 and KI 10.

That is a total of 16 needles, with all of them being needled only on the left side. There are plenty of situations where I will put needles in on the right side as well, which would require me to reconsider some of the needles mentioned as I would prefer not to exceed 16 needles in the treatment.

There are also situations where I might needle on the forearm as a mirror image of the lower leg. There are even a couple of other approaches that I might employ. You will get a very good sense of how I treat as you work your way through this book.

My local points will work on the injured site; they are working on clearing out the old/unhealthy Vital Substances that have collected there since the injury occurred. This is what I call 'working from the inside-out'.

My distal points are designed to move fresh/healthy Vital Substances to the injury site. This is what I call 'working from the outside-in'. Distal points are also used to help clear away the old/unhealthy Vital Substances.

My adjacent points are there to aid in the transfer of fresh/healthy Vital Substances into the injured area, as well as to help clear away the old/unhealthy Vital Substances. This is what I call 'working in harmony with local and distal'.

This is where the analogy of the donut and a cricket ball/baseball comes in. By working from the inside-out, as well as the outside-in, I am breaking down the stagnation more effectively. I'm also providing an avenue for the escape of the old/unhealthy Vital Substances. This results in the donut image.

If I only worked on the injury from the outside-in, I get my cricket ball/baseball image.

Which of these could you easily crush in your hand? The donut is the winner here, and we want that because this means that the patient can heal faster. The donut analogy gets the old/unhealthy Vital Substances out of the injured area, thereby allowing for a more effective transfer of fresh/healthy Vital Substances into the injury; this will speed up the healing process, whereas the cricket ball/baseball will not.

You can still get adequate results if you only work from the outside-in, but it will be slower and your patient may not hang around long enough for you to reach the results you were both hoping for.

There are exceptions to this rule but, for the most part, I treat local, adjacent and distal.

7. Summary of good/bad acupuncture point combinations

Good and bad acupuncture point combinations will tend to follow the approaches shown in Boxes 2.1 and 2.2 (these are just a snapshot of what was previously spoken about).

Box 2.1 Summary of good acupuncture point combinations

- They will have points on multiple channels traveling in different directions. This will ensure the Vital Substances have the best chance of getting to an area, as well as moving out of an area.

- They will be scattered all over the body. This provides the opportunity for Vital Substances to bash through unseen stagnations, as well as ensuring they are continually moving everywhere, all the time.

- They will ensure the Vital Substances are traveling to the organs as well as the extremities. This is important because the organs are where the Vital Substances are made, and the extremities are where we perform our action (both physical and mental).

- They will have either a single-minded purpose or a multifaceted approach. This has to be determined before the point combination is worked out.

- They will target the relevant function of each point (this is particularly important when the point has multiple functions). As stated with SP 6 earlier, some points do a lot of things in the body, and it's our job to make the point target-specific.

- They will enhance the relevant function of each point. This is done by putting additional points in the combination that target the same diagnosis, sign or symptom.

- They will make each of the points in the combination work stronger, better, faster. When you have a good point combination, the points will work so much better than they would if they were trying to do it all on their own. For example, LI 4 is an excellent point for all types of headaches.[23] I often show my patients where that point is, so they can push on it at home when they have a headache.

- But LI 4 will be so much better for headaches if it is used with other points that also treat headaches. These might include, but wouldn't be limited to, SI 3, LR 3, GB 20, M-HN-3 (Yìn Táng), BL 60 and GB 41.[24]

Box 2.2 Summary of bad acupuncture point combinations

- Obviously bad acupuncture point combinations will be those that don't adhere to the principles above. For example, a bad combination will be one that stacks all points in the same area.

- Although that might seem like a good approach, particularly for musculoskeletal disorders, it's still a much better idea to include points at a distance to the local points.

- The same applies for combinations that have one part of it working on a particular action, with another part of the combination opposing that action.

- For example, your patient has been diagnosed with Stomach Fire Blazing and so you have points such as ST 44, TE 5 and LI 11, which would be sound choices.[25] But then you included CV 2, which would be the wrong choice as it won't treat Stomach Fire Blazing and, instead, will treat Lower Jiāo organs, in particular Kidney Jīng Xū.[26]

---

8. Shapes, designs, patterns

Acupuncture point combinations will often end up in different shapes, designs or patterns. These may or may not have been done on purpose but they are in a pattern nonetheless. My two favorites are the Triangle of Power/Influence and the Figure Eight. Each of these shapes will be discussed in more detail in Chapters 6 and 7 respectively.

I will, however, briefly discuss the Triangle of Power. As the name suggests, the shape is a triangle made with three needles. These three needles generate an immense amount of power, but this influence isn't contained to the Triangle's two dimensions.

The power generated within the Triangle forces the Vital Substances to move into a three-dimensional pyramid design. Depending on where the Triangle is positioned, these substances can move more effectively up and down the body, or in and out (front to back) of the body.

Other shapes, designs and patterns that I like include a plus sign (typically four or five needles), an asterisk or star (typically eight or nine needles), a square (four or five needles), a pentagon (five or six needles) and a hexagon (six or seven needles).

As you may have worked out, the extra needle used in each of the above examples would be a needle directly in the middle of the shape.

Regardless of the design used, each of the acupuncture point combinations will be enhanced via the shape chosen. One could argue that this is because of the points chosen and has nothing to do with the shape (which is purely coincidental). Everybody is entitled to their own opinion, of course. In the end, you will come to your own conclusion about this, and the many other conflicting opinions we face in Chinese medicine. And should we really be surprised? After all, we have more than 2000 years of history to work from, don't we?

9. Does it matter in what order the points are needled?

As stated in Chapter 1, I don't personally think it matters in what order you needle the points. On occasion I may want to calm my patient by putting a needle or two in at the beginning that will achieve that purpose. But other than that, I can only think of one other situation where I need to needle points in a certain order, and that is when I want to open the Eight Extraordinary Vessels.

Throughout this book, if I feel that a point combination requires to be needled in a certain order, I will specify it and provide the sequence, as well as the reason for it. If the reason is a particular author's recommendation, then I will reference accordingly.

10. Cautions and contraindications with acupuncture point combinations

As with any acupuncture book, it is a good idea to highlight potential cautions and contraindications with needling.[27] See Appendix 4 for a thorough list.

When it comes to constructing point combinations for different aspects of a patient's illness, you need to be careful that the combination doesn't have one part of it working on a particular action, with another part of the combination opposing that action.

Although it's quite difficult to manage this, it's definitely possible. Maciocia (2015, pp.1178–1184) discusses this very possibility when he talks about treating

External Pathogenic Factor (EPF) invasion. As you probably know, this is typically what we refer to as a common cold in Western medical terms.

Maciocia discusses this by asking the reader if we are planning to tonify Zhèng Qì, expel the EPF or try to do both in the same treatment. I typically try to do both in the same treatment as I've found this to be more effective than focusing purely on one or the other.

The difficulty is that if you are not careful, you might inadvertently tonify the EPF when you tonify the Zhèng Qì. Another possibility is that while expelling the EPF, you end up sedating Zhèng Qì as well. So please be very aware of the point combination you are constructing.

I like to discuss this scenario with my students (and sometimes my patients) by getting them to visualize a battle. One of those traditional-style battles with the two armies facing one another across 'no man's land'. The EPF is one army and the Zhèng Qì is the other army.

Both armies are fairly evenly matched. If the EPF army wins, then the pathogen will move from the exterior to the interior of the body (bad news). If the Zhèng Qì wins, then the EPF will be kicked out of the exterior of the body (good news). So I want to do everything in my power to aid the Zhèng Qì.

To do that, I need to tonify the Zhèng Qì, which will provide additional soldiers to the Qì army. I also need to sedate the EPF. In this scenario I explain that my Qì army has successfully flanked the EPF army; therefore, the EPF army is being cut down from every direction, with the end result that the Zhèng Qì army will win.

So how do we do that? One of my favorite acupuncture point combinations to ensure victory over the EPF, as well as give the Zhèng Qì a nice boost, is set out in Table 2.3.

Table 2.3 Tonify Zhèng Qì and sedate EPF treatment[28]

Location of point	Point	Reasoning
Head/face/neck	GB 20 LI 20	Clears the EPF from the body and sense organs Clears the EPF from the sense organs
Trunk (back)	BL 12 BL 13	Clears the EPF and tonifies Zhèng Qì Clears the EPF and tonifies Zhèng Qì
Arms/hands	LU 7 LI 4 LI 11	Clears the EPF and tonifies Zhèng Qì Clears the EPF and tonifies Zhèng Qì/treats sense organs Clears the EPF and tonifies Zhèng Qì
Legs/feet	ST 36	Clears the EPF and tonifies Zhèng Qì
Total points needled		16 needles used bilaterally

Another clinical situation where you need to be careful (that you don't have one part of your treatment working on a particular action, with another part of the combination opposing that action) is when a patient has an underlying deficiency but also has an excess or stagnant musculoskeletal complaint. A really good example of this came a few years ago from the student clinic that I often supervise at Endeavour College of Natural Health (ECNH) in Brisbane, Queensland, Australia.

CASE STUDY 2.2 A 55-YEAR-OLD FEMALE (HS) WITH CHRONIC LEFT KNEE PAIN AND SWELLING

HS had never received acupuncture before and was referred to the student clinic via a friend.

She described the knee pain as being either sharp and stabbing or dull and throbbing. She couldn't always isolate when each type of pain was more prevalent. But HS did add that the sharp and stabbing pain would arrive suddenly but didn't linger for long (five minutes to a couple of hours usually), whereas the dull and throbbing pain would have a more gradual onset and could hang around for days at a time.

The left knee was something that had been bothering her for nearly 12 months but had never been a problem prior to that. HS had tried physiotherapy and massage with minimal improvement. She had not seen a specialist.

The pain was throughout the entire knee joint and didn't radiate away from the knee. Sometimes the knee would swell and create stiffness and clicking when bending or straightening the knee. This tended to occur in the summer months when the weather was humid and hot.

The knee was aggravated by overuse, which was a concern because HS liked to keep fit. Her preference was to do personal training classes which did include a portion of higher-impact exercises on her knee. As stated above, her knee was also aggravated by hot and humid weather. However, hot and dry weather could trigger the sharp and stabbing pain, whereas damp and humid weather would trigger the dull and throbbing pain. HS could even predict when it was going to rain or when a severe humid heatwave was coming, because her knee would play up.

After gathering this information, the student practitioner proceeded to ask her additional questions to identify her Zàng Fǔ pattern diagnosis. This quickly became problematic because the patient only wanted her knee treated and didn't think the additional questioning was necessary. What the student did manage to obtain was that HS suffered from some low back pain/discomfort, got occasional swollen and stiff ankles, and had suffered from some night sweats and hot flushes/flashes throughout her menopause (she was at the back end of her menopause, which she had been managing with herbal medicine and dietary assistance via a naturopath).

Because of the length of time it took the student to gather the information on the knee, as well as the obvious aggravation shown by the patient, my student didn't obtain any further signs and symptoms other than tongue and pulse. The student described the pulse as being strong, fast and full, and the tongue as being red and dry.

Upon presentation to me, the student explained all of the above information and diagnosed HS as having a Damp Heat Bì in the left knee along with a mild Kidney Xū. I had not seen the patient and therefore had also not taken the pulse or looked at the tongue. I accepted the diagnosis and the accompanying 15-needle treatment, which was:

- Bilateral – KI 3, SP 9, GB 34, LI 10 and LI 11.

- Unilateral (left side only) – SP 10, ST 34, ST 36, GB 33 and M-LE-27 (Hè Dǐng).

The reasons for the point choices were:[29]

- KI 3 – local point for the ankles and was used bilaterally for Kidney Xū.

- SP 9 – local point for the knee which was used bilaterally to move Damp.

- LI 11 – used bilaterally to clear Heat, and because the elbow is the 'mirror image' of the knee.

- GB 34 – local point for the knee which was used bilaterally to move Damp Heat. It was also used to flush the extremities (legs).

- LI 10 – used to flush the extremities (arms).

- The unilateral points – all chosen as local points for the knee.

As is usually the case in the student clinic, I go in and check the tongue and pulse and check needle location. The only issue I could see at the time was that the pulse wasn't strong, fast and full. It was fast, but it was floating and empty rather than strong and full. Unfortunately, the student had missed the rather rare Kidney Yīn Xū pulse, where it floats superficially but then becomes empty at the middle pressure before re-emerging as a thin pulse at the deep level. But more on that shortly.

HS said she began to feel better the second she got off the table and started walking. To say she was pleased would be an understatement. She was seriously happy and kept bending and straightening her leg in the reception area. The follow-up appointment was booked in for five days' time.

This is where the case gets interesting. Three days after her treatment, HS calls up the student clinic to complain of intense fatigue and lethargy, along with a deep ache in every bone and joint in her body, which began two days after the treatment. The receptionist did, however, get the patient to acknowledge that her knee and ankles had felt great for two days post-treatment but had been bad for the past 24 hours or so. This turned out to be the only reason she agreed to come back – the two days of relief for her knee and ankles.

HS agreed to come in for another treatment that same day, and it turned out to be purely coincidental that I was the clinic supervisor on that day. However, the student practitioner was different. Upon arriving for my clinic shift, I was informed of the situation with HS, and so I got her file out and studied it.

As soon as I saw her age and that she was post-menopausal, I had a fair idea of what we had missed in the first treatment. This was pretty much confirmed when I was reminded of her misdiagnosed floating, empty and fast pulse, as well as the low back pain/discomfort, swollen/stiff ankles, and that she had suffered from night sweats and hot flushes/flashes throughout menopause.

When HS arrived, I went in with the student and explained that acupuncture can sometimes give mixed messages post-treatment. I also told the patient that the improvement she got was pleasing and that if she persevered for a few more treatments, she was unlikely to continue getting the worsening of symptoms.

I also explained to HS that we needed to ask more questions in order to get the most accurate diagnosis we could; her answers of late-afternoon fevers, a dry throat and some mild dizziness confirmed the diagnosis of Kidney Yīn Xū.

Her knee diagnosis of Damp Heat Bì remained. This time, however, we changed the treatment slightly, which was crucial in the context of the new diagnosis. I got rid of the extremity flushing points of GB 34 and LI 10 because these points were too draining for her underlying Kidney Yīn Xū. Then we added KI 6 and SP 6 to tonify Kidney Yīn.[30]

Although HS didn't have as much instant improvement in her knee (compared with her first appointment), she also didn't have any worsening of symptoms three days later.

HS had five more weekly appointments, by which stage she had minimal knee pain/swelling, her ankles and low back were symptom-free, and her residual menopause symptoms had also virtually ceased.

Since then HS has referred the student clinic more than a dozen new patients. At last check she was still visiting the student clinic once every four weeks for maintenance and had virtually no complaints.

To remind you, I mention this case because of the fact that HS had an underlying deficiency with an excess/stagnant musculoskeletal complaint. The points chosen were not perfect because the extremity flushing points were too draining and this negatively impacted on her underlying Kidney Yīn Xū.

The extremity flushing points are very good at moving the Vital Substances, but the minute you move them, you burn them up. It's like petrol/gas in your car. If the car sits idle and unused, the petrol/gas does likewise. The minute you turn on the car, however, you start burning up the petrol/gas. The same principle applies with the extremity flushing points, and that's why they were inappropriate for HS.

Remember that when it comes to constructing point combinations for different aspects of a patient's illness, you need to be careful that the combination doesn't have one part of it working on a particular action, with another part of the combination opposing that action. My hope is that by the time you have worked your way through this book, there won't be any possibility of this occurring.

11. Treat the person, not the disease

One of the first things I was taught in my Chinese medicine studies was that our medicine treats the person, not the disease!

Western medical practitioners, on the other hand, appear to do the opposite. But aren't we also doing something similar when we diagnose our patients with Zàng Fǔ patterns (or whatever diagnostic method you use) and then treat them via a learned treatment?

There are two ways to ensure this never happens in your clinic. One is to think for yourself, and the second is to use sticky labels. Allow me to explain.

Think for yourself

This book will teach you how to think for yourself by giving you the tools (the learning) to construct treatments. In that way you are allowing your treatment to be malleable because it's rare for your patient to be a perfect fit diagnostically, regardless of your diagnostic preference.

I will give an example by using the Zàng Fǔ patterns. In my clinic I regularly diagnose my patients as having Liver Qì Stagnation – in fact, it's the most common diagnosis in my clinic. This pattern obviously has a set list of points, which are typically LR 3, LR 13, LR 14, GB 34, PC 6 and LI 4.[31]

These are good points to use, but what happens if the patient isn't completely Liver Qì Stagnant? What if the patient also complains of a poor appetite, lethargy, abdominal bloating and loose stools? Seems to me that they also have some Spleen Qì Xū, which also has a set list of points – typically, SP 3, SP 6, ST 36, BL 20, CV 12 and LR 13.[32]

I now have too many points as I prefer to use 8–16 needles, so I need to edit, and this is where I become an acupuncture chef (of sorts). So how would I edit this treatment?

- For starters, I look for any points that are mentioned in both lists as I will definitely use those. Only LR 13 is in both point formulas.

- I don't like to flip a patient mid-treatment, so I can eliminate any points that are not on the same side. Looking at the points listed above, there are ten points that I can needle face up and eight that I can needle face down.

- Since LR 13 is a definite, and also located on the front of the body, I will do a face-up treatment. This means I won't be using BL 20.

- I like to have treatments that utilize points on all parts of the body, meaning I like to use the head/face, trunk, arms/hands and legs/feet. I don't like stacking points in one or two areas only.

- I consider the acupuncture points' areas of location and look to remove some points from stacked areas. Table 2.4 shows how that would look.

Table 2.4 Acupuncture point locations

Location of points	Points	
Head/face/neck	None	
Trunk (front)	LR 13 LR 14	CV 12
Arms/hands	PC 6	LI 4
Legs/feet	LR 3 GB 34 SP 3	SP 6 ST 36

Then I see which points combine well and which don't. Reminding myself that I am treating a patient with Liver Qì Stagnation and Spleen Qì Xū, I go through each point as follows:

- LR 13 is the Front Mù Collecting point of the Spleen[33] and is also on the Liver channel, so it's a keeper.

- LR 14 is the Front Mù Collecting point of the Liver and is a meeting point for the Liver and Spleen channels,[34] but it doesn't necessarily treat the Spleen; in fact, it tends to be better for Liver and Stomach disharmonies, so I'm going to dump it.

- CV 12 is the Front Mù Collecting point of the Stomach and is also an excellent point to harmonize the Middle Jiāo.[35] Since both the Spleen and Liver are located in the Middle Jiāo, and as it's also a terrific point in combination with LR 13, PC 6, SP 3, SP 6 and ST 36, it's a keeper.

- PC 6 moves Liver Qì and harmonizes the Spleen,[36] and therefore it's a keeper.

- LI 4 and LR 3 'open the Four Gates',[37] so they both have to be considered. This combination will be discussed in more detail in Chapter 6; suffice to say that it moves Qì, sedates excess conditions and can tonify deficiencies. So this combination is a keeper.

- GB 34 moves Liver Qì[38] but doesn't tonify Spleen Qì, so I'm dumping it.

- SP 3 is the Yuán Source point of the Spleen as well as being the Shù Stream and Earth point on the Spleen channel.[39] It is also a Horary point, which is a double-up of the element[40] – in this case, the Earth point on an Earth channel. So although this point is excellent to tonify Spleen Qì, it doesn't move Liver Qì and I'm dumping it.

- SP 6 is the 'Three Leg Yīn Connector'.[41] This means that it connects the Spleen, Liver and Kidney channels. It's also an excellent point to tonify Spleen Qì and move Liver Qì, so it's a keeper.

- ST 36 is, in my opinion, one of the top five best points on the body. There is not much it can't do and it happens to be terrific when combined with the majority of the points in my list, so it's a keeper.

Table 2.5 gives a summary of which points I am keeping and which I am dumping.

Table 2.5 Acupuncture point locations – keep or dump?

Location of points	Points	Keep or dump?
Trunk (front)	LR 13 LR 14 CV 12	Keep Dump Keep
Arms/hands	PC 6 LI 4	Keep Keep
Legs/feet	LR 3 GB 34 SP 3 SP 6 ST 36	Keep Dump Dump Keep Keep

This gives me a final list of LR 13, CV 12, PC 6, LI 4, LR 3, SP 6 and ST 36. They are scattered all over the body and they total 13 needles when needled bilaterally. I have also listed the combinations from the treatment in Table 2.6.

Table 2.6 Acupuncture point combinations

Point	Combines with	
LR 13	CV 12 PC 6 LR 3	SP 6 ST 36
CV 12	LR 13 PC 6	SP 6 ST 36
PC 6	LR 13 CV 12 LR 3	SP 6 ST 36
LI 4	LR 3 SP 6	ST 36
LR 3	LR 13 PC 6	LI 4 SP 6
SP 6	LR 13 CV 12 PC 6	LI 4 LR 3 ST 36
ST 36	LR 13 CV 12 PC 6	LI 4 SP 6

Sticky labels

The other way to ensure that you always treat the person and not the disease is to give each patient a metaphorical sticky label.

Regardless of the type of diagnostic method you use, a sticky label will work. Using my preferred Zàng Fǔ patterns method, it goes something like this:

- My patient comes in and I ask a series of questions in order to gather a diagnosis. This diagnosis isn't binding, and in order to remind myself of this fact, I put a pretend sticky label on to my patient's forehead.

- If I use my previous example, then my patient's sticky label would read 'Liver Qì Stagnation with Spleen Qì Xū'. This label allows me to work out my treatment.

- I perform the treatment. Then, when I remove the needles, I also remove the sticky label and put it into the patient's file next to the date of treatment.

- The patient makes another appointment and then leaves the clinic without the sticky label attached to their forehead, which means they leave the clinic as themselves. It's important that they don't leave the clinic with their diagnosis still attached, because the last thing we want to do as Chinese medicine practitioners is to give our patients disease labels. If we do, then we are effectively treating the disease and not the person.

- Upon the patient's return to our clinic for a follow-up treatment, they once again arrive as themselves and not their disease.

- Repeat the previous steps.

You might find that the patient is diagnosed the same way for multiple sessions and that's perfectly okay. Just remember to always remove the sticky label after every treatment. As I stated just before, we never want patients to become accustomed to their disease label. I see this happen all the time with Western disease labels. I honestly believe that the more we label our diseases, the more we become our diseases. So my advice to you is always to use metaphorical sticky labels!

Notes

1 Wu 1993, p.191. *The Spiritual Pivot* (Líng Shū) was written somewhere between 200 and 0 BCE.
2 McDonald and Penner 1994, pp.142–147, 166–168.
3 Ellis, Wiseman and Boss 1989, p.162.
4 Marchment 2004, p.147.
5 Maciocia 2015, p.75.
6 Ibid., p.43.
7 Ibid., p.409.
8 Some of the more famous modern-day authors who share my view are Giovanni Maciocia (2015, pp.1191–1207), Jeremy Ross (1995) and Ellis, Wiseman and Boss (1991, pp.443–446).
9 Deadman, Al-Khafaji and Baker 2007, pp.580–581. There are some books that also recommend M-UE-24 (Luò Zhěn) for diarrhea and stomach pain, but I don't personally use this point for those conditions.
10 Deadman *et al.* 2007, pp.158–161.
11 Hartmann 2009, p.106.

12 Ibid., p.73.
13 Ibid., p.174.
14 Ibid., p.48.
15 Deadman *et al.* 2007, pp.112, 396.
16 Maciocia 2015, pp.986, 997.
17 Hartmann 2009, p.5.
18 Sun 2011, p.422.
19 Hecker *et al.* 2005, p.53; www.betterhealth. vic.gov.au/health/conditionsandtreatments/ acupuncture.
20 Ellis *et al.* 1991, pp.448–449.
21 Ibid., pp.447–448; Maciocia 2015, pp.1173–1178; Ni 1995, pp.231–234: 65th chapter.
22 Ellis *et al.* 1991, p.443; Maciocia 2015, pp.1195–1198; Ross 1995, pp.50–51.
23 Deadman *et al.* 2007, p.104.
24 Hartmann 2009, p.73.
25 Ibid., p.20.
26 Maciocia 2015, p.1130.
27 Ni 1995, pp.187–189: 52nd chapter. *The Yellow Emperor's Classic (Inner Canon of the Yellow Emperor/*Huáng Dì Nèi Jīng) was written somewhere between 200 and 0 BCE. In the 52nd chapter there was a brief discussion on contraindications when needling, specifically (but not entirely) into organs.
28 Hartmann 2009, p.44.
29 Deadman *et al.* 2007, pp.111–112, 340; Shi 2007, pp.139, 217, 283.
30 Ross 1995, pp.171–172, 214–215.
31 Ibid., p.9.
32 Ibid., p.18.
33 O'Connor and Bensky 1981, pp.181–182.
34 Ibid., p.181.
35 Li 2007, p.813.
36 Deadman *et al.* 2007, p.377.
37 Wang and Robertson 2008, p.563.
38 Deadman *et al.* 2007, p.451.
39 Ellis *et al.* 1991, p.150.
40 Hicks, Hicks and Mole 2010, pp.284–285.
41 Deadman *et al.* 2007, pp.189–190.

Part 2

The Framework of Acupuncture Point Combinations

There is a method to book learning. Simply scrub clean the mind, then read. If you don't understand the text, put it down for the moment, wait until your thoughts have cleared, then pick it up and read it again. Now we can speak about the need to open up our minds. The mind, how can we open it? We just have to take it and keep it focused on the text.

Zhū Xī/朱熹 (1130–1200 CE)[1]

Welcome to Part 2 of *The Principles and Practical Application of Acupuncture Point Combinations*. Over the following five chapters I will be taking you through the basics of how to combine acupuncture points. This will include three chapters that look at different point combinations from the classics (both ancient and modern classics) and from my own experience. Some of these point combinations will be small and some will be large, with each of the combinations discussed in depth.

In almost every single situation, I will be explaining why/how the points work together, helping to guide you to construct your own point combinations in the future in your own clinic.

Note

1   Liang 1996, p.153. Zhū Xī (1130–1200 CE) was a Neo-Confucian marvel and was a leading intellectual of his time. He was also directly responsible for the canonization of the 'Four Books' (*Confucian Analects*, the *Mencius*, *The Great Learning*, *The Doctrine of the Mean*). He was a serious philosophical superstar!

Nature produces those things which, being continually moved by a certain principle contained in themselves, arrive at a certain end.

Aristotle (384–322 BCE)[1]

The highest good is the nature. Originally the nature has not the least evil. Therefore it is called the highest good. To abide by it is simply to recover one's original state.

Wáng Yángmíng/王陽明 (1472–1529 CE)[2]

3

How to Combine Acupuncture Points

This chapter is dedicated to discussing how to combine acupuncture points. The sections below include local and distal points on the same channel, Wǔ Xíng point combinations, Six Division partnerships, points that treat the same Zàng Fǔ patterns as well as signs and symptoms.

1. Local and distal points on the same channel

This is a point combination that many of you are probably familiar with. As the name suggests, you choose a point that is local to the patient's complaint and then you deliberately choose a distal point on the same channel to act as a support.

This is a very simple combination but also very effective. The local point will immediately start to treat the area of concern in two ways:

- It will try to move and then clear any local stagnation.

- It will try to draw fresh Vital Substances to the local area for healing.

The local stagnation is counterproductive as it is old, toxic and taking up space. Because of this, the stagnation needs to be cleared out to make room for the fresh Vital Substances to enter the area for healing.

The distal points in this combination also work on two things:

- They try to send Vital Substance reinforcements to the local area to assist with the healing process.

- They try to drag/pull/draw/push the stagnation away from the area of concern.

Let me give you two examples.

Blocked nose

- Local point = LI 20

- Distal point = LI 4

According to Deadman, Al-Khafaji and Baker (2007, pp.104, 120), LI 20 is 'the foremost local point for treating all disorders of the nose'. Further, LI 4 'is the single most important point to treat disorders of the face and sense organs'.[3]

Acting together, LI 4 and LI 20 are excellent at treating all nose disorders, not just a blocked nose.

This combination uses the popular theme of having distal points on the limbs for disorders on the head, face or trunk – more specifically, points on the limbs that are below the elbows or knees.[4]

Swollen ankles and feet

- Local point = SP 3

- Distal point = SP 9

According to Maciocia (2015, p.997), '[an] important function of this point [SP 3] is to resolve Dampness, for which it is a major point'. Further, Deadman *et al.* (2007, p.194) advise that SP 9 treats edema and swelling of the legs and feet.

First of all, both these points are good at transforming and transporting the Jīn Yè.[5]

Second, I wanted to show a local-and-distal combination that worked in the opposite manner to the previous example of a blocked nose. Here, I have used a distal point above the local point, whereas in the previous example I had a distal point below the local point. In this example, I am referring to the term distal as being 'at a distance' from the local injury; I'm not referring to distal as the opposite of proximal.

Third, this is a great combination to drag Jīn Yè up the leg, which is an impressive feat considering how heavy it can be. This forces the acupuncture points to fight against this heaviness, as well as fighting against gravity too.

If the patient had edema in other areas of the body as well, there are a couple of other considerations with this example:

- There is no reason you couldn't contemplate using additional points on the Spleen channel to enhance the effects of SP 3 and SP 9, particularly if the patient had swelling in the feet, ankles, knees and abdomen. For example, you could add in SP 6 and SP 15, which are also effective in transforming and transporting Jīn Yè.[6]

- You could, of course, add points on other channels to create a more balanced point combination too. Some possible additions include CV 9, ST 36, LU 7, KI 7 and BL 21.[7]

As the previous examples showed, it is common practice to use local and distal points on the same channel, just as it is common to use local and distal points that aren't on the same channel. For a more in-depth discussion on the local and distal points that aren't on the same channel, see Chapter 5.

2. Yīn and Yáng partners – Wǔ Xíng

The Yīn and Yáng Wǔ Xíng pairings are another fantastic way to combine acupuncture points with a number of safe and effective point combinations. These include using a range of special point categories such as:

- Luò Connecting points

- Horary points

- Front Mù Collecting points – if they are on the Yīn and Yáng channel pairings[8]

- Yuán Source points.

There are also some more obscure pairings for the Yīn and Yáng partners, which include:

- points that treat the same Zàng Fǔ patterns

- points that treat the same signs/symptoms

- points on the channels that are in close proximity

- a local point on one channel with a distal point on its paired channel

- points with similar Pīn Yīn names/meanings.

Table 3.1 lists the Yīn and Yáng pairings according to the Wǔ Xíng.

Table 3.1 Wǔ Xíng Yīn and Yáng partners[9]

Wǔ Xíng	Yīn organ/channel	Yáng organ/channel
Wood	Liver	Gall Bladder
Fire	Heart Pericardium	Small Intestine Sān Jiāo
Earth	Spleen	Stomach
Metal	Lungs	Large Intestine
Water	Kidneys	Urinary Bladder

For each of the six Yīn and Yáng Wǔ Xíng pairings I will provide a few examples. Throughout I will ensure that the different combination options mentioned above are covered. Each of the different point combinations discussed are effective for at least one but usually numerous reasons.

Wood element – Liver and Gall Bladder
Example 1: LR 14 and GB 24
This point combination takes advantage of the following aspects:

- Both Front Mù Collecting points.

- Points that treat the same Zàng Fǔ patterns.

  Among others, these points are great for treating Damp Heat in the Liver and Gall Bladder.[10]

- Points on the channels that are in close proximity.

  In addition, LR 14 and GB 24 are also Jiāo Huì Meeting/Intersecting points with the Spleen, thereby making them an effective combination for treating the Spleen.[11]
  LR 14 is also a Jiāo Huì Meeting/Intersecting point with the Yīn Wéi Mài, where GB 24 is the Jiāo Huì Meeting/Intersecting point with the Yáng Wéi Mài.[12] This combination is effective to help your patient live in the now, as opposed to living in the past or future.[13]

  The Yang Wei and Yin Wei channels link different transitions or milestones in our life. People can invest their qi, blood, and essence (Jing) in reliving past moments or living a fantasy of the future. Being out of the present moment can be draining. The Wei channels can assist in releasing these attachments. (Twicken 2013, p.37)

Example 2: LR 3 and GB 40
This point combination takes advantage of the following aspects:

- Both Yuán Source points.

- Points that treat the same Zàng Fǔ patterns.

  Among others, these points are great for treating Liver Xuè Xū with Gall Bladder Xū.[14]

- Points on the channels that are in close proximity.

  While not technically side by side, these points are roughly 3 cùn away from one another.

Example 3: LR 2 and GB 1

This point combination takes advantage of the following aspects:

- Points that treat the same signs/symptoms.

  Among others, these points are great for treating eye disorders, namely red, dry, gritty and bloodshot.[15]

- A local point on one channel (GB 1) with a distal point on its paired channel (LR 2) for treating eye disorders.

Fire element – Heart and Small Intestine

Example 1: HT 5 and SI 7

This point combination takes advantage of the following aspects:

- Both Luò Connecting points.

- Points that treat the same Zàng Fǔ patterns.

  Among others, these points are great for Calming the Shén.[16, 17]

- Points with similar Pīn Yīn names/meanings.

  #### HT 5 (Tōng Lǐ)
  Tōng = connect or communicate; Lǐ = village crossroads or interior.[18]
      This is likely to mean a crossroads that connects the Heart and Small Intestine channels because it is the Luò Connecting point.

  #### SI 7 (Zhī Zhèng)
  Zhī = a branch; Zhèng = correct or to put right.[19]
      This is likely to mean a branch or connection, and because it is the Luò Connecting point, it's probably referring to the connection between the Small Intestine and Heart channels.

Example 2: HT 8 and SI 5

This point combination takes advantage of the following aspects:

- Both Horary points (Fire points on Fire channels).

- Points that treat the same Zàng Fǔ patterns.

  Among others, these points are great for clearing Heat to calm the Shén.[20]

- Points on the channels that are in close proximity.

Example 3: HT 7 and SI 4

This point combination takes advantage of the following aspects:

- Both Yuán Source points.

- Points that treat the same signs/symptoms.

  Among others, these points are great for treating Throat Painful Obstruction (Hóu Bì). This is usually defined as swelling, pain and congestion of the throat.[21]

- Points on the channels that are in close proximity.

Fire element – Pericardium and Sān Jiāo

Example 1: PC 6 and TE 5

This point combination takes advantage of the following aspects:

- Both Luò Connecting points.

- Points on the channels that are in close proximity.

- Points with similar Pīn Yīn names/meanings.

  #### PC 6 (Nèi Guān)

  Nèi = inner or inside; Guān = pass or gate.[22]
  PC 6 is located on the inner side of the forearm, and is a pass or gateway to the Sān Jiāo channel because it's the Luò Connecting point of the Pericardium channel.

  #### TE 5 (Wài Guān)

  Wài = outer or outside; Guān = pass or gate.[23]
  TE 5 is located on the outer side of the forearm, and is a pass or gateway to the Pericardium channel because it's the Luò Connecting point of the Sān Jiāo channel.

  Interestingly, both these points are opening/confluent points for two of the Eight Extraordinary Vessels. PC 6 opens the Yīn Wéi Mài, and TE 5 opens the Yáng Wéi Mài.[24] This combination is effective to help your patient live in the now, as opposed to living in the past or future.[25]

  > Are you always thinking of the future? If you are, it is a Yang Wei issue… Are you living in the past? If you are, it is a Yin Wei issue. (Twicken 2013, p.98)

Example 2: PC 8 and TE 6

This point combination takes advantage of the following aspects:

- Both Horary points (Fire points on Fire channels).

- Points that treat the same signs/symptoms.

  Among others, these points are great for treating Heart/chest pain with chest oppression.[26]

Example 3: PC 7 and TE 4
This point combination takes advantage of the following aspects:

- Both Yuán Source points.

- Points that treat the same signs/symptoms.

  Among others, these points are great for treating wrist problems.[27]

- Points on the channels that are in close proximity.

Earth element – Spleen and Stomach
Example 1: SP 3 and ST 36
This point combination takes advantage of the following aspects:

- Both Horary points (Earth points on Earth channels).

- Points that treat the same Zàng Fǔ patterns.

  Among others, these points are great for treating Spleen and Stomach Qì Xū.[28]

Example 2: SP 1 and ST 3
This point combination takes advantage of the following aspects:

- Points that treat the same signs/symptoms.

  Among others, these points are great for treating nose bleeds.[29]

- A local point on one channel (ST 3) with a distal point on its paired channel (SP 1) for treating nose disorders.

Example 3: SP 4 and ST 40
This point combination takes advantage of the following aspects:

- Both Luò Connecting points.

- Points that treat the same Zàng Fǔ patterns.

  Among others, these points are great for assisting the Spleen to transform and transport ('T & T') the Jīn Yè.[30]

Metal element - Lungs and Large Intestine
Example 1: LU 5 and LI 11
This point combination takes advantage of the following aspects:

- Points that treat the same signs/symptoms.

  Among others, these points are great for treating tennis elbow/lateral epicondylitis.[31]

- Points on the channels that get close to one another.

- Points with similar Pīn Yīn names/meanings.

LU 5 (Chǐ Zé)
Chǐ = a Chinese measurement which equals about one foot; Zé = marsh.[32]

LU 5 is located about one foot from the wrist crease pulse. It is also a Water point and Hé (Uniting) Sea point on the Lung channel, thereby explaining the reference to a marsh.

LI 11 (Qū Chí)
Qū = bent or crooked; Chí = pool or pond.[33]

LI 11 is located at the bend of the elbow. It is also the Hé (Uniting) Sea point on the Large Intestine channel, thereby explaining the reference to a pool or pond of water.

Example 2: LU 9 and LI 4
This point combination takes advantage of the following aspects:

- Both Yuán Source points.

- Points that treat the same Zàng Fǔ patterns.

  Among others, these points are great for clearing External Pathogenic Factors, specifically Wind, as well as to strengthen Wèi Qì.[34]

- Points on the channels that are in close proximity.

Example 3: LU 10 and LI 18
This point combination takes advantage of the following aspects:

- Points that treat the same signs/symptoms.

  Among others, these points are great for treating throat problems and/or loss of voice.[35]

- A local point on one channel (LI 18) with a distal point on its paired channel (LU 10) for treating throat disorders.

Water element – Kidneys and Urinary Bladder
Example 1: KI 2 and BL 66
This point combination takes advantage of the following aspects:

- Points that treat the same signs/symptoms.

  Among others, these points are great for treating various sweating disorders.[36]

- Points with similar Pīn Yīn names/meanings.

  KI 2 (Rán Gǔ)
  Rán = burn; Gǔ = valley.[37]
      KI 2 is located in a valley on the foot. It is also the Yíng Spring (Fire clearing) point on the Kidney channel, thereby explaining the reference to burning.

  BL 66 (Zú Tōng Gǔ)
  Zú = foot or leg; Tōng = connect; Gǔ = valley.[38]
      BL 66 is located in a valley on the foot and connects the Urinary Bladder channel to the Kidney channel, through BL 67 and KI 1, before reaching KI 2.

Example 2: KI 4 and BL 58
This point combination takes advantage of the following aspects:

- Both Luò Connecting points.

- Points that treat the same Zàng Fǔ patterns.

  Among others, these points are great for strengthening the Kidneys.[39]

- Points that treat the same signs/symptoms.

  Among others, these points are great for treating low back pain.[40]

Example 3: KI 11 and BL 67
This point combination takes advantage of the following aspects:

- Points that treat the same signs/symptoms.

  Among others, these points are great for treating nocturnal emissions.[41]

- A local point on one channel (KI 11) with a distal point on its paired channel (BL 67) for treating urinary disorders.

3. Yīn/Yīn partners – Six Divisions

The Yīn/Yīn or Six Division pairings are another fantastic way to combine acupuncture points with a number of safe and effective point combinations. These include using a range of special point categories such as:

- Yuán Source points.

- Wŭ Xíng partnered points.

- Top and bottom.

- Corresponding/mirroring on the paired channels.

There are also some more obscure pairings for the Yīn/Yīn partners which include:

- Points that treat the same Zàng Fŭ patterns.

- Points that treat the same signs/symptoms.

- Points on the channels that are in close proximity.

- A local point on one channel with a distal point on its paired channel.

- Points with similar Pīn Yīn names/meanings.

Table 3.2 lists the Yīn/Yīn pairings according to the Six Divisions.

Table 3.2 Six Division Yīn/Yīn partners[42]

Six Divisions	Arm/hand Yīn channel	Leg/foot Yīn channel
Tài Yīn (Greater Yīn)	Lungs	Spleen
Shào Yīn (Lesser Yīn)	Heart	Kidneys
Jué Yīn (Terminal Yīn)	Pericardium	Liver

For each of the three Yīn/Yīn Six Division pairings I will provide a few examples. Throughout I will ensure that the different combination options mentioned above are covered. Each of the different point combinations discussed are effective for at least one but usually numerous reasons.

Tài Yīn – Lungs and Spleen
Example 1: LU 9 and SP 3
This point combination takes advantage of the following aspects:

- Both Yuán Source points.

- A top-and-bottom point combination.

    LU 9 is the top/higher point and SP 3 is the bottom/lower point.

- Points that treat the same Zàng Fǔ patterns.

  Among others, these points are great to strengthen/tonify Lung and Spleen Qì.[43]

Example 2: LU 1 and SP 20
This point combination takes advantage of the following aspects:

- Points that treat the same signs/symptoms.

  Among others, these points are great for treating chest fullness/distension, cough and shortness of breath.[44]

- Points on the channels that are in close proximity.

  LU 1 is also a Jiāo Huì Meeting/Intersecting point between the Lung and Spleen channels.[45] In this case, the link is between LU 1 and SP 20.

Example 3: LU 6 and SP 8
This point combination takes advantage of the following aspects:

- A top-and-bottom point combination.

  LU 6 is the top/higher point and SP 8 is the bottom/lower point.

- Corresponding/mirroring on the paired channels.

  Both points are located midway up the forearm and lower leg on the anterior lateral aspect of the limb (when the body is in the correct anatomical position).

  Corresponding points can be effective to treat the local area. This is done by having a local and a distal point that mirror each other. In this example it can work two ways: (1) a patient complains of shin splints with pain radiating up the Spleen channel (inside/medial side of the tibia). In this example, SP 8 would act as the local point, and LU 6 would be the distal mirror; (2) a patient complains of tennis elbow (lateral epicondylitis) which radiates distally along the Lung channel (the anterior lateral aspect of the forearm). In this example, LU 6 would act as the local point, and SP 8 would be the distal mirror.

  Interestingly, both points are also Xì Cleft points. As Xì Cleft points are used to move stagnations along a channel as well as to help reduce pain,[46] LU 6 and SP 8 would have that additional benefit when treating shin splints and tennis elbow.

Shào Yīn - Heart and Kidneys
Example 1: HT 7 and KI 3
This point combination takes advantage of the following aspects:

- Both Yuán Source points.

- A top-and-bottom point combination.

  HT 7 is the top/higher point and KI 3 is the bottom/lower point.

- Corresponding/mirroring on the paired channels.

  Both points are located at the wrist and ankle (mirrored joints) on the anterior medial aspect of the limb (when the body is in the correct anatomical position).

- Points that treat the same Zàng Fǔ patterns.

  Among others, these points are great to treat a Shào Yīn Imbalance.[47]

- Points that treat the same signs/symptoms.

  Among others, these points are great for treating nocturnal emissions.[48]

Example 2: HT 7, KI 10, KI 22 and KI 25
This point combination takes advantage of the following aspects:

- A top-and-bottom point combination.

  HT 7, KI 22 and KI 25 are the top/higher points, whereas KI 10 is the bottom/lower point.

- Points that treat the same Zàng Fǔ patterns.

  Among others, these points are great to balance the Fire and Water element connection. How does that work exactly?

  HT 7 is the Yuán Source point on the Heart channel. As such, it regulates any Heart imbalance. The Heart is a part of the Fire element, plus, according to the 8th chapter of *The Yellow Emperor's Classic* (Huáng Dì Nèi Jīng/黄帝內經), it is considered the Emperor/Sovereign organ;[49] therefore, the Heart channel points are very important to balance out the Fire element.

  KI 10 is the Horary point on the Kidney channel (Water point on a Water channel). As such, it regulates the Water element.[50]

KI 22 (Bù Láng)
Bù = walk or step; Láng = veranda or corridor. Translates as 'Veranda/Corridor Walk'.[51]

Meaning/interpretation – the Water element (Yīn) loves serenity and security and the home is where we often feel safest. The Fire element (Yáng) loves getting out in the world, being around lots of people.

A veranda is that middle ground between the security of one's house and the big wide world. It's a place of moderation, where the Fire and Water elements feel equally valued and nourished.

Therefore, KI 22 treats the Water and Fire elements.[52]

KI 25 (Shén Cáng)

Shén = spirit; Cáng = storehouse. Translates as 'Spirit Storehouse'.[53]

Meaning/interpretation – the Shén encompasses every one of the Seven Emotions, which are anger, joy, pensiveness, worry, sadness, fear and shock. The Shén also incorporates every one of the Wǔ Shén, which are called the Hún, Shén, Yì, Pò and the Zhì. Granted, these are all stored in different organs, but the primary organ that controls them all is the Heart Shén.[54]

At KI 25 the Heart Shén can access all emotions and spirits to encourage emotional health and wellbeing.

> It is perhaps the point of choice in situations when the intensity of feelings of rejection and loneliness have devastated the stability and strength of a person's *shen*. (Hicks, Hicks and Mole 2010, p.324)

Therefore, KI 25 treats the Fire element.[55]

- Two local points (KI 22 and KI 25) with a distal point on the same channel (KI 10) as well as a distal point on its Shào Yīn paired channel (HT 7).

- Points with similar Pīn Yīn names/meanings.

 HT 7 (Shén Mén) translates as Spirit Gate, and KI 25 (Shén Cáng) translates as Spirit Storehouse. Both of these points are effective to regulate the Heart Shén.[56]

 In this example, KI 10 and KI 22 don't apply as their Pīn Yīn names aren't similar.

Example 3: HT 3 and KI 10

This point combination takes advantage of the following aspects:

- A top-and-bottom point combination.

 HT 3 is the top/higher point and KI 10 is the bottom/lower point.

- Corresponding/mirroring on the paired channels.

 Both points are located at the elbow and knee (mirrored joints) on the medial aspect of the limb.

Corresponding points can be effective to treat the local area. This is done by having a local and a distal point that mirror each other. In this example it can work two ways: (1) a patient complains of knee pain radiating along the medial aspect of the knee along the Kidney channel. In this example, KI 10 would act as the local point, and HT 3 would be the distal mirror; (2) a patient complains of golfer's elbow (medial epicondylitis) which radiates along the Heart channel (the medial aspect of the elbow/arm). In this example, HT 3 would act as the local point, and KI 10 would be the distal mirror.

- Points that treat the same signs/symptoms.

  Among others, these points are effective at treating mania.[57] Although not stated in the reference, the reason for this effect is that both HT 3 and KI 10 are Water points. Since manic behavior is almost always as a result of too much Fire, using Water (points) can put out the fire.

Jué Yīn - Pericardium and Liver
Example 1: PC 7 and LR 3
This point combination takes advantage of the following aspects:

- Both Yuán Source points.

- A top-and-bottom point combination.

  PC 7 is the top/higher point and LR 3 is the bottom/lower point.

- Points that treat the same signs/symptoms.

  Among others, these points are particularly effective at treating insomnia plus a range of chest disorders, including chest and lateral costal pain/fullness/distension, shortness of breath with sighing, and breast pain/swelling.[58]

Example 2: PC 6 and LR 14
This point combination takes advantage of the following aspects:

- A top-and-bottom point combination.

  LR 14 is the top/higher point and PC 6 is the bottom/lower point.

- Points that treat the same Zàng Fǔ patterns.

  Among others, these points are great to treat Liver Qì Stagnation.[59]

- A local point on one channel (Liver – LR 14) with a distal point on its paired Jué Yīn channel partner (Pericardium – PC 6) for treating the Liver.

Example 3: PC 8, PC 9, LR 1 and LR 2

This point combination takes advantage of the following aspects:

- Wǔ Xíng partnered points.

  This point combination uses Horary points on each of the channels, as well as the partnered Wǔ Xíng point on each channel: PC 8 is the Horary point on the Pericardium channel (Fire point on a Fire channel). As such, it regulates the Fire element;[60] LR 1 is the Horary point on the Liver channel (Wood point on a Wood channel). As such, it regulates the Wood element;[61] PC 9 is the Wood point on the Pericardium channel (Wood point on a Fire channel). As such, it regulates the connection between the Wood and Fire elements;[62] LR 2 is the Fire point on the Liver channel (Fire point on a Wood channel). As such, it regulates the connection between the Fire and Wood elements.[63]

  To summarize, this combination of points is very effective at regulating any imbalance between the Wood and Fire elements.

- A top-and-bottom point combination.

  PC 8 and PC 9 are the top/higher points, whereas LR 1 and LR 2 are the bottom/lower points.

- Points that treat the same Zàng Fǔ patterns.

  Among others, these points are great to sedate Fire Blazing, particularly when it gets into the head and Heart Shén.[64] Of the wide range of signs and symptoms this implies, these points are effective for loss of consciousness, dizziness/collapse, hypertension,[65] fever/heat/sweats, headaches, anger/irritability,[66] manic behavior/agitation, epilepsy/convulsions and Wind Stroke/Wind Strike (Zhōng Fēng).[67]

4. Yáng/Yáng partners – Six Divisions

The Yáng/Yáng or Six Division pairings are another fantastic way to combine acupuncture points with a number of safe and effective point combinations. These include using a range of special point categories such as:

- Yuán Source points.

- Lower Hé (Uniting) Sea points.

- Wǔ Xíng partnered points.

- Top and bottom.

- Corresponding/mirroring on the paired channels.

There are also some more obscure pairings for the Yáng/Yáng partners, which include:

- Points that treat the same Zàng Fǔ patterns.

- Points that treat the same signs/symptoms.

- Points on the channels that are in close proximity.

- A local point on one channel with a distal point on its paired channel.

- Points with similar Pīn Yīn names/meanings.

Table 3.3 lists the Yáng/Yáng pairings according to the Six Divisions.

Table 3.3 Six Division Yáng/Yáng partners[68]

Six Divisions	Arm/hand Yáng channel	Leg/foot Yáng channel
Tài Yáng (Greater Yáng)	Small Intestine	Urinary Bladder
Yáng Míng (Bright Yáng)	Large Intestine	Stomach
Shào Yáng (Lesser Yáng)	Sān Jiāo	Gall Bladder

For each of the three Yáng/Yáng Six Division pairings I will provide a few examples. Throughout I will ensure that the different combination options mentioned above are covered. Each of the different point combinations discussed are effective for at least one but usually numerous reasons.

Tài Yáng - Small Intestine and Urinary Bladder
Example 1: ST 39 and BL 40
This point combination takes advantage of the following aspects:

- Both Lower Hé (Uniting) Sea points.

  ST 39 is the Lower Hé (Uniting) Sea point for the Small Intestine, and BL 40 is the Lower Hé (Uniting) Sea point for the Urinary Bladder.[69]

- Points that treat the same signs/symptoms.

  Among others, these points are effective at treating lower back pain that radiates up the back, down the legs and around to the groin.[70]

Example 2: SI 14, SI 15, BL 11 and BL 41
This point combination takes advantage of the following aspects:

- Points that treat the same signs/symptoms.

  Among others, these points are effective at treating shoulder, upper back and neck disorders involving the spine and/or muscles.[71]

- Points on the channels that are in close proximity.

- Points with similar Pīn Yīn names/meanings.

  SI 14 (Jiān Wài Shū) translates as Outer Shoulder Point, and SI 15 (Jiān Zhōng Shū) translates as Middle Shoulder Point. As their names suggest, both of these points are effective to treat the shoulder region.[72]
  In this example, BL 11 and BL 41 don't apply as their Pīn Yīn names aren't similar.

Example 3: SI 2, SI 5, BL 60 and BL 66
This point combination takes advantage of the following aspects:

- Wǔ Xíng partnered points.

  This point combination uses Horary points on each of the channels, as well as the partnered Wǔ Xíng point on each channel: SI 5 is the Horary point on the Small Intestine channel (Fire point on a Fire channel). As such, it regulates the Fire element;[73] BL 66 is the Horary point on the Urinary Bladder channel (Water point on a Water channel). As such, it regulates the Water element;[74] SI 2 is the Water point on the Small Intestine channel (Water point on a Fire channel). As such, it regulates the connection between the Water and Fire elements;[75] BL 60 is the Fire point on the Urinary Bladder channel (Fire point on a Water channel). As such, it regulates the connection between the Fire and Water elements.[76]
  To summarize, this combination of points is very effective at regulating any imbalance between the Water and Fire elements.

- A top-and-bottom point combination.

  SI 2 and SI 5 are the top/higher points, whereas BL 60 and BL 66 are the bottom/lower points.

- Corresponding/mirroring on the paired channels.

  SI 2 and BL 66 are located near the fifth metacarpophalangeal and metatarsophalangeal joints of the hands and feet.

  SI 5 and BL 60 are located on the wrist and ankles.

- Points that treat the same signs/symptoms.

  Among others, these points work well together to treat neck pain/stiffness/swelling, visual dizziness (Mù Xuàn),[77] red/painful eyes, epistaxis (nosebleed),[78] febrile diseases including malaria, madness/mania[79] and headaches.[80, 81]

- Points with similar Pīn Yīn names/meanings.

This doesn't apply here even though three of the four points have Gǔ in their name. Gǔ means valley, which is purely to signify these points are located in little grooves. This similarity doesn't indicate these points could or should be used together. Their combination is, however, useful via the examples discussed above.

Yáng Míng – Large Intestine and Stomach
Example 1: ST 37 and ST 36
This point combination takes advantage of the following aspects:

- Both Lower Hé (Uniting) Sea points.

    ST 37 is the Lower Hé (Uniting) Sea point for the Large Intestine, and ST 36 is the Lower Hé (Uniting) Sea point for the Stomach.

- Points that treat the same Zàng Fǔ patterns.

    Among others, these points are very good at treating Yáng Míng Fire Blazing.[82]

- Points that treat the same signs/symptoms.

    With regard to Yáng Míng Fire Blazing, that would represent such signs and symptoms as constipation, diverticulitis, irritable bowel syndrome, heartburn, frontal headaches and halitosis/bad breath.[83]
    If we look at ST 37 and ST 36 without the Zàng Fǔ pattern diagnosis, and just look at other signs and symptoms that these points treat, they include diarrhea, dysentery, epigastric/abdominal issues such as bloating/distension/pain, hemiplegia and lower limb painful obstruction syndrome.[84]

Example 2: LI 10 and ST 36
This point combination takes advantage of the following aspects:

- A top-and-bottom point combination.

    LI 10 is the top/higher point and ST 36 is the bottom/lower point.

- Corresponding/mirroring on the paired channels.

    Both points are located just distal to the elbow and knee (mirrored joints) on the anterior lateral aspect of the limb.

- Points that treat the same Zàng Fǔ patterns.

    Among others, these two points are effective at regulating the Large Intestine and Stomach (Yáng Míng) organs.[85]

- Points that treat the same signs/symptoms.

Typically, these relate to the regulating of the Large Intestine and Stomach organs. These signs and symptoms include, but are not limited to, epigastric and abdominal distension/fullness/pain, and digestive problems ranging from vomiting to heartburn to poor assimilation of food to bowel issues such as constipation and/or diarrhea.[86]

LI 10 and ST 36 can also do what I call an extremity flush. What I mean by this is that LI 10 will flush the upper extremities and ST 36 will flush the lower extremities.[87] This is particularly good for arm and leg musculoskeletal complaints. Basically, it's giving the limbs a huge Qì boost to help clear out any stagnation. A word of warning, though: when you move Qì, you burn up the Qì. So don't use this method on someone who is underlying deficient/Xū.

- Points with similar Pīn Yīn names/meanings.

Shǒu = Arm/Hand; Zú = Leg/Foot; Sān = Three; Lǐ = Miles/Measurement.

LI 10 (Shǒu Sān Lǐ) translates as 'Arm/Hand Three Miles/Measurement', and ST 36 (Zú Sān Lǐ) translates as 'Leg/Foot Three Miles/Measurement'. According to Ellis, Wiseman and Boss (1989, pp.45–46, 90–91), this is because both points are located on the arms (Shǒu) and legs (Zú) and are roughly three (Sān) equal measurements (Lǐ) from the tip of the elbow and the lower border of the patella/knee cap.[88]

I'm sure most of you have just done a double take after reading that last sentence! 'Hang on a minute! LI 10 is only two equal measurements from the elbow,' I hear you say, and you would be absolutely correct. But this explanation is referring to the elbow tip or olecranon, which definitely is closer to three equal measurements.[89]

Example 3: LI 1, LI 11, ST 36 and ST 45
This point combination takes advantage of the following aspects. They are:

- Wǔ Xíng partnered points.

This point combination uses Horary points on each of the channels, as well as the partnered Wǔ Xíng point on each channel: LI 1 is the Horary point on the Large Intestine channel (Metal point on a Metal channel). As such, it regulates the Metal element;[90] ST 36 is the Horary point on the Stomach channel (Earth point on an Earth channel). As such, it regulates the Earth element;[91] LI 11 is the Earth point on the Large Intestine channel (Earth point on a Metal channel). As such, it regulates the connection between the Earth and Metal elements;[92] ST 45 is the Metal point on the Stomach channel (Metal point on an Earth channel). As such, it regulates the connection between the Metal and Earth elements.[93]

To summarize, this combination of points is very effective at regulating any imbalance between the Metal and Earth elements.

- A top-and-bottom point combination.

  LI 1 and LI 11 are the top/higher points, whereas ST 36 and ST 45 are the bottom/lower points.

- Points that treat the same Zàng Fŭ patterns.

  The main area these four points treat is to Clear Heat from the upper portion of the channels, which is the neck and head.[94]

- Points that treat the same signs/symptoms.

  Among others, these points work well together to restore consciousness,[95] treat Throat Painful Obstruction,[96] toothache, Wind Stroke/Wind Strike, febrile diseases including malaria, chest fullness/pain/obstruction, madness/mania[97] and jaw problems including lockjaw.[98, 99]

Shào Yáng - Sān Jiāo and Gall Bladder
Example 1: TE 4 and GB 25
This point combination takes advantage of the following aspects:

- Points that treat the same Zàng Fŭ patterns.

  Among others, these two points are effective at strengthening Yuán Qì.[100]
  GB 25 is the Front Mù Collecting point of the Kidneys. With the Yuán Qì housed in the Kidneys, this point is a logical choice as a local point.
  TE 4 is not as straightforward, so we need to refer back to *The Classic of Difficulties* (Huáng Dì Bā Shí Yī Nán Jīng/黃帝八十一難經) to make sense of it. In the 66th difficulty, Flaws (2004, p.121) translates the text as: 'The triple burner [Sān Jiāo] is the special messenger of this original [Yuán] qi.' Unschuld (1986, p.561) translates the text as: 'The Triple Burner is the special envoy that transmits the original influences.'
  Therefore, the Sān Jiāo is directly responsible for moving our Yuán Qì.
  TE 4 is also the Yuán Source point on the Sān Jiāo channel. Yuán Source points are where the Yuán Qì can be activated,[101] thereby making it potentially the most effective point in the entire body to move the Yuán Qì.

- A local point on one channel with a distal point on its paired channel.

  As discussed above, combining TE 4 distally and GB 25 locally works well for strengthening Yuán Qì.

Example 2: TE 21 and GB 2
This point combination takes advantage of the following aspects:

- Points that treat the same signs/symptoms.

Since both of these points are located just anterior to the ear, they are very effective local points for all ear disorders.[102]

- Points on the channels that are in close proximity.

  Both points are located in the hollow between the tragus of the ear and the condyloid process of the mandible.[103]

- Points with similar Pīn Yīn names/meanings.

  TE 21 (ĚR MÉN)
  Ěr = ear; Mén = gate.[104]

  GB 2 (TĪNG HUÌ)
  Tīng = hearing; Huì = meeting.[105]

Example 3: TE 2 and GB 43

This point combination takes advantage of the following aspects:

- A top-and-bottom point combination.

  TE 2 is the top/higher point and GB 43 is the bottom/lower point.

- Corresponding/mirroring on the paired channels.

  Both points are located just proximal to the margin of the web of the fourth and fifth digits; TE 2 is just proximal to the margin of the web of the fourth and fifth fingers, whereas GB 43 is just proximal to the margin of the web of the fourth and fifth toes.

- Points that treat the same Zàng Fǔ patterns.

  The primary focus of TE 2 and GB 43 is to clear heat from the top of their channels; in this case, that is the head. This is because they are Yíng Spring points, which are very effective at clearing heat quickly from the opposite ends of their channels.[106]

- Points that treat the same signs/symptoms.

  TE 2 and GB 43 are a great distal point combination to treat all ear disorders. In addition, they are also effective at treating headache, red/dry eyes, madness/mania and febrile diseases including malaria.[107]

5. Points that treat the same Zàng Fǔ patterns

As you will have seen from earlier in the book, and particularly in this chapter, I have started to include the Zàng Fǔ patterns in my point combinations. These have typically only been with between two and four points listed.

As you progress further into the book, more and more points will be added into the combinations. When this happens, there will be continued discussion as to why the points are combined in that manner so that you can continue to learn from this book.

To give you a better understanding of what is to come with the Zàng Fǔ patterns, I will include another case study.

CASE STUDY 3.1 A 19-YEAR-OLD MALE (CH) WITH SYMPTOMS OF HEADACHES, SORE EYES AND ANGER ISSUES

CH was a new patient with the primary complaints of severe splitting headaches that started at the back of his neck (left GB 20) which then traveled right through the head to just behind, and slightly above, the left eye. His other main complaints were red/painful/dry/gritty/itchy eyes and anger issues.

I asked him whether he was aware of any triggers and he suggested it was because of a lack of alcohol consumption, and then he laughed uproariously and smacked me on the leg. I asked him what is not enough and he told me he had to get 'maggot drunk', which usually meant a bottle of rum plus some beers in a single drinking session.

I advised CH that, in my medical opinion, this is too much alcohol in a single sitting and asked why he thought he needed that much. He answered that alcohol helped keep him calm, jovial and happy, and helped him to sleep. When he doesn't drink, he is generally very quick to anger and has regular outbursts. He also pointed out that when he gets angry he also gets quite dizzy with a very hot face and has an intense aversion to heat.

CH was an apprentice plumber by trade and said that he got extremely stressed, irritable and frustrated, and felt overwhelmed. He also advised me that he 'hated' his job but didn't know how to change careers.

CH also complained of tight neck and shoulders and violent dreams while sleeping, which he says are eliminated after a heavy drinking session. His tongue was, not surprisingly, red, especially on the sides, and his pulse incredibly wiry and strong.

I diagnosed CH with Liver Fire Blazing and wrote the point combination shown in Table 3.4 down in his file:

Table 3.4 Liver Fire Blazing treatment[108]

Location of points	Points	
Head/face/neck	GV 14 GV 20 GB 13 GB 14	GB 20 BL 2 M-HN-9 (Tài Yáng)
Trunk (back)	BL 18	

Arms/hands	LI 4 LI 11	TE 5
Legs/feet	LR 2 LR 3	GB 37
Total points needled	26 needles used bilaterally	

Even though I wrote all those points down, I had no intention of needling them all. For starters, it was CH's first-ever acupuncture appointment and I didn't want to scare him off with so many needles. Second, I rarely needle more than 16 points on any patient as I consider it to be too many, for reasons already discussed. Third, I don't like flipping my patient halfway through a session (as also previously discussed), so I would need to trim this list anyway because it has both front and back points.

I had pretty much made up my mind to needle CH face up, so the first thing to do is look to see what points couldn't be needled in that position. As it turns out, only GV 14 and BL 18 can't be needled in CH when he lies face up, and that only brings the needle number down from 26 to 23 needles. Still too many. So I have two more strategies to get the points down to 16 or fewer:

- Look at the diagnosis again.

- Look at the point combinations.

LOOK AT THE DIAGNOSIS AGAIN
With Liver Fire Blazing, CH has too much Heat in his head; therefore, I would want to use points that were predominantly away from the head to drag the heat out. At the moment I have 11 needles scheduled for his head, which is almost half the prescription. Too much!

LOOK AT THE POINT COMBINATIONS
Probably the best way to explain this is to do it in segments. I will also consider the fact that I have too many points in the head in my comments.

GB 13, GB 14, GB 20 and GB 37
All of the points are on the Gall Bladder channel, making them excellent to use together. But there are too many in the head/neck region. GB 13 would probably be the one to remove as it's further from CH's main complaints than GB 14 and GB 20.

GB 37 is a keeper because it is an excellent distal point for eye disorders.[109] Also, I don't have too many points in the legs anyway.

LR 2 and LR 3

These are both located on the lower limb and both on the Liver channel, so I would probably keep both of these points.

The Liver and Gall Bladder are Wood element organs. As such, their sense organ of choice is the eyes, and their emotion is anger.[110] They also both treat the type of headache described. This makes these points extremely important for CH.

LI 4, LI 11 and TE 5

All three points are located on the arms and all help to clear heat from the head.[111] However, I am still conscious that I need to remove some points from my prescription, so I need to dig a little deeper into these points and their functions.

LI 4 has to be a keeper as it is the best point on the entire body for headaches and is also a terrific point to treat all of the sense organs.[112] It will also 'open the Four Gates', along with LR 3, which is an excellent combination to sedate excess patterns.[113]

LI 11 clears heat from the eyes but it doesn't treat headaches. TE 5 treats Liver Fire Blazing headaches but doesn't treat the eyes.

Since CH's primary complaint is his headache, I would probably keep TE 5 and dump LI 11. But as LI 4 does combine quite well with both points, it wouldn't really matter which one I chose; besides, I could alternate the points for the follow-up appointment anyway.

GV 20, BL 2 and M-HN-9 (Tài Yáng)

These are the remaining local points on offer. At this stage I have pretty much locked away 14 points to be needled, so I probably need to dump one or two more local points from the list above.

GV 20 is a point that divides opinions. Some say it draws energy up the body, some say it sends energy down, and some have the view that it can do both. I believe it can do both, depending on what points you combine it with. Deadman *et al.* (2007, p.553) agree: 'Baihui Du-20 is located at the apex of the head, the highest and hence most yang point of the body. It therefore has a profound effect on regulating yang, both to descend excess yang and to raise deficient yang.'

GV 20 will therefore drop the Liver Fire out of the head. But it also has two more benefits for CH: it can treat the eyes and can also calm his anger, stress, irritability, frustration and feeling overwhelmed.[114] Therefore, it's a keeper.

So that leaves BL 2 and M-HN-9 (Tài Yáng). My point prescription is now down to 15 needles, so I don't really have to keep either of these points. Plus, I have five points in the head/neck already. Finally, CH has never had acupuncture before, so I would prefer to do less rather than more in a first session. So I am going to dump both of them. This leaves me with the final tally shown in Table 3.5.

Table 3.5 Liver Fire Blazing - final selection of points

Location of points	Points	
Head/face/neck	GV 20 GB 14	GB 20[115]
Arms/hands	LI 4	TE 5
Legs/feet	LR 2 LR 3	GB 37
Total points needled	15 needles used bilaterally	

Overall, it's a good combination because I have points in the feet, legs, hands, arms, neck, head and face. Most importantly, however, the points work well together - they aren't just random points chosen without any relationship to each other.

6. Points that treat the same signs/symptoms

Similar to the Zàng Fǔ patterns in Section 5 above, the signs and symptoms have already been included but with no more than two to four points listed.

What I want to do here is to give you a point combination for a common disorder seen in clinic and then explain how those points work together.

In my clinic in Australia, one of the most commonly seen signs/symptoms is stress. One of my favorite point combinations for stress is shown in Table 3.6.

Table 3.6 Stress treatment[116]

Location of points	Points	
Head/face/neck	GV 20 M-HN-3 (Yìn Táng)	GB 20
Trunk (front)	CV 17	
Arms/hands	LI 4 HT 3	IIT 7 PC 6
Legs/feet	LR 3	GB 34
Total points needled	17 needles used bilaterally	

I'm unlikely to needle all 17 of those points in one session, but they are a good bunch of points to have in mind when treating stress.

So, if we get rid of GB 20, LI 4 and LR 3 (we talked about these in the previous Zàng Fǔ patterns section), that would leave us with 11 needles. In all likelihood I would actually use those points for stress.

Table 3.7 shows which of the points combines well with the others.

Table 3.7 Stress point combinations

Point	Combines with	
GV 20	M-HN-3 (Yìn Táng) CV 17 HT 3	HT 7 PC 6
M-HN-3 (Yìn Táng)	GV 20 CV 17 HT 3	HT 7 PC 6
CV 17	GV 20 M-HN-3 (Yìn Táng) HT 3	HT 7 PC 6
HT 3	GV 20 M-HN-3 (Yìn Táng) CV 17	HT 7 PC 6
HT 7	GV 20 M-HN-3 (Yìn Táng) CV 17	HT 3 PC 6
PC 6	GV 20 M-HN-3 (Yìn Táng) CV 17	HT 3 HT 7 GB 34
GB 34	PC 6	

Let's look more closely at some (but not all) of the combinations.

GV 20 and M-HN-3 (Yìn Táng)

Both points are located on the head as well as on the midline of the body and are very effective to calm the Shén.[117] A person with a calm Shén will be significantly less stressed and will be able to cope with a lot more life challenges. Therefore, irrespective of the Chinese medicine cause of the stress, a calm Shén leads to a more relaxed and calm approach to life in general.

GV 20 and CV 17

Both points are located on the midline of the body and are very effective to calm the Shén.[118] Typically, points located on the head/face, on the chest/upper back (over the Heart organ) and on the Heart and Pericardium channels are excellent to calm the Shén. Obviously, not all the points in those regions have Shén-calming qualities, but they are more likely than on other areas/channels of the body. Why?

The Heart organ houses the Shén,[119] so nearly every point located over the Heart will activate the Shén.

Our brain is also heavily involved with the Shén; therefore, a lot of points located over/adjacent to the brain will also be effective to treat the Shén.[120]

As I said above, the Heart organ houses the Shén, and the Pericardium encircles the Heart. Therefore, both the Heart and Pericardium channels will also be effective to treat the Shén.[121]

GV 20 and HT 3

With a point on the head and then a bilateral point on the arms, this combination is another excellent one to calm the Shén. The points are also part of another combination type called the Triangle of Power, which will be discussed in Chapter 6.

GV 20 and HT 3 are also an effective combination to stimulate endorphins, which helps the person to cope better with stress and to feel calm, relaxed, happy and even euphoric.

GV 20 and HT 7

Similar to the previous combination, this combination has a point on the head and then a bilateral point on the arms, and is excellent to calm the Shén. The points also make the Triangle of Power.

GV 20 and HT 7 are an exceptionally good combination for calming the Shén for the following reasons:

- HT 7 advises such in its name. Shén Mén = Spirit Gate; this essentially tells us that the point is an access area (gateway) straight to the Shén. So regardless of why the Shén isn't balanced, HT 7 can regulate the cause, leading to a decrease in stress.

- GV 20 regulates energy up and/or down the body, as stated earlier. When the Shén isn't balanced, this can cause (or be caused by) excess or deficiency in the head. Regardless of the cause of the imbalance, GV 20 can rebalance the Shén, leading to a decrease in stress.

GV 20 and PC 6

Although this might be getting a little repetitive, this combination has a point on the head and then a bilateral point on the arms, and is also excellent for calming the Shén.[122] The points also make the Triangle of Power.

PC 6 and GB 34

An excellent combination to ensure the smooth flow of Qì. From a Chinese medicine perspective, this is the single biggest cause of stress; but the opposite also applies: stress leads to the stagnation of Qì.[123] These stresses are typically emotional, such as frustration, repressed anger, irritability, resentment, moodiness and depression.[124]

But why are Qì Stagnation and stress so inherently linked?

- The Liver ensures the smooth flow of Qì in every direction. When Qì is flowing smoothly, the other Vital Substances will also be smooth flowing. This is because the Qì drives the other Vital Substances, which are typically slower. But also because the other Vital Substances are just different types of Qì.[125]

When the Vital Substances are flowing smoothly, there is minimal disease, including stress. From an internal perspective, this is because the Vital Substances are ensuring the body is moving healthy material to all places, which then pushes the unhealthy content out of the body. From an external perspective, strong Vital Substances ensure that no External Pathogenic Factors can invade the body because our defenses are strong.

According to Chapter 62 of *The Yellow Emperor's Classic* (Huáng Dì Nèi Jīng/ 黃帝內經), 'When the qi and blood are not regulated, illness occurs' (Ni 1995, pp.215–216).

There is only so much room available in the body. When unhealthy material is allowed to build up in certain areas (e.g. via stress), it creates a block because it takes up space; this hinders the flushing of the area with the Vital Substances. Therefore, the area needs to be flushed of unhealthy material, which in turn creates the opposite effect: the area is now full of clean/healthy material, which takes up space, thereby not allowing the unhealthy to get in.

- The Shén is also just an immaterial form of Qì.[126] Therefore, if there is stagnation of Qì, then the Shén will be obstructed. Conversely, if the Shén is unbalanced, this can create an imbalance in Qì. Both of these scenarios can lead to stress.

Stress in the body can lead to internal imbalance or invasion from External Pathogenic Factors. However, if the Shén and Qì are strong, this is unlikely to occur. *The Yellow Emperor's Classic* says it perfectly in chapter 73: 'Therefore, when the qi and shen are present and sound, no pathogen can invade a person, even when the cycles of nature are disruptive and plagues are near' (Ni 1995, p.279).

There are other point combinations that haven't been discussed from Table 3.7 above. Most of those relationships act in a similar manner to the ones already analyzed – that is, they calm the Shén to reduce stress or to minimize the likelihood of stress occurring in situations where it might normally.

Notes

1   From 'Physics' written in 350 BCE. Aristotle (384–322 BCE) would probably have to be considered the most famous philosopher of all time (Western or Eastern). He was prolific in his writing, theorizing and philosophizing.

Quotation taken from https://todayinsci.com/A/Aristotle/Aristotle-Quotations.htm.

2   Liang 1996, p.111. Wáng Yángmíng (1472–1529 CE) tended to buck the trend of the time, which encouraged rote learning of the Four

Books (*Confucian Analects*, the *Mencius*, *The Great Learning*, *The Doctrine of the Mean*) as a means for individual philosophical evolution. He advised, instead, to actively participate in day-to-day life and, in that space, learn to find the Way (Dào). What a brilliant concept!

3 Deadman *et al.* (2007, p.104) reference *The Classic of the Jade Dragon* (Bian Que's *Spiritual Guide to Acupuncture and Moxibustion, Jade Dragon Classic*/Biǎn Què Shēn Yīng Zhēn Jiǔ Yù Lóng Jīng) written by Wang Guo Rui in 1329 CE. The quotation used is: 'Hegu LI-4 treats all diseases of the head, face, ears, eyes, nose, cheeks, mouth and teeth.' I regularly tell my students that LI 4 is in my top five favorite points to use in clinic. It treats so much, and not just the head and face as quoted above.

4 Maciocia 2006, pp.180–181.

5 McDonald 1986, pp.25, 31.

6 Ellis *et al.* 1991, pp.151, 157.

7 Yang 2011, p.89. Yue Lu translated *The Great Compendium – Volume VIII* (*The Great Compendium of Acupuncture and Moxibustion*/Zhēn Jiǔ Dà Chéng) in 2011. The original text was written by Jizhou Yang in 1601 CE.

8 Only the Wood element has Front Mù Collecting points on both of its Yīn and Yáng partnered channels: the Liver (LR 14) and Gall Bladder (GB 24) channels. None of the other element partners do.

9 Maciocia 2015, p.169; Mi 2004, p.5: *The Systematic Classic of Acupuncture and Moxibustion* (Zhēn Jiǔ Jiá Yǐ Jīng) was written by Huang Fu Mi in 282 CE.

10 McDonald and Penner 1994, p.133.

11 Deadman *et al.* 2007, p.54.

12 Ellis *et al.* 1991, pp.314, 343.

13 Twicken 2013, pp.37, 98.

14 Hartmann 2009, pp.2, 9.

15 O'Connor and Bensky 1981, p.293; Shi 2007, p.259.

16 The Shén is translated as spirit or mind. It is essentially everything related to our memory (short-term and long-term memory in the context of studying, concentrating and recalling information), consciousness (fully alert, semi-conscious, unconscious), thinking, sleep, emotions and our Wǔ Shén. It is also our focus, drive and determination. It is also involved with how we handle stress, anxiety, frustration, irritability and feeling overwhelmed.

17 Maciocia 2009, pp.252, 255.

18 Ellis *et al.* 1989, pp.123–124; Lade 1989, pp.339, 347.

19 Ellis *et al.* 1989, p.133.

20 Maciocia 2009, pp.253–254.

21 Deadman *et al.* 2007, pp.219, 235, 632.

22 Ellis *et al.* 1989, pp.227–228.

23 Ibid., p.235.

24 Ross 1995, p.102.

25 Twicken 2013, pp.37, 98.

26 Maciocia 2015, pp.1084–1085, 1092–1093. Maciocia (2015, p.1093) references *An Explanation of Acupuncture Points*/Jīng Xué Jiě written by Yue Han Zhen in 1654 CE. The quotation used is: 'The Triple Burner [Sān Jiāo] channels go to the centre of the chest, when there is stagnation, there is a feeling of oppression of the chest and the point TB-6 [TE 6] should be reduced to relieve the feeling of oppression. When there is heart pain, the Pericardium channel's Qi rebels upwards and this point should be reduced.'

27 Legge 2011, p.220.

28 Hartmann 2009, pp.18, 20.

29 Deadman *et al.* 2007, pp.132, 182.

30 Ibid., pp.166, 186–187.

31 Legge 2011, p.209.

32 Ellis *et al.* 1989, pp.28–29.

33 Ibid., pp.46–47.

34 Ellis *et al.* 1991, pp.85, 95; Hartmann 2009, p.129.

35 Shi 2007, pp.90, 104.

36 Deadman *et al.* 2007, pp.325, 338.

37 Lade 1989, p.180.

38 Ellis *et al.* 1989, p.413; Lade 1989, p.177.

39 Maciocia 2015, pp.1055, 1066.

40 Ellis *et al.* 1991, pp.230, 249.

41 Shi 2007, pp.214, 223.

42 Wang and Robertson 2008, p.18.

43 Li 2007, pp.52, 246–247.

44 Deadman *et al.* 2007, pp.76, 204.

45 Ellis *et al.* 1991, p.80.

46 Ross 1995, p.64.

47 A Shào Yīn Imbalance is a term to describe a disease that is affecting both the Heart and Kidneys. In regard to the Zàng Fǔ patterns, that could result in a variety of patterns, including, but not limited to, Heart and Kidney Yīn Xū; Heart and Kidney Yáng Xū; Heart Fire Blazing with Kidney Yīn Xū; and Heart Fire Blazing with Kidney Yáng Xū.

48 Wang and Robertson 2008, p.119.

49 Ni 1995, p.34: 8th chapter. *The Yellow Emperor's Classic* (*Inner Canon of the Yellow Emperor*/Huáng Dì Nèi Jīng) was written somewhere between 200 and 0 BCE.

50 Hicks *et al.* 2010, p.323.

51 Ellis *et al.* 1989, pp.217–218.

52 Hicks *et al.* 2010, p.323.

53 Ellis *et al.* 1989, p.220.

54 Hicks *et al.* 2010, pp.323–324.

55 Twicken 2013, p.61.

56 Hicks *et al.* 2010, pp.314, 323–324.

57 Deadman *et al.* 2007, pp.214–215, 350–351.

58 Ibid., pp.379, 477.

59 Hartmann 2009, p.9.

60 Hicks *et al.* 2010, p.327.

61 Ibid., p.335.

62 Ibid., p.327.

63 Ibid., p.335.

64 Deadman *et al.* 2007, pp.381–382, 473–475; Lade 1989, pp.199–200; McDonald 1986, p.40;

McDonald 1989, pp.49–50; Maciocia 2015, pp.1085, 1120–1121.

65   Although none of the references state that LR 1 treats hypertension, Liver Fire Blazing is one of the main Zàng Fǔ patterns that is diagnosed with hypertension (O'Connor and Bensky 1981, pp.596–599; Hartmann 2009, p.81). LR 1 is a Jǐng Well point, so it can treat acute Fire Blazing flare-ups of hypertension fast, thereby making it a point to consider when treating certain types of hypertension.

66   Similar to my previous point, none of the references suggest LR 1 can treat anger/irritability. However, anger is very common in cases of Liver Fire Blazing because anger is associated with the Liver in Wǔ Xíng theory. Often anger and/or irritability can come on rapidly, leading to an acute rage/rant episode. In this instance, needling or applying Tuī Ná massage to LR 1 can have a quite profound effect, helping to bring down that rage fast. This is because LR 1 is a Jǐng Well point and they work on acute-stage disorders quickly.

67   Wind Stroke or Wind Strike (Zhōng Fēng) is essentially just a stroke from a Western medical perspective.

68   Wang and Robertson 2008, p.18.

69   Lower Hé (Uniting) Sea points regulate the organ they are associated with, thereby making them excellent points to use for any disease of their associated organ.

70   Deadman et al. 2007, pp.164, 300.

71   Soulie de Morant 1994, pp.407–408, 415, 426–427.

72   O'Connor and Bensky 1981, pp.195, 310.

73   Hicks et al. 2010, pp.315–316.

74   Ibid., p.320.

75   Ibid., p.315.

76   Ibid., p.320.

77   Visual dizziness (Mù Xuàn) is where the person gets cloudy vision that precedes the dizziness, as opposed to the person getting dizzy first and then getting cloudy vision.

78   Although none of the references state that SI 5 treats nosebleed, the point is effective at clearing heat out of the head. Generally speaking, however, this tends to be more for the eyes, ears, jaw, mouth, tongue and teeth. Therefore, I would personally recommend choosing a different point for epistaxis.

79   Similar to my previous point, none of the references suggest SI 2 can treat madness/mania. Having said that, SI 2 is the Yíng Spring point on the Small Intestine channel, thereby making it a fast-acting point to clear heat from the top ends of the channel. Second, the Small Intestine organ is the Yáng partner to the Heart (which is the most important organ to calm the Shén). Third, because they are both part of the Fire Element of which mania is a key component in Wǔ Xíng theory, I might consider using SI 2 for madness/mania. But only for the

acute fast-acting calming effect, and not for the chronic root cause of the madness/mania.

80   SI 5 wasn't mentioned as a point that could treat headaches other than in Hecker et al. (2005, p.168) where they mentioned it was a good point to treat 'headaches associated with the common cold'.

81   Deadman et al. 2007, pp.232–233, 236–237, 318–319, 324–325; Ellis et al. 1991, pp.177–180, 231, 235; Maciocia 2015, pp.1016–1017, 1019, 1056–1057, 1059–1060; O'Connor and Bensky 1981, pp.282, 309, 319.

82   Hartmann 2009, p.20.

83   Ibid.

84   Deadman et al. 2007, pp.158–163.

85   Ibid., pp.111–112, 158–161.

86   Ellis et al. 1991, pp.99, 132–133.

87   Bisio 2004, pp.208–209.

88   I was also told by one of my lecturers (his name omitted for obvious reasons) that the meaning was slightly different. His version suggested that LI 10 connected the Three Arm Yáng channels of the Large Intestine, Small Intestine and Sān Jiāo, and that these generated heaps of power which resulted in the Vital Substances traveling great distances (Lǐ). The same applied to ST 36 with the Three Leg Yáng channels of the Stomach, Urinary Bladder and Gall Bladder connecting and sending the Vital Substances great distances (Lǐ). Although I like the sound of this theory, I haven't seen anything written to suggest his statement is accurate, but that doesn't mean I've ruled it out. After all, I haven't read everything written on Chinese medicine. I wish!

89   You will have noticed that I haven't used the word 'cùn' when describing these points, and instead have used the word 'measurement'. This is because it's a better English translation of Lǐ.

90   Hicks et al. 2010, p.301.

91   Ibid., p.307.

92   Ibid., p.303.

93   Ibid., p.308.

94   Deadman et al. 2007, pp.100, 112, 158, 172; Ellis et al. 1991, pp.93, 100, 133, 139.

95   Although none of the references state that LI 11 restores consciousness, if the cause is from too much heat in the head, then LI 11 would be a good point to choose. If, however, it's from a deficiency, then I wouldn't use LI 11.

96   Throat Painful Obstruction (Hóu Bì) is a blanket term to describe throat pain/swelling/congestion.

97   None of the references advise the use of LI 1 for madness/mania. Having said that, the use of Jǐng Well points are effective at treating acute emotional turmoil, although typically LI 1 wouldn't be near the top of the list when treating madness/mania.

98   I couldn't find any mention of LI 11 treating jaw problems. However, it is a distal point on a channel that passes through the jaw, so in theory LI 11 could treat the jaw.

99 Deadman *et al.* 2007, pp.100–101, 112–114, 158–161, 172–173; Ellis *et al.* 1991, pp.93, 99–100, 132–133, 139; Lade 1989, pp.37, 46–47, 72–74, 84; Maciocia 2015, pp.962, 967, 985–987, 991–992; O'Connor and Bensky 1981, pp.230–231, 271–272, 308, 315.

100 Deadman *et al.* 2007, pp.442–443; Maciocia 2015, p.1090.

101 Maciocia 2015, p.845.

102 Shi 2007, pp.257, 260.

103 There are three points located in the space between the tragus of the ear and the condyloid process of the mandible – TE 21, SI 19 and GB 2. When I teach point location to my students, I give them a tip to help them remember which point is located where and what number they are. In Australia we have a 'Goods and Services Tax' or GST. Using that acronym and working from the bottom up, you have the Gall Bladder channel first (represented by the 'G'), then we have the Small Intestine channel (represented by the 'S'), and at the top is the Triple Energizer channel (represented by the 'T'). So, you have the GST letters running from bottom to top. Teaching them the numbers of the points works as well. If you work from the bottom up, you have GB 2 plus SI 19 = TE 21 (2 + 19 = 21).

104 Ellis *et al.* 1989, p.248.

105 Ibid., p.253.

106 Deadman *et al.* 2007, p.33.

107 Ibid., pp.392–393, 462–463.

108 Hartmann 2009, pp.9, 60.

109 Ellis *et al.* 1989, p.283.

110 Ni 1995, p.16: 4th chapter.

111 Deadman *et al.* 2007, pp.103–105, 113, 396–397.

112 Ibid., pp.103–104.

113 Ross 1995, p.249.

114 Maciocia 2015, p.1155.

115 GB 20 can be needled with the patient laying face up. With them lying down, you turn their head to one side and needle the point obliquely, ensuring the needle handle lies flat against the pillow when they turn their head back to the center position. Repeat for the other side. These needles will now be hidden from view, so don't forget to take them out at the end of the appointment.

116 Hartmann 2009, p.149.

117 Ellis *et al.* 1991, pp.383, 399.

118 Ross 1995, pp.140–141, 160–161.

119 Matsumoto and Birch 1983, p.10.

120 Maciocia 2015, p.112.

121 Ibid., p.171.

122 Lade 1989, pp.196, 288.

123 Maciocia 2015, pp.532–533.

124 McDonald and Penner 1994, p.119; Maciocia 2015, pp.532–533.

125 Maciocia 2015, p.43.

126 Rossi 2007, p.51.

The mind is the ruler of the soul. It should remain unstirred by agitations of the flesh – gentle and violent ones alike. Not mingling with them, but fencing itself off and keeping those feelings in their place. When they make their way into your thoughts, through the sympathetic link between mind and body, don't try to resist the sensation. The sensation is natural. But don't let the mind start with judgements, calling it 'good' or 'bad'.

Marcus Aurelius (121–180 CE)[1]

4

Using Similar Pīn Yīn Names/ Meanings When Combining Acupuncture Points

In Australian colleges and universities, acupuncture point names are given to students through a combination of channel and number – for example, Large Intestine 4 or its abbreviation, LI 4. Some colleges and universities will include the Pīn Yīn, along with the English translation, as well as the Chinese characters for the points (traditional and/or simplified).

When I was studying, I was required to learn the channel/number system as well as the Pīn Yīn. The only problem was we weren't told what the Pīn Yīn names meant. It became a rote learning exercise, and soon after I graduated I forgot the Pīn Yīn names.

It wasn't until I started teaching Chinese medicine that I slowly began to relearn the Pīn Yīn names. This time, however, I learned their English translation as well. This provided me with a much greater understanding of the acupuncture points and their meanings, which the channel/number system doesn't provide.

As I learned the Pīn Yīn names and their English translation, I provided these to my students so that they could have a better understanding of the points and their meanings. I even rewrote the point location subject to include the nomenclature for the Pīn Yīn point names.[2] I included examples of Pīn Yīn names that referred to water, mountains, valleys, animals, plants, architecture, astronomy, anatomy and therapeutic properties. Some of these included:

- HT 3 (Shào Hǎi) – Shào = Lesser; Hǎi = Sea. Meaning of Lesser Sea.[3]

  HT 3 is a Hé (Uniting) Sea point and is part of the Shào (Lesser) Yīn Six Division partnership with the Kidney. Hence the name, Lesser Sea.

- LU 10 (Yú Jì) – Yú = Fish; Jì = Border. Meaning of Fish Border.[4]

The area where LU 10 is located looks similar to a fish belly, with the scales and the smoothness being like the border of the red and white skin of the hand, or the smooth flesh and the hairy flesh.

- HT 7 (Shén Mén) – Shén = Spirit; Mén = Gate. Meaning of Spirit Gate.[5]

The Heart houses the Shén. The Pīn Yīn name of HT 7 implies that it is a great point to access the Shén. Using the point will open a gateway directly to the Shén.

- GB 24 (Rì Yuè) – Rì = Sun; Yuè = Moon. Meaning of Sun and Moon.[6]

Classical Chinese texts call the left eye sun and the right eye moon. The eyes are associated with the liver, and, through exterior–interior relationship, with the gall bladder. This name Sun and Moon reflects the relation of GB 24 to the eyes by way of association with the liver. (Ellis *et al.* 1989, p.273)

- SI 14 (Jiān Wài Shū) – Jiān = Shoulder; Wài = Outer; Shū = Acupuncture Point. Meaning of Outer Shoulder Point.[7]

SI 14 is an acupuncture point located on the outside (posterior aspect) of the shoulder.

- BL 1 (Jīng Míng) – Jīng = Eye; Míng = Bright. Meaning of Eyes Bright.[8]

BL 1 is located in the eye socket and is a great point to brighten the eyes and aid in all eye disorders.

1. Pīn Yīn point combinations

This was introduced in Chapter 3 but not in great depth, so I have included some additional examples of how points with similar Pīn Yīn names/meanings can be used in point combinations. We will start with small point combinations before expanding to include larger ones.

2. SP 6 (Sān Yīn Jiāo) and TE 8 (Sān Yáng Luò)

SP 6 – Sān = three; Yīn = Yīn; Jiāo = intersect, join or meet.[9]

TE 8 – Sān = three; Yáng = Yáng; Luò = connect or mesh.[10]

SP 6 connects the Three Leg Yīn channels of Spleen, Liver and Kidney. TE 8 connects the Three Arm Yáng channels of Large Intestine, Small Intestine and Sān Jiāo.

This point combination is very effective if your patient has problems that are across the Middle Jiāo and the Lower Jiāo. The two points will treat the Middle Jiāo organs of Spleen and Liver as well as the Lower Jiāo organs of Kidney, Large

Intestine and Small Intestine. Plus, the Middle and Lower Jiāos will be linked via the Sān Jiāo.

Signs and symptoms could be mild or severe, including:[11]

- epigastric and abdominal pain/bloating/distension/tightness

- poor digestion

- bowel problems including constipation, diarrhea, dysentery, irritable bowel syndrome, diverticulitis, Crohn's disease or ulcerative colitis

- urinary problems including increased urinary output, minimal urination, blood/stones in the urine, pain on urination or urinary tract infections

- menstrual/reproductive/genital problems including amenorrhea, dysmenorrhea, infertility, endometriosis, spermatorrhea, impotence or polycystic ovary syndrome.

From a Zàng Fǔ pattern perspective, this could include:[12]

- Spleen Damp Accumulation with Liver Qì Stagnation

- Spleen Invaded by Liver Qì

- Spleen and Liver Xuè Xū

- Spleen and Kidney Yáng Xū

- Liver and Kidney Yīn Xū

- Sān Jiāo Not Communicating[13]

- imbalances in the Large Intestine and/or the Small Intestine with either the Spleen, Liver or Kidneys.

3. LR 3 (Tài Chōng) and ST 42 (Chōng Yáng)

LR 3 – Tài = great or supreme; Chōng = surge, rush or thoroughfare.[14]

ST 42 – Chōng = surge, rush or thoroughfare; Yáng = Yáng.[15]

As the names suggest, there is a lot of power available at these points. LR 3 has a supreme amount of surging Qì it can access. This makes sense when you consider that LR 3 is one of the best points to move Qì through the body.[16]

ST 42 is similar in that it can access surging Yáng Qì and rush it through the body.[17]

These points are also Yuán Source points. As such, they are potentially the best point on the channel to treat the organ.[18] Therefore, when a patient has an imbalance between the Liver and Stomach organs, this point combination would be perfect because it will generate surging Qì flow to the troubled area to help heal it faster.

The force generated between these two points is immense. One is driving Qì up the body, and one is driving Qì down the body. This powerful force comes from the channels flowing in different directions and along different aspects of the body. But the force also comes from the function of the two points; and the Pīn Yīn names/ meanings of the points tell you that.

One of the best Zàng Fǔ patterns that LR 3 and ST 42 will treat is Liver Qì Invading the Stomach. The signs and symptoms of this pattern include, but are not limited to:[19]

- epigastric and hypochondriac pain/distension, belching, nausea and possible acid regurgitation or vomiting, depression, irritability, and irregular menstruation in women.

Some Western diseases that can also be diagnosed as a result of Liver Qì Invading the Stomach include, but are not limited to:[20]

- gastric or duodenal ulcers

- gastritis

- hepatitis

- cirrhosis of the liver.

4. BL 17 (Gé Shū) and BL 46 (Gé Guān)

BL 17 – Gé = diaphragm; Shū = transport.[21]

BL 46 – Gé = diaphragm; Guān = pass.[22]

Both points are located level with the lower border of the seventh thoracic vertebra (T7). BL 17 is 1.5 cùn lateral to the midline; BL 46 is located 3 cùn lateral to the midline.

Both points will regulate the diaphragm, which is:

the dome-shaped sheet of muscle and tendon that serves as the main muscle of respiration and plays a vital role in the breathing process. Also known as the thoracic diaphragm, it serves as an important anatomical landmark that separates the thorax, or chest, from the abdomen.[23]

From a Chinese medicine perspective, the diaphragm lies between the Upper and Middle Jiāos. As such, BL 17 and BL 46 can:[24]

- regulate the Middle Jiāo

- descend Lung Qì Rebellion

- descend Stomach Qì Rebellion

- stop bleeding.

The signs and symptoms of these can include:[25]

- cough, dyspnea, belching, nausea/vomiting, acid reflux, indigestion, hiccup, chest pain/oppression, vomiting blood (hematemesis).

5. GB 15 (Tóu Lín Qì) and GB 41 (Zú Lín Qì)

GB 15 – Tóu = head; Lín = overlook or arrive; Qì = tears.[26]

GB 41 – Zú = foot or leg; Lín = overlook or arrive; Qì = tears.[27]

As can be seen from the names, GB 15 and GB 41 are an excellent point combination to regulate the fluid in the eyes. As Deadman *et al.* (2007, p.433) advise, 'GB-15 is indicated for lacrimation as well as for redness and pain of the eyes and superficial visual obstruction. In this respect it mirrors Zulinqi [GB 41].'

6. KI 18 (Shí Guān) and CV 5 (Shí Mén)

KI 18 – Shí = stone; Guān = pass.[28]

CV 5 – Shí = stone; Mén = gate.[29]

Both points are effective at breaking through stagnant barriers, including stones in the body, such as gall stones, kidney stones or abdominal masses.

But stagnations aren't always stones, and in Chinese medicine terms we might refer to stagnations as being Xuè Stasis, Qì Stagnation and/or Phlegm Accumulation. If we look at each of them and provide a Western example, it might clarify the wide range of signs and symptoms that this point combination treats:[30]

- Xuè Stasis – pooled blood in the uterus, uterine bleeding, endometriosis, infertility, severe and specific abdominal pain, and/or constipation with blood in the stools on voiding

- Qì Stagnation – vague abdominal pain over a large area, pre-menstrual tension/stress (PMT/PMS), irregular menstruation, gas/wind, constipation and/or diarrhea

- Phlegm Accumulation – polycystic ovarian syndrome, infertility, edema, diarrhea, abdominal distension/bloating, leucorrhea and/or thrush.

KI 18 and CV 5 can also treat Painful Urinary Dysfunction (Lín Zhèng), which is typically defined as any urinary issue that relates to 'urinary difficulty, urgency and frequency' (Deadman *et al.* 2007, p.630).

7. BL 21 (Wèi Shū) and BL 50 (Wèi Cāng)

BL 21 – Wèi = stomach; Shū = transport.[31]

BL 50 – Wèi = stomach; Cāng = granary.[32]

Both points are located level with the lower border of the twelfth thoracic vertebra (T12). BL 21 is 1.5 cùn lateral to the midline; BL 50 is located 3 cùn lateral to the midline.

Both points will regulate the Stomach organ, as well as the other Middle Jiāo organs. Because they are located side by side on the back of the trunk, I would ideally like to see some distal points and/or points on the front of the trunk to further enhance the point combination. Possible point inclusions to consider are:[33]

- main – ST 21, ST 36, CV 12 and SP 4

- secondary – SP 6, ST 25, ST 42, BL 20 and LR 13.

8. LI 8 (Xià Lián) and ST 39 (Xià Jù Xū)

LI 8 – Xià = lower; Lián = angle or ridge.[34]

ST 39 – Xià = lower; Jù = great; Xū = hollow or void.[35]

According to Deadman *et al.* (2007, p.110), LI 8 and ST 39 reflect each other. ST 39 is the Lower Hé (Uniting) Sea point of the Small Intestine[36] and is located on the lower leg. Its effects can be enhanced by using LI 8, which is its corresponding/mirrored point on the arms.

LI 8 and ST 39 can therefore be used to regulate the Small Intestine organ.

Interestingly, in volume 1.34 of *The Classic of Supporting Life*, ST 39 is described as having two Pīn Yīn names. One is Xià Jù Xū, but the other is actually Xià Lián (the same name as LI 8). The way the author Zhízhōng Wáng chooses to differentiate these two points is to call LI 8 Xià Lián and ST 39 Zú Xià Lián – as in Lower Angle and Leg Lower Angle.[37]

If one felt so inclined, one could go further and write LI 8 as Shǒu Xià Lián, or Arm Lower Angle.

9. LI 9 (Shàng Lián) and ST 37 (Shàng Jù Xū)

LI 9 – Shàng = upper; Lián = angle or ridge.[38]

ST 37 – Shàng = upper; Jù = great; Xū = hollow or void.[39]

Similar to the previous combination, Deadman *et al.* (2007, p.110) state that LI 9 and ST 37 reflect each other. ST 37 is the Lower Hé (Uniting) Sea point of the Large Intestine[40] and is located on the lower leg. Its effects can be enhanced by using LI 9, which is its corresponding/mirrored point on the arms.

LI 9 and ST 37 can therefore be used to regulate the Large Intestine organ.

Interestingly, in volume 1.34 of *The Classic of Supporting Life*, ST 37 is described as having two Pīn Yīn names. One is Shàng Jù Xū, but the other is actually Shàng Lián (the same name as LI 9). The way the author Zhízhōng Wáng chooses to differentiate these two points is to call LI 9 Shàng Lián and ST 37 Zú Shàng Lián – as in Upper Angle and Leg Upper Angle.[41]

As with the previous combination, if one felt so inclined one could go further and write LI 9 as Shǒu Shàng Lián, or Arm Upper Angle.

10. KI 24 (Líng Xū) and HT 4 (Líng Dào)

KI 24 – Líng = Yīn spirit; Xū = burial ground or ruins.[42]

HT 4 – Líng = Yīn spirit; Dào = path, road or way.[43]

KI 24 works on ensuring that our Shén is harmonious in its Yīn Yáng qualities. A Shén that is clogged/blocked/filled to capacity will not be a harmonious one. When we refuse to let things go emotionally and hold on to them, it fills up space in our Shén. If we do this a lot, then there won't be any more room left for new, and healthy, emotional responses to enter. This is where KI 24 can help.[44]

This point can help us to remove something we have been hanging on to that is old and no longer self-serving. This process will work regardless of whether:

- we are aware of it and want to do something about it

- we are aware of it but don't want to do anything about it

- we are totally oblivious to it.

In the first instance, the person has made an active effort to clear some emotional clutter but has reached an impasse. KI 24 will help them move through that impasse.

The second instance suggests that while the person is aware of the emotional baggage, they actually don't want to do anything about it. This might occur, for example, when a person continues to grieve long after the death of a loved one. If the grief is no longer self-serving, then KI 24 can help them through that process.

The third instance suggests that the person's oblivious nature has resulted in the build-up of old emotionally toxic material. Therefore, the person's Shén is about to force the ending (death) of that stagnant emotion. If that is the case, then KI 24 can ease them through that phase more gently.

Regardless of the type of emotional build-up, the old waste has to be removed to make space for healthy emotions to come in and recreate a harmonious Yīn Yáng spirit.

> When we are resigned, low in spirits, or have suffered a long hard road, then this point [KI 24] re-establishes contact with our inner strength and brings back our vital reserves. Here our spirit can be resurrected and we can again experience the riches of life, joy, enthusiasm, hope and meaning. (Kaatz 2005, p.539)

HT 4 is a point that helps us to reconnect or stay in line with our true path or journey. If we feel as if we have lost our way, this point can redirect us back on to the right path.[45] Maciocia (2009, p.252) suggests that HT 4 is good for 'sadness, fear, anxiety and mental restlessness'.

Perhaps you have a patient/family member/friend who questions why they are even on planet Earth? They might say things like 'What's the point to life?' or 'Why am I even here?' or 'Nothing ever seems to work out for me. I might as well just give up.' If that is the case, then HT 4 is one of the key points to access.[46]

As you can see, these points are quite amazing on their own. But how do KI 24 and HT 4 work together in a combination?

When our Shén is toxic, it's very hard to find our way in life. Everything seems too difficult and nothing seems to work out anyway. This negative cycle bleeds into everything we do and everything that we are. No longer are we following the Dào.

Interestingly, this negative loop can lead to a toxic Shén, or the opposite can occur, with a toxic Shén leading to the person losing their way (Dào) in life. Regardless of the original cause, KI 24 and HT 4 can help.

Finally, if the person is in quite a chronic state, you should consider additional points to add to the combination. The best ones would be dependent on what diagnosis you use for your patient.

11. CV 18 (Yù Táng), CV 21 (Xuán Jī) and BL 9 (Yù Zhěn)

CV 18 – Yù = jade; Táng = ancestral hall or palace hall.[47]

CV 21 – Xuán = a type of fine jade; Jī = pearl or pivot.[48]

BL 9 – Yù = jade; Zhěn = pillow.[49]

The Chinese say that jade symbolizes the great human virtues of courage, intelligence and purity. (Kaatz 2005, p.454)

CV 18 is where we can reconnect to our ancestral heritage, which allows us to access our ancestors' wisdom or knowing.[50] Another way of putting it is that this is our Pre-Heaven Intellect. This is the stuff we know without ever having remembered that we learned it in the first place. We didn't need to learn it because our ancestors already learned it and they passed that intellect on to us at conception. I typically explain this to my students the following two ways:

- I have owned a couple of blue heelers (Australian cattle dogs) over the years. These dogs are excellent at herding cattle, with a particular characteristic of nipping at cows' heels if they start to stray. I got these puppies early, when they were only about 8–12 weeks old. I took them home and before long they started nipping at my heels with their sharp puppy teeth. My blue heelers weren't taught that by their parents because they were taken from them before they learned it. So how did they know how to do it?

- I have also owned a couple of border collies (sheep dogs). When they were puppies, they used to try to herd small children into the corners of the room. It was the funniest thing to watch. This is once again a characteristic of sheep dogs – to herd the sheep into a pen or paddock. My border collies were trying to herd my friend's kids into the corners of the room. This is another example of Pre-Heaven Intellect or ancestral wisdom/knowing.

CV 21 allows us to access our inner beauty and permit it to shine like a piece of jade or a pearl. Our true inner beauty can only emerge if we show faith, humility, benevolence and moderation.[51]

A lot of ancient Chinese philosophies – in particular Confucianism, when taught by Confucius (Kǒng Zǐ) and Mencius (Mèng Zǐ) – believed that everyone is born good. This inner goodness can always be accessed even if the world/environment made us bad (nature versus nurture). This inner goodness is therefore our inner beauty. If we show faith, humility, benevolence and moderation, we can gain access to our inner beauty or goodness.

BL 9 is where we lay our head. Here we can dream and inspire ourselves to be more benevolent, more righteous, more virtuous, more honest, more correct and more humble – more like jade.[52]

Using CV 18, CV 21 and BL 9 together[53] gives us access to our ancestor's knowledge and our inner beauty/goodness. This will prompt us to be better people. Better to those around us but also better to ourselves.[54]

> Jade will always be beautiful… It reveals its flaws openly, giving it the qualities of radiance, brightness, loyalty and faith. (Kaatz 2005, p.51)

Jade is perfectly imperfect – just like the human race!

12. Fēng points

GB 20 – Fēng = wind; Chí = pool.[55]

BL 12 – Fēng = wind; Mén = gate.[56]

GV 16 – Fēng = wind; Fǔ = palace.[57]

GB 31 – Fēng = wind; Shì = market.[58]

All four of these points have the ability to eliminate wind from the body. Of the four, only GB 20 and GV 16 can clear both External Wind and Internal Wind. BL 12 only clears External Wind, and GB 31 clears External Wind or aids in the signs and symptoms of Wind Stroke/Wind Strike, which can include hemiplegia, muscle atrophy, numbness of the legs and/or knee rigidity.[59]

Therefore, as a point combination, GB 20, BL 12, GV 16 and GB 31 will help to clear External Pathogenic Wind. The signs and symptoms of this can include chills and fevers, aversion to wind, cough, sore throat, nasal congestion and/or runny nose, headache, body aches and pains, red eyes and/or teary eyes, and facial swelling.[60]

13. Shén points

Of the wide range of Shén points available, I will be discussing HT 7, BL 44, KI 23, KI 25, GB 13, GV 11 and GV 24.

> HT 7 – Shén = spirit; Mén = gate.[61]
>
> BL 44 – Shén = spirit; Táng = hall or temple.[62]
>
> KI 23 – Shén = spirit; Fēng = seal.[63]
>
> KI 25 – Shén = spirit; Cáng = storehouse.[64]
>
> GB 13 – Běn = root; Shén = spirit.[65]
>
> GV 11 – Shén = spirit; Dào = path, road or way.[66]
>
> GV 24 – Shén = spirit; Tíng = court or courtyard.[67]

HT 7

HT 7 is the Spirit Gate. The Heart houses the Shén, which therefore means that points on the Heart channel will be effective at balancing Shén-based disorders. HT 7 is the pick of the bunch as it's the gateway to the Shén.

HT 7 will regulate everything attributed to the Shén, which includes all the emotions and all of the Wǔ Shén, our memory, consciousness, thinking and sleep.[68]

One could even argue that HT 7 is the single best point on the entire body to balance the Shén.[69]

BL 44

BL 44 is located lateral to the Back Shù Transporting point of the Heart (BL 15). As already stated, the Heart houses the Shén, and therefore the proximity of BL 44 to BL 15 makes it an excellent point to treat the Heart Shén.[70]

Interestingly, in ancient times the Chinese character for Táng (堂) would have been more accurately translated as temple. Emperors were often buried in temples, and their spirits continued to reside there.[71] Interesting because the Emperor organ in Chinese medicine is the Heart and the spirit is translated as Shén.

> BL-44 calms the Mind [Shén]. Its indications include depression, insomnia, anxiety, mental restlessness, sadness, grief and worry… BL-44 can also stimulate the Mind's clarity and intelligence. (Maciocia 2009, p.258)

KI 23

Similar to a Chinese emperor stamping his wax seal on important documents, KI 23 has access to where we have stamped our Shén. This is where we identify with our true spiritual identity.[72]

This point is often effective when a person feels they have lost their way in life, either a sense of direction or a sense of self.

KI 23 regulates the Earth element.[73] Earth, being in the center, is directly responsible for the balancing of all things. It thrives on the 'Knowing' even if we don't know that we know. KI 23 can treat our internal spiritual environment and look to balance out any excesses or deficiencies in our Shén that we might be unaware of, especially if they are affecting our sense of self.[74]

KI 25

KI 25 regulates the Fire element.[75] As mentioned on previous pages, our Shén is every single emotion, which includes anger, joy, pensiveness, worry, sadness, fear and shock. Our Shén is also all of the Wǔ Shén, which are the Hún, Shén, Yì, Pò and Zhì. Granted, these are all stored in different organs, but the primary organ that controls them all is the Heart, and the Heart is a Fire element organ.

> It is perhaps the point [KI 25] of choice in situations when the intensity of feelings of rejection and loneliness have devastated the stability and strength of a person's shen. (Hicks *et al.* 2010, p.324)

GB 13

GB 13 is another excellent point to regulate the Shén. This can be for emotional turmoil such as anxiety, fear, mania, worry and pensiveness. The point can also be used to treat willpower, memory problems, jealousy, suspicion and even schizophrenia.[76]

GB 13 has the capacity to get down into the deepest aspect of emotional turmoil to find the root cause. Ellis *et al.* (1989, p.263) state: 'GB-13 is utilized in treating spirit [Shén] disorders, and treating the spirit is known as treating the source (root) of a disease.'

GV 11

GV 11 is located medial to the Back Shù Transporting point of the Heart (BL 15). As already stated, the Heart houses the Shén; therefore the proximity of GV 11 to BL 15 makes it an excellent point to treat the Heart Shén, as confirmed by Ellis *et al.* (1989, p.336):

GV-11 is located between the two associated-shu points of the heart [BL 15]; the heart can be treated through this point. Because the heart stores the spirit [Shén], GV-11 can be said to be a path to the spirit or a 'spirit path' [Shén Dào].

GV 24

GV 24 is yet another excellent point to balance the Shén. It has the ability either to raise the Vital Substances into the head in cases of deficiency or to descend excess energies out of the head.[77]

As you can see from the above point descriptions, HT 7, BL 44, KI 23, KI 25, GB 13, GV 11 and GV 24 are effective at balancing the Shén. Regardless of the sign or symptom, everything related to the Shén can be treated using this combination.

Similar to the 'Figure Eight' point combination I will be discussing later in the book (Chapter 7), this combination is effective to balance singular or multiple emotional disturbances.

But the other really amazing thing is that this combination can also have an impact on our personality traits. The idea is that we can get our internal spiritual environment back into a harmonious balance, and I'm sure that's something that a lot of our patients would benefit from!

But is it possible to needle all of these points at the same time? The short answer is no,[78] so you have two choices to make. The first is that you do a face-up and face-down treatment in the one session. Or you could alternate the points across two separate treatments. Let's look at where these points are located using Table 4.1.

Table 4.1 Location of the Shén combination points

Location of points	Points	
Head/face/neck	GB 13	GV 24
Trunk (front)	KI 23	KI 25
Trunk (back)	BL 44	GV 11
Arms/hands	HT 7	
Total points needled	12 needles used bilaterally	

As you know by now, I'm not a fan of flipping my patients halfway through a treatment. However, if I did decide to do that in this instance, I would take my time with the session. Assuming the patient wasn't in a rush, I would extend the appointment to accommodate a minimum of 15–20 minutes with all the needles in a face-up position and then repeat the 15–20 minutes when they are face down. Table 4.2 shows how that treatment would look.

Table 4.2 Shén point combination treatment

Face up		Face down	
KI 23	GB 13	HT 7	GV 11
KI 25	GV 24	BL 44	
Total of 7 needles used bilaterally		Total of 5 needles used bilaterally	

If, however, you are like me and prefer not to flip your patient during the session, then you will have to needle the points across two separate treatments. With these two treatments you may even decide to add in a few additional points to help round out the treatment. As you are probably aware, there are a stack of other points in the body that can balance the Shén. My *Acupoint Dictionary* has the following ten points for treating the Shén:[79]

- Main points – HT 3, HT 7, BL 15, BL 44 and PC 6.

- Secondary points – GV 20, GB 20, BL 10, M-HN-3 (Yìn Táng) and CV 15.

Of these points, only HT 7 and BL 44 are already included as part of this Shén point discussion. Therefore, if we added the new group of points into the original treatment shown in Table 4.1, we could have more substantial treatment options; two options in fact – one that is entirely face up (see Table 4.3) and one that is entirely face down (see Table 4.4).

Table 4.3 Edited Shén point combination: Session 1 – face up

Location of points	Points	
Head/face/neck	GB 13	GV 24
	GV 20	M-HN-3 (Yìn Táng)
Trunk (front)	KI 23	CV 15
	KI 25	
Arms/hands	HT 7	
Total points needled	12 needles used bilaterally	

Table 4.4 Edited Shén point combination: Session 2 – face down

Location of points	Points	
Head/face/neck	GB 20	BL 10
Trunk (back)	BL 15	GV 11
	BL 44	
Arms/hands	HT 3	PC 6
Total points needled	13 needles used bilaterally	

Finally, if I chose to do these treatments, I would need to look at the two different point combinations to see if there is a balanced distribution of needles. As Tables 4.3 and 4.4 show, there is a good, and sensible, scattering of needles over a large area of the body.

Regardless of your decision (from the multiple options discussed above), all of the treatments have the potential to be good for your patients.

14. Tiān points

Tiān = celestial, Heaven, sky.[80]

There are a lot of acupuncture points that refer to Tiān in their Pīn Yīn name. Table 4.5 lists these points in terms of their location, abbreviated English name and their Pīn Yīn name/meaning.

Table 4.5 Pīn Yīn point name/meaning

Location of points	Points	Meaning[81]
Head/face/neck	BL 7 (Tōng Tiān) BL 10 (Tiān Zhù) GB 9 (Tiān Chōng) TE 16 (Tiān Yǒu) SI 16 (Tiān Chuāng) SI 17 (Tiān Róng) LI 17 (Tiān Dǐng) CV 22 (Tiān Tú)	Tōng = connection; Tiān = celestial Tiān = celestial; Zhù = pillar Tiān = celestial; Chōng = hub Tiān = celestial; Yǒu = window Tiān = celestial; Chuāng = window Tiān = celestial; Róng = countenance Tiān = celestial; Dǐng = tripod Tiān = celestial; Tú = chimney
Trunk (front)	SP 18 (Tiān Xī) ST 25 (Tiān Shū) PC 1 (Tiān Chí)	Tiān = celestial; Xī = ravine Tiān = celestial; Shū = pivot Tiān = celestial; Chí = pool
Trunk (back)	TE 15 (Tiān Liáo) SI 11 (Tiān Zōng)	Tiān = celestial; Liáo = bone-hole Tiān = celestial; Zōng = gathering
Arms/hands	LU 3 (Tiān Fǔ) PC 2 (Tiān Quán) TE 10 (Tiān Jǐng)	Tiān = celestial; Fǔ = storehouse Tiān = celestial; Quán = spring Tiān = celestial; Jǐng = well

Of the 16 points listed above that have Tiān in their name, seven of them are referred to as the 'Window of Heaven' or 'Windows of the Sky' points. These points were first referred to in the 2nd and 21st essays of *The Spiritual Pivot* (Líng Shū/靈樞) but were not classified as Window of Heaven points at that stage.[82]

If we look at the 16 points from an anatomical perspective, we find the following:

- All of the points are located above the umbilicus and above the elbow.

- Of the 16 points, eight are on the neck or head. In Chinese medicine the head is closest to Heaven. Further, if we look at the body as a microcosm of the Universe, then the head is the Heavenly aspect.

What do we find if we explore the Chinese medicine perspective?

- All six of the Yáng channels have at least one point on them in this combination – BL 7, BL 10, GB 9, TE 10, TE 15, TE 16, SI 11, SI 16, SI 17, LI 17 and ST 25.

- Three of the Yīn channels have at least one point in this combination – LU 3, PC 1, PC 2 and SP 18. Plus, the Yīn governor (Rèn Mài) has a point – CV 22.

Most importantly, however, these points all have a common theme: they all have Tiān in their name. As stated above, Tiān translates as celestial, Heaven or sky, but what does that mean when it comes to using this point combination in clinical practice? These points can be effective in the following Chinese medicine scenarios:[83]

- Reconnecting the head with the body

- Descending Rebellious Qì

- Descending Rising Yáng

- Clearing Damp or Damp Heat

- Heart Shén-based disorders

- Treating the sense organs.

Let's look at each of these scenarios in a little more detail, bearing in mind that every single Chinese medicine treatment (provided in Tables 4.6–4.15) has been referenced from the same sources.[84]

Reconnecting the head with the body

The head is a very heavy part of our anatomy and can weigh 5–10% of our body weight.[85] This weight is supported by a very thin neck, but as long as the head sits square on its axis (neck), then this doesn't usually cause any dramas.

But when the head falls off its neck axis, the muscles in the neck and upper back have to work extra hard to support it. This is when drama starts and local Qì and Xuè stagnates. This stagnation negatively affects the flow of Vital Substances into and out of the head, which can lead to a disconnection between the head and the body.

This combination can help to reconnect the head and the body, thereby correcting the flow of the Vital Substances.

Signs and symptoms of this disharmony can include poor memory, difficulty learning, foggy/fuzzy head, headache, dizziness, vertigo, sense organ problems, plum-stone throat (Méi Hé Hóu),[86] a lack of 'sense of self', redness and/or swelling of the face.

Of the options available to us from the Tiān points, Table 4.6 is a point combination you could consider to help reconnect the head with the body.

Table 4.6 Tiān point combination – reconnecting the head with the body

Location of points	Points	
Head/face/neck	BL 10 GB 9	TE 16 SI 16
Arms/hands	LU 3	TE 10
Total points needled	12 needles used bilaterally	
Method of needling	The best approach would be to lay the patient face down with the arms resting in an arm cradle below the face-hole.	

Descending Rebellious Qì

Qì is supposed to move in all directions throughout the body, including upwards. Sometimes, however, too much Qì ascends to the detriment of every other direction (particularly down) and it accumulates in the chest, head and neck regions.

Signs and symptoms of this complaint are wide and varied but can include cough, asthma, wheezing, shortness of breath, nausea, vomiting, heartburn, acid reflux, indigestion, dizziness, vertigo, headache, plum-stone throat and/or a stiff neck.[87]

It turns out that all of the points, apart from BL 7, can descend Rebellious Qì. Therefore, a good approach would be to use these points over two separate treatments, one face up and one face down. Two possible options are in Tables 4.7 and 4.8.

Table 4.7 Tiān point combination – descending Rebellious Qì: Session 1 – face up

Location of points	Points	
Head/face/neck	SI 16 SI 17	CV 22
Trunk (front)	SP 18 ST 25	PC 1
Arms/hands	PC 2	TE 10
Total points needled	15 needles used bilaterally	
Method of needling	The best approach would be to lay the patient face up with the hands clasped over the epigastric region.	

Table 4.8 Tiān point combination – descending Rebellious Qì: Session 2 – face down

Location of points	Points	
Head/face/neck	BL 10 GB 9	TE 16 LI 17
Trunk (back)	TE 15	SI 11
Arms/hands	LU 3	
Total points needled	14 needles used bilaterally	
Method of needling	The best approach would be to lay the patient face down with the arms resting in an arm cradle below the face-hole.	

Descending Rising Yáng

Yáng is heat, and just like heat in nature, Yáng rises. Most of the time this is tempered with Yīn acting as a balance, but sometimes when Yáng is too powerful for Yīn, it rises out of control. This is particularly prevalent if Yīn is deficient.

Signs and symptoms of Yáng rising are also wide-ranging, but are, typically, fever, headaches/migraines, red face, red/dry/painful eyes, nose bleeds, tinnitus (sharp and intense), dizziness, dry mouth/throat, anger, irritability and even rage or mania.[88]

A total of ten points (out of the 16 Tiān points) can be used to descend Yáng Rising. If used bilaterally, that's 20 needles. Therefore, it would probably make sense to separate the points across two treatments, one face up and one face down. Two possible options are in Tables 4.9 and 4.10.

Table 4.9 Tiān point combination – descending Rising Yáng: Session 1 – face up

Location of points	Points	
Head/face/neck	BL 7 GB 9	SI 16
Trunk (front)	ST 25	PC 1
Arms/hands	LU 3	TE 10
Total points needled	14 needles used bilaterally	
Method of needling	The best approach would be to lay the patient face up with the hands clasped over the epigastric region.	

Table 4.10 Tiān point combination – descending Rising Yáng: Session 2 – face down

Location of points	Points	
Head/face/neck	BL 10 GB 9	TE 16
Trunk (back)	TE 15	
Arms/hands	LU 3	TE 10
Total points needled	12 needles used bilaterally	
Method of needling	The best approach would be to lay the patient face down with the arms resting in an arm cradle below the face-hole.	

Clearing Damp or Damp Heat

Sometimes Damp can accumulate in the upper regions of the body. This is not particularly common because Damp is heavy and therefore tends to accumulate lower down the body, particularly in the abdomen and the joints in the extremities. Having said that, it can occasionally accumulate swiftly and this tends to lock the Damp into a region. This then negatively affects the flow of Vital Substances through that region. When this happens, the Damp gets stuck and strong, and with no stronger force to shift it, the Damp stays put.

Signs and symptoms of Damp accumulation that occurs higher up the body include a heavy head, unclear thought, vagueness, poor memory, swollen throat, throat nodules, weeping eyes, blocked ears, headaches, fuzzy/foggy head, mouth ulcers and swollen lips.[89]

Although the previous scenario is uncommon, Damp Heat is not, but this is still dependent on whether Damp or Heat is dominant. If Damp is stronger than Heat, then Damp Heat will typically accumulate lower down the body in the abdomen and the joints in the extremities. However, if Heat is dominant, then Damp Heat will rise up the body and accumulate in the chest, neck and head.

Signs and symptoms of Damp Heat accumulation that occurs higher up the body include fever, yellow/sticky exudation from the throat/nose/ears, red/shiny face, severe headaches/migraines, restlessness, mental derangement (e.g. manic depression), insomnia, chest infections, swollen/painful throat, throat nodules, plum-stone throat and memory problems.[90]

A total of 11 points (out of the 16 Tiān points) can be used to clear Damp or Damp Heat. If used bilaterally that's 21 needles. Therefore, it would probably make sense to separate the points across two treatments, one face up and one face down. Options for this are shown in Tables 4.11 and 4.12.

Table 4.11 Tiān point combination – clearing Damp or Damp Heat: Session 1 – face up

Location of points	Points	
Head/face/neck	BL 7 GB 9	SI 17 CV 22
Trunk (front)	ST 25	PC 1
Arms/hands	LU 3	TE 10
Total points needled	15 needles used bilaterally	
Method of needling	The best approach would be to lay the patient face up with the hands clasped over the epigastric region.	

Table 4.12 Tiān point combination – clearing Damp or Damp Heat: Session 2 – face down

Location of points	Points	
Head/face/neck	BL 10 GB 9	TE 16
Trunk (back)	TE 15	
Arms/hands	LU 3	TE 10
Total points needled	12 needles used bilaterally	
Method of needling	The best approach would be to lay the patient face down with the arms resting in an arm cradle below the face-hole.	

Heart Shén-based disorders

Regardless of the cause of the Shén imbalance, these points can also be effective in assisting a range of different Shén-based disorders. Why? Well, as you can see from the different causes already discussed, this point combination can regulate the flow of Vital Substances in and out of the head.

Although there will be a range of Shén-based disorders that are unique to each point, some of the more commonly seen are insomnia, restlessness, memory problems, foggy/fuzzy head, melancholy and sadness.

Of the options available to us from the Tiān points, Table 4.13 is a point combination you could consider to treat Heart Shén-based disorders.

Table 4.13 Tiān point combination – Heart Shén-based disorders

Location of points	Points	
Head/face/neck	BL 10 GB 9	SI 16
Trunk (front)	ST 25	
Arms/hands	LU 3 PC 2	TE 10
Total points needled	14 needles used bilaterally	
Method of needling	The best approach would be to lay the patient face up with the hands clasped over the epigastric region or the groin region.[91]	

Treating the sense organs

Each of the 16 Tiān points has the ability to treat sense organ problems. Some of the more common problems include blurry vision, red/painful eyes, tinnitus, deafness, nasal congestion, speech problems involving the tongue, swollen/painful throat and plum-stone throat.[92]

Therefore, it would probably make sense to separate the points across two treatments, one face up and one face down. Two options are shown in Tables 4.14 and 4.15.

Table 4.14 Tiān point combination – treating the sense organs: Session 1 – face up

Location of points	Points	
Head/face/neck	BL 7 GB 9	SI 17 CV 22
Trunk (front)	PC 1	
Arms/hands	LU 3 PC 2	TE 10
Total points needled	15 needles used bilaterally	
Method of needling	The best approach would be to lay the patient face up with the hands clasped over the epigastric region.	

Table 4.15 Tiān point combination – treating the sense organs: Session 2 – face down

Location of points	Points	
Head/face/neck	BL 10	TE 16
	GB 9	SI 16
Trunk (back)	TE 15	
Arms/hands	LU 3	TE 10
Total points needled	14 needles used bilaterally	
Method of needling	The best approach would be to lay the patient face down with the arms resting in an arm cradle below the face-hole.	

Notes

1   Aurelius 2004, p.70. Marcus Aurelius wrote *Meditations* around 170 CE while he was Emperor of Rome. A lot of what he wrote was not original. Having said that, he was one of the most powerful people on the planet at the time, so when he spoke, people listened. Therefore, he was able to bring previous philosophical ideas to the forefront of people's thinking.

2   This was when I was head of the Chinese medicine department, and chief subject developer/writer at the Australian Institute of Applied Sciences (2003).

3   Ellis *et al.* 1989, p.122.

4   Ibid., p.34.

5   Lade 1989, p.105.

6   Ellis *et al.* 1989, pp.272–273.

7   Ibid., p.138.

8   Ibid., pp.143–144.

9   Ibid., p.105.

10   Ibid., pp.237–238.

11   Chen 2004, pp.177–185, 198–209, 211–216. Not all of the signs and symptoms listed are in the reference provided.

12   McDonald and Penner 1994, pp.189–190, 202–203; Maciocia 2015, pp.560–562, 616–619.

13   Sān Jiāo Not Communicating is a Zàng Fǔ pattern that I have created to help explain diseases and patients that are 'unexplainable'. This pattern encompasses patients with acute and/or chronic disease that is complicated, stubborn and confusing. The patient has a myriad of signs and symptoms and it is impossible to isolate one or two Zàng Fǔ patterns that are a true representation of their disease. By diagnosing them as Sān Jiāo Not Communicating, I have accepted that my patient is an extremely difficult case and I need to create some sort of balance in the body first by encouraging the production and movement of Vital Substances. Once I have created more balance by recommunicating the Sān Jiāo, my patient's follow-up treatments will make more sense.

In addition, the patient's pulse quality will be quite unique. When the Sān Jiāo is out of balance, it shows up in the pulse as an 'uneven' quality. Although this is not one of the standard 28 pulse qualities, it is one that you will almost certainly have felt in your clinic and struggled to explain within the confines of the 28 qualities. An uneven pulse feels unbalanced with the cùn, guān and chǐ pulse positions all beating out of time. They are 'consistently inconsistent'. This is an uneven pulse quality and is used to determine the diagnosis of Sān Jiāo Not Communicating.

Sān Jiāo Not Communicating, along with the uneven pulse, will likely be only short-term labels because the patient typically responds fast to treatment. The newer signs and symptoms clear away, exposing the previous mysteries of their internal environment. This gives you access to much more accurate Zàng Fǔ pattern diagnosis, and its subsequent treatment plan.

14   Ellis *et al.* 1989, pp.292–293.

15   Ibid., pp.96–97.

16   Deadman *et al.* 2007, p.478.

17   Lade 1989, p.81.

18   Ross 1995, pp.61–62.

19   McDonald and Penner 1994, p.125.

20   Ibid.

21   Lade 1989, pp.334, 345.

22   Ibid., pp.334–335.

23   www.innerbody.com/image/musc06.html.

24   Deadman *et al.* 2007, pp.273–274, 306.

25   Ibid.

26   Ellis *et al.* 1989, pp.264–265.

27   Ibid., pp.286–287.

28   Lade 1989, pp.335, 344.

29   Ibid., pp.340, 344.

30   Maciocia 2015, pp.471–475, 478–481. This reference doesn't include all of the conditions I have listed.

31   Lade 1989, pp.345, 348.

32   Ibid., pp.330, 348.

33   Hartmann 2009, p.19.
34   Ellis *et al.* 1989, pp.43–44, 379.
35   Ibid., pp.93–94.
36   O'Connor and Bensky 1981, p.315.
37   Wang 2014, pp.100, 130–131. Yue Lu translated *The Classic of Supporting Life* (*The Classic of Supporting Life with Acupuncture and Moxibustion*/Zhēn Jiǔ Zī Shēng Jīng) in 2014. The original text was written by Zhízhōng Wáng somewhere between 1180 and 1195 CE.
38   Ellis *et al.* 1989, pp.44, 379.
39   Ibid., pp.91–92.
40   O'Connor and Bensky 1981, p.273.
41   Wang 2014, pp.101, 132.
42   Ellis *et al.* 1989, pp.219–220.
43   Ibid., pp.122–123.
44   Hicks *et al.* 2010, p.323.
45   Kaatz 2005, p.245.
46   Ibid.
47   Ibid., p.51.
48   Ellis *et al.* 1989, p.323.
49   Ibid., p.150.
50   Kaatz 2005, p.51.
51   Ibid., p.54.
52   Ibid., p.454.
53   This point combination can all be done together. Either the patient lies on their side or you needle BL 9 transversely and then gently lay the patient on their back, ensuring the needles stay flat on the pillow. I would also encourage the patient not to move their head around too much while the needles are in.
54   In Confucianism terms, this would be a sage (Jūn Zǐ), or perfect person.
55   Lade 1989, pp.331, 333.
56   Ibid., pp.333, 340.
57   Ibid., pp.333–334.
58   Ibid.
59   Deadman *et al.* 2007, pp.266, 437, 449, 548–549.
60   Chen 2004, p.154; Maciocia 2015, pp.727–732.
61   Ellis *et al.* 1989, p.125.
62   Ibid., p.175.
63   Ibid., p.218.
64   Ibid., p.220.
65   Ibid., p.262.
66   Lade 1989, p.281.
67   Ellis *et al.* 1989, p.347.
68   Dechar 2006, pp.170–175.
69   Deadman *et al.* 2007, p.220.
70   Ellis *et al.* 1989, p.175.
71   Ibid.
72   Kaatz 2005, p.538.
73   Twicken 2013, p.61.
74   Hicks *et al.* 2010, p.323.
75   Ibid., pp.323–324.
76   Maciocia 2009, pp.268–270.
77   Ibid., p.279.
78   Technically, you could lay your patient on their side and be able to needle all of these points. However, this is problematic because, from experience, it's quite difficult to needle the back points and upper chest points accurately when they are lying on their sides.
79   Hartmann 2009, p.139.
80   Ellis *et al.* 1989, p.396.
81   All Pīn Yīn translations are referenced using Ellis *et al.* 1989, pp.396–397.
82   Wu 1993, pp.12, 98–99. *The Spiritual Pivot* (Líng Shū) was written somewhere between 200 and 0 BCE.
83   Deadman *et al.* 2007, pp.48–50; Maciocia 2015, pp.860–861.
84   Deadman *et al.* 2007, pp.78–79, 118, 148–149, 202–203, 241–242, 244–246, 260–261, 263–264, 370–371, 402–403, 406–407, 428, 522–523; Ellis *et al.* 1991, pp.81–82, 104, 126–127, 158–159, 183, 186–187, 198–200, 269–270, 285–286, 288–289, 305, 363; Maciocia 2015, pp.951–952, 969, 980–981, 1021–1022, 1024–1025, 1029–1031, 1080–1081, 1094–1096, 1102–1103, 1144.
85   www.reference.com/science/much-human-head-weigh-e88885d350f7b71b.
86   Plum-stone throat (Méi Hé Hóu) is a term that describes a feeling of something stuck in the throat. This is typically considered 'substantial' or 'non-substantial'. Substantial plum-stone is real phlegm that the patient is able to cough up (often with difficulty). Non-substantial plum-stone is a false read. This is because there isn't anything real stuck in the throat but it still feels as if there is. This is actually Qì and it is often stuck there because the patient can't/won't/shouldn't express their emotions. Therefore, you need to establish whether the plum-stone is substantial or non-substantial because each requires a different treatment.
87   Maciocia 2015, pp.425–438, 471–472.
88   Chen 2004, p.139.
89   Ibid., p.156; Maciocia 2015, pp.737–743.
90   Maciocia 2015, pp.737–743, 745–750.
91   In this instance I would needle BL 10 in the following manner. Get the patient to turn their head to one side. Needle BL 10 in a transverse manner and then gently turn the patient's head back to the center. If everything feels okay, get them to gently turn their head to the other side. Repeat the process. Once the patient has their head back to center and they are comfortable, you can proceed to needle the remaining points.
92   All of the points on the Yáng channels can treat the sense organs because the channels pass through/beside every single one of the sense organs.

[Gong-sun Chou said], 'May I ask what this "flood-like ch'i [Qì]" is?'

[Mencius replied], 'It is difficult to explain. This is a ch'i [Qì] which is, in the highest degree, vast and unyielding. Nourish it with integrity and place no obstacle in its path and it will fill the space between Heaven and Earth. It is a ch'i [Qì] which unites rightness and the Way [Dào].'

Mencius/Mèng Zǐ/孟子 (371–289 BCE)[1]

5

Strategies/Types of Acupuncture Point Combinations

The previous two chapters were designed to give examples of how to combine acupuncture points. The next three chapters are taking it a step further and will provide a framework for point combinations.

There are a number of different ways that you can combine points in acupuncture treatments. Some of these are pre-designed for us via a particular diagnosis (discussed shortly); some are points that you have found to be effective via empirical evidence; and some are chosen via other means. I even know therapists who choose different points depending on the time of the day and the time of year. They call this chrono-acupuncture, or the ten heavenly stems and twelve earthly branches.[2]

As I have already stated, I choose my points primarily according to the patient's main complaints and the subsequent Zàng Fǔ patterns. But that's only stage one of my final point selection because the points I ultimately choose need to have a strong relationship to one another; they also need to be scattered (sensibly) all over the body to ensure good movement of Vital Substances (Qì, Xuè, Jīn Yè and Jīng). I also need to consider the patient in the process.

Throughout the next three chapters I will be incorporating acupuncture point combinations that follow those rules – unless, of course, they are point combinations that I reference directly from the classics – ancient and modern.

This chapter focuses on the more basic point combinations, and then Chapter 6 starts to discuss more complex and slightly bigger combinations, followed by Chapter 7, which incorporates the largest and most complex point combinations. It is worth noting that not every combination is likely to be effective every time and so I will include a comment on factors that could negate the effect, where relevant.

1. Top and bottom

The top-and-bottom method is designed to get the Vital Substances moving at great lengths along the body with the furthest point combination moving Vital Substances from the top of the head to the bottom of the feet.

In effect, each end acts as an anchor for the other, creating a pulling force towards its opposite. This is very effective if, for example, the patient has Yáng Rising into the throat and head, because the bottom/lower point will help to drag the Yáng back down. The opposite is also true if the patient has Qì Sinking because the top/higher point will help to raise the Qì.

Essentially, the top-and-bottom method ensures a better overall balance, with the movement and distribution of Vital Substances throughout the body flowing to where they are most needed, regardless of the direction.

The top-and-bottom method can be used in six different ways by choosing points:

- on the head/face and the legs/feet

- on the head/face and the arms/hands

- on the head/face, legs/feet and the arms/hands

- on the arms/hands and the legs/feet

- on the trunk (front/back) and the legs/feet

- on the trunk (front/back), legs/feet and the arms/hands.

Below are some examples of the top-and-bottom method with explanations on what the points treat as well as how/why the points combine well together.

Head/face and legs/feet

Let me give a simple, but extremely effective, point combination to start:

- GV 20 and KI 1.

This combination is using the highest point (GV 20) and lowest point (KI 1) on the body.[3]

Both points have a natural affinity for the upward movement of Vital Substances. Having said that, both points can be manipulated to encourage movement in the opposite direction. We see this when KI 1 is used to treat hypertension[4] by draining the point, forcing the descending of the Vital Substances.

GV 20 can also be manipulated in order to descend Vital Substances. An example of this effectiveness is that it can 'extinguish liver wind and subdue liver yang' (Ellis, Wiseman and Boss 1991, p.383).

When GV 20 and KI 1 are used together, they have the ability to help the body decide whether the Vital Substances need to move up or down; this combination also has the capacity to do both in the same treatment, if required.

As with most point combinations that use only a few points, it's generally a good idea to supplement the combination with additional points. This will give the body a lot more ammunition to assist in your patient's healing.

Head/face and arms/hands

- M-HN-3 (Yìn Táng), N-HN-54 (Ān Mián) and HT 7.

Useful for calming the Shén in the treatment of insomnia.[5] There are a number of different types, and causes, of insomnia in Chinese medicine which require different point selections. Having said that, you can use M-HN-3 (Yìn Táng), N-HN-54 (Ān Mián) and HT 7 for all types of insomnia.

M-HN-3 (Yìn Táng) acts as a sedative, helping the patient's mind to settle, thereby making it a very effective point for insomnia.[6]

N-HN-54 (Ān Mián) actually means 'Peaceful Sleep'. Ān = peaceful or calm; Mián = sleep.[7]

HT 7 is the Yuán Source point of the Heart and is also a very good point to calm the Shén and treat insomnia.[8]

To have all of these points needled at the same time, position the patient supine (lying on their back). Needle N-HN-54 (Ān Mián) by gently rolling their head to one side. Repeat for the other side. The needles can be inserted in any order depending on your own preference.[9]

Head/face, legs/feet and arms/hands

Apart from the point combination for calming the Shén and insomnia (above), there are two additional insomnia combinations:

- N-HN-54 (Ān Mián), PC 6 and SP 6.[10]
- M-HN-3 (Yìn Táng), HT 7 and SP 6.[11]

Both of these point combinations are to be considered when your patient presents with insomnia. These two combinations are effective for treating insomnia of any cause.[12]

It wouldn't even be too much to consider needling all of the points listed in the 'head/face and arms/hands' and 'head/face, legs/feet and arms/hands' sections above. After all, it's only nine needles; plus, they are scattered over the head, face, arms, hands and legs, which makes for a good point combination.

Arms/hands and legs/feet

- HT 6, HT 7, KI 6 and KI 7.

For use in Kidney Yīn and Yáng Xū night sweats and hot flushes/flashes.[13] Although I don't run into a lot of menopausal women who are diagnosed with Kidney Yīn Xū and Kidney Yáng Xū, I have had some over the years. As you can imagine, they make for quite a long-term patient, especially if you don't quite get the diagnosis correct and instead focus more on just Kidney Yīn Xū or Kidney Yáng Xū.

HT 6 treats Heart Yīn Xū and also the symptoms of night sweats, hot flushes/flashes and late-afternoon fevers.[14]

HT 7 is the Yuán Source point on the Heart channel, which makes it effective to tonify the Heart. As the Heart is the Emperor organ, and the Heart is the partner of the Kidneys (Shào Yīn), it can aid the Kidneys by strengthening their deficiency.

KI 6 is typically needled for Kidney Yīn Xū and also the symptoms of night sweats, hot flushes/flashes and late-afternoon fevers.[15]

KI 7 is typically needled for Kidney Yáng Xū and for regulating the water passages (Jīn Yè), which will make it an effective point to treat night sweats, hot flushes/flashes and late-afternoon fevers.[16]

The Kidney channel was chosen because it activates the Kidneys and they are the site of our 'Yuán Yīn' and 'Yuán Yáng'. Boosting this original or primary Yīn and Yáng can aid in the tonification of the Kidney Xū.

The Heart channel was selected as it combines very well with the Kidney channel (via Shào Yīn), especially in times of great need; and let's face it, any patient diagnosed with a Yīn and Yáng Xū are in great need.

Trunk (front/back) and the legs/feet

- ST 25 and ST 37.

These two points are the Front Mù Collecting and Lower Hé (Uniting) Sea points of the Large Intestine organ respectively. As a collective, these points are excellent to regulate/balance the Large Intestine.

Trunk (front/back), legs/feet and arms/hands

- CV 4, CV 12, CV 17, ST 36, SP 6, LI 10, TE 8, LU 9 and HT 7.

This combination is a little more complex. It connects the Three Arm Yáng channels (twice), Three Leg Yáng channels and the Three Leg Yīn channels, as well as activating the Lung and Heart/Pericardium organs (which are associated with the Three Arm Yīn channels); this has a balancing effect on all of the organs in the body. It is worth noting here that the function of this combination is somewhat debatable and I will leave it up to you to decide as to its validity. Personally, I have had good success with it but that doesn't necessarily mean it worked because of the function stated above. Let me explain.

CV 4 is effective at balancing out the organs in the Lower Jiāo. CV 12 does likewise for the Middle Jiāo organs, and CV 17 regulates the Upper Jiāo organs.[17]

SP 6 definitely connects the Three Leg Yīn channels, and TE 8 definitely connects the Three Arm Yáng channels.[18] The debate comes when we discuss ST 36 and LI 10.

ST 36 translates as Leg Three Miles/Measurement, and LI 10 translates as Arm Three Miles/Measurement.[19] These names suggest that there is a connection for ST 36 with the Three Leg Yáng channels, and the same applies for LI 10 with the Three Arm Yáng channels. Having said that, I have never seen anything written on this – ever! But I have heard it mentioned by a prominent lecturer when I was studying more than 20 years ago.

LU 9 is the Yuán Source point of the Lungs, and HT 7 is the Yuán Source point of the Heart. These two points are the best points on their channels to treat their organs. They also have an excellent, but indirect, link to CV 17.

To date, my view is still an open one. I'm not sure if this combination works because of these connections, or whether it works at balancing out the organs and channels simply because of the choice of points – because, let's face it, that is an excellent point combination!

When might the top-and-bottom point combination not be effective?

Having points at great distances from one another is problematic when there is stagnation between the points because it negatively impacts on the effectiveness of Vital Substance flow.

This leaves you with two choices. The first is to choose a different combination; the second is to include some local points around the stagnation. I appreciate that this changes the combination from a true top-and-bottom method. It would now be called top, bottom and local, but this adjustment to the method has the potential to make it effective, when otherwise it wouldn't have been.

An example of this is when you want to use GV 20 and KI 1 to regulate the flow of Vital Substances up and down the body (see the 'head/face and legs/feet' section above) but there is localized stagnation of the trapezius and levator scapula muscles of the neck. As a result, you include the local points of GB 20, BL 10, SI 14 and M-HN-30 (Bǎi Láo).

The example above does result in an increase in the number of points used to 11 needles, but the local neck points will have the effect of improving the flow of Vital Substances between GV 20 and KI 1, which is ultimately what you are wanting with that top-and-bottom combination in the first place.

2. Corresponding/mirroring

The corresponding, or mirroring, combination is a popular one that has found a new lease of life thanks to the Dr Tan method of treatment. I won't be going into his method of treatment, however, and will be sticking to just the corresponding/mirroring combination.

The idea is that your arms and legs are mirror images of each other, as in:

- fingers and toes

- hands and feet

- wrists and ankles

- forearm and lower leg

- elbow and knee

- upper arm and upper leg

- shoulders and hips.

Therefore, you can choose a point on the lower or upper limb to mirror the point you have already decided to use. In this way, the point on the other limb acts as a support, with the hope that it will enhance the treatment. Theoretically, this method can be useful for a lot of signs and symptoms.

You can use this method either as a bilateral pairing or as an opposite-side unilateral pairing. Personally, I like using bilateral needling whenever I can.

An example of this pairing would be using SI 8 and BL 40 bilaterally (four needles) for the treatment of knee or elbow disorders.

An example of a unilateral pairing using just two needles would be LI 11 on the left side for tennis elbow (lateral epicondylitis) with a mirrored support on the right knee via ST 35.

Below are examples of the corresponding/mirroring method with explanations on what the points treat as well as how/why the points combine well together.

Fingers and toes

- LU 11 and SP 1.

These two points are Sūn Sī Miǎo Ghost points, Jǐng Well points and Tài Yīn (Six Division) partners.[20] Therefore LU 11 and SP 1 are an effective combination in three different ways.

Sūn Sī Miǎo Ghost points

The Ghost points are effective at treating various emotional imbalances. As a combination, LU 11 and SP 1 can be used together to treat manic depression (Diān Kuáng).[21]

Jǐng Well points (see Chapter 8)

According to the 68th difficulty (Flaws 2004, p.123) in *The Classic of Difficulties* (*Canon of the Yellow Emperor's Eighty-One Difficult Issues*/Huáng Dì Bā Shí Yī Nán Jīng/黃帝八十一難經), 'The wells [Jǐng Well points] rule fullness below the heart.'

LU 11 and SP 1 as a combination can treat fullness of the Heart (and below the Heart) with sweating. They can also treat Heart agitation with cough and dyspnea and heat/fullness in the chest.[22]

Jǐng Well points can also be used for acute-stage disorders.[23] In this case that would be acute disorders of the Lung and Spleen organs and their associated channels. This can include, but would not be limited to:

- LU 11 – asthma, wheezing, sore throat, runny nose, nosebleed, mania and vomiting[24]

- SP 1 – nosebleed, fever, diarrhea, vomiting (possibly with blood), agitation and mania.[25]

TÀI YĪN PARTNERS

Maciocia (2015, pp.760–761) suggests that when the Tài Yīn division is injured, it shows signs and symptoms of abdominal fullness, feeling cold, vomiting, no appetite, diarrhea, no thirst and tiredness (similar to Spleen Yáng Xū). Although LU 11 and SP 1 cannot treat most of these signs and symptoms, they are an effective combination for treating vomiting.[26]

Wang and Robertson (2008, pp.63–64) also talk about the Tài Yīn being good for regulating nutrition and dampness. While SP 1 definitely treats both those areas, LU 11 does not.

Hands and feet

- TE 3 and GB 42.

These two points are excellent distal points to treat various head, eye and ear disorders. These include but aren't limited to:[27]

- head disorders – headaches that are typically one-sided and located around the ears, temples and eyes; dizziness or vertigo; red face; fevers

- eye disorders – pain, redness, swelling, itching, blurry vision

- ear disorders – tinnitus, deafness, ear infections, blocked ears, pain.

Wrists and ankles

- TE 4 and KI 3.

These points are an effective combination for strengthening the Yuán Qì and Jīng.[28]

Both points are Yuán Source points, which is where the Yuán Qì can be activated.[29]

TE 4 is probably not a point that you might automatically think is high on the list for treating Yuán Qì, so you have to go back to *The Classic of Difficulties*. The 66th difficulty tells us that the Sān Jiāo is directly responsible for moving our Yuán Qì.[30]

As TE 4 is also the Yuán Source point of the Sān Jiāo, it makes it potentially the most effective point in the entire body to move the Yuán Qì.

KI 3 is the Yuán Source point of the Kidneys, and the Kidneys store the Yuán Qì and Jīng.[31]

By combining TE 4 and KI 3, you have an excellent treatment for strengthening Yuán Qì and Jīng.

Forearm and lower leg

- PC 5 and ST 40.

This is an excellent combination to transform Phlegm.[32] Deadman *et al.* (2007, p.375) state: 'Together with Fenglong ST-40 it [PC 5] is one of the two main acupuncture points to treat phlegm disorders.'

ST 40 is the Luò Connecting point of the Stomach channel.[33] Luò Connecting points treat diseases of their exteriorly–interiorly related partner, which in this case is the Spleen. The Spleen organ is directly responsible for the transformation and transportation of the Jīn Yè.[34] If the Spleen is not functioning well, then this negatively impacts on body fluid breakdown and distribution, which can lead to Phlegm accumulating.

PC 5 is another terrific point to transform Phlegm, particularly in the Upper Jiāo. However, it can work on Phlegm anywhere in the body because it is the Yīn partner of the Sān Jiāo, which aids in regulating Fire and Water everywhere. This is because the Sān Jiāo encompasses all the organs in the body.[35]

Elbow and knee

- PC 3 and LR 8.

    PC 3 – Qū = bend or crook; Zé = marsh.[36]

    LR 8 – Qū = bend or crook; Quán = spring.[37]

PC 3 and LR 8 treat chronic Jué Yīn disease because they are both Hé (Uniting) Sea points on the Jué Yīn paired channels.

Hé (Uniting) Sea points

The Hé (Uniting) Sea points (see Chapter 8) are terrific points to treat chronic diseases of their associated organ.

According to the 68th difficulty (Flaws 2004, p.123) in *The Classic of Difficulties*, 'the uniting [Hé Sea points] rule counterflow qi and discharge [or diarrhea]'.

PC 3 and LR 8 as a combination can treat counterflow Qì and discharge. Signs and symptoms of this can include diarrhea (may contain undigested food, pus or blood), dysentery, seminal emission, urinary enuresis, uterine prolapse, headache, mania, nosebleed, dyspnea, cough, fever, heatstroke, dry mouth with thirst, and/or vomiting (which may contain blood).[38]

Hé (Uniting) Sea points can also be used for chronic-stage disorders of the internal organs. In this case, that would be chronic disorders of the Pericardium/Heart and Liver organs and their associated channels. This can include, but would not be limited to:

- PC 3 – heart pain, palpitations, pounding sensation below the heart[39]

- LR 8 – swelling/masses in the hypogastric region, eye disorders including visual dizziness, pain, swelling and heat. The Liver channel also has a large influence on the Lower Jiāo and LR 8 is great for clearing Damp Heat in the genito-urinary and bowel regions. This can include swelling/itching of the genitals, impotence, urinary difficulties, diarrhea (may include undigested food, pus or blood), infertility and amenorrhea.[40]

JUÉ YĪN PARTNERS

Maciocia (2015, pp.762–763) suggests that when the Jué Yīn division is injured, it shows signs and symptoms of emaciation, persistent thirst, rushing feeling in the chest, pain and heat in the heart region, hunger but no desire to eat, cold limbs, diarrhea and vomiting (characterized by heat above and cold below).

Of these disorders, PC 3 and LR 8 can treat persistent thirst, rushing feeling in the chest, pain and heat in the heart region, diarrhea and vomiting.[41]

Wang and Robertson (2008, pp.151–155) also talk about the Jué Yīn being good for regulating External and Internal Wind, Xuè and Yīn. It also fosters the Xuè/Qì relationship and calms the Shén. Having said that, PC 3 and LR 8 don't really combine well together for any of those. Although they can technically treat any chronic Jué Yīn condition because they are Hé (Uniting) Sea points, you don't see that happen much for this point combination clinically.

Upper arm and upper leg

- LU 3 and LR 9.

This combination ensures a solid connection between the Hún and Pò.[42]

The Hún and Pò will be discussed in more detail in Chapter 13. The Hún is our Heavenly/Ethereal/Dream-Big soul, and the Pò is our Earthly/Corporeal/Do-Big soul. The Hún is necessary because that is where we come up with new dreams/ideas, and the Pò is needed because it takes those dreams and makes them reality.

The Hún and Pò connection is extremely important in the body, with each acting as an anchor for the other. Neither can work on its own. LU 3 and LR 9 can help ensure that the Hún and Pò stay in a balanced state by working for each other. This should also guarantee a more balanced Shén.

The Lungs house the Pò, and the Liver houses the Hún.[43] Although LU 3 is predominantly used to access the Pò, it also has the ability to access the Hún. The same applies for LR 9, which is predominantly used to access the Hún, although it can also access the Pò.[44]

Kaatz (2005, pp.226, 404) says it best when she states: 'Here [LU 3] within us is the light of heaven that can revitalize and rejuvenate our life bringing courage, purpose and strength... Yin Bao [LR 9] is a place of protection where we can rest and be nourished by our inner vision.'

Shoulders and hips

- TE 14 and GB 29.

This combination can be used for lateral hip/shoulder problems according to the cutaneous region of Shào Yáng.[45]

Via the Shào Yáng cutaneous region, TE 14 and GB 29 are mirrored points on the shoulders and hips. Therefore, they can be used to treat the other; in this way, the point on the other limb acts as a support, with the hope being that it will enhance the treatment.

As I stated earlier, you can use this pairing as bilateral or unilateral needling. Bilateral needling is self-explanatory: you use both shoulders and both hips regardless of which shoulder/hip is the main complaint. With the unilateral method, you tend to use the opposite side as the support. I will give two examples below:

- Right deltoid shoulder pain and stiffness: TE 14 is used on the right shoulder as the local point, and GB 29 is used on the left hip as its distal mirror.

- Right hip pain and stiffness: GB 29 is used on the right hip as the local point, and TE 14 is used on the left shoulder as its distal mirror.

When might the corresponding/mirroring point combination not be effective?

As with any treatment combination, sometimes they don't work as well as you would expect, and this method is no different. Personally, I don't generally use the corresponding/mirroring method until I have exhausted other combinations.

This is partly because it wasn't a main focus of treatment taught to us when I studied and I haven't seen it mentioned much in my research either. Therefore, it's definitely a more recent 'rediscovery-of-sorts' for me. This means that I have a lot of other reliable treatment formulas that I use first before I consider trying the corresponding/mirroring method.

Maybe in a few years' time, once I have used this method more, I will be more convinced as to the benefits.

3. Local and distal[46]

This point combination is one of the most common types discussed in this book. As the name suggests, you choose a point that is local to the patient's complaint and then you deliberately choose a distal point to act as a support. I used some examples of this method in Chapter 3 when I discussed local and distal points that are on the same channel.

This section is dedicated to local and distal points that are not on the same channel.

The local-and-distal method is a very simple combination but also very effective. The local point will immediately start to treat the area of concern in two ways:

- It will try to move and then clear any local stagnation.

- It will try to draw fresh Vital Substances to the local area for healing.

The local stagnation is counterproductive as it is old, toxic and taking up space. The stagnation needs to be cleared out to make room for the fresh Vital Substances to enter the area for healing.

The distal points in this combination also work on two things:

- They try to send Vital Substance reinforcements to the local area to assist with the healing process.

- They try to drag/pull/draw/push the stagnation away from the area of concern.

You can use the local-and-distal method on so many different parts of the body. Let me give you four examples:

- eyes

- nose

- acute low back pain/tension with sciatica

- tennis elbow (lateral epicondylitis).

Eyes[47]

Local points – BL 1, BL 2, ST 2, GB 1.

Distal points – LR 3, GB 37, LI 4, BL 18.

If you were to use all the points above, that would be a total of 16 needles if used bilaterally: eight local and eight distal.

The local point functions are self-explanatory: all local points around the eye will treat the eye. The points selected cover three different channels that travel along separate pathways on the body, which allows for more holistic Vital Substance flow.

Having said that, BL 1, BL 2, ST 2 and GB 1 are all on channels that travel from the head down to the feet.

The distal points need a little bit more explanation.

The Wood element organs are the Liver and Gall Bladder. The sense organ for these organs is the eyes.[48]

LR 3 is the Yuán Source point of the Liver, thereby making it one of the best points on the channel to treat the organ. By treating the Liver organ, you treat the eyes as well.

BL 18 is the Back Shù Transporting point of the Liver, thereby making it the best point on the back of the body to treat the organ. By treating the Liver organ, you treat the eyes.[49]

GB 37 is the Luò Connecting point on the Gall Bladder channel, which connects to the Liver channel.[50] This connection between the two Wood element organs makes it an excellent point to nourish the organs and treat the eyes. Further, the traditional Chinese characters for Guāng Míng (光明) can be used to describe the eyes – the name for GB 37 is often translated as 'Eyes Bright'.[51] However, the Pīn Yīn is typically translated as 'Bright Light' (Guāng = light; Míng = bright).[52]

LI 4 is another excellent point to treat the eyes; in fact, it treats every sense organ.[53] It's also a good choice in this combination because it's the only point on the upper extremities, thereby allowing for a more balanced treatment.

LR 3 and LI 4 are also important in this combination because they are the only points on channels that travel up the body.

The local points of BL 1 and BL 2 link directly with the distal point BL 18. The same applies to GB 1 and GB 37.

Finally, there are points located on the face, trunk (back), the arms and the legs, which are excellent for strong Vital Substance flow.

Nose[54]

Local points – LI 20, M-HN-14 (Bí Tōng) and M-HN-3 (Yìn Táng).

Distal points – LI 4 and LU 7.

Adjacent points – GB 20 and BL 7.

If you were to use all the points above, that would be a total of 13 needles if used bilaterally: five local, four distal and four adjacent.

The local point functions are self-explanatory: all local points around the nose will treat the nose.

The distal points to treat the nose are located on the Lung and Large Intestine channels. These channels belong to the Metal element, of which the sense organ is the nose.[55]

LI 4 is an excellent distal point to treat the nose; in fact, it treats every sense organ.[56]

LU 7 is also a great distal point for the nose[57] for two reasons:

- It is the Luò Connecting point on the Lung channel, which connects to the Large Intestine channel.[58] The Large Intestine channel finishes next to the nose.

- Both the Lung and Large Intestine organs belong to the Metal element, of which the sense organ is the nose. Because of this, in theory, every Lung channel point can treat the nose.

I have also included GB 20 and BL 7 as adjacent points. These aren't technically local or distal to the nose. They are located on the head/neck regions and both are excellent adjacent points to treat the nose.[59]

Acute low back pain/tension with sciatica[60]

Local points – BL 23, BL 25, GB 30, GV 3 and GV 4.

Distal points – BL 40, BL 60, N-UE-19 (Yāo Tòng Xué) and GB 34.

As you can see from the combination above, there are 18 points if needled bilaterally: eight local and ten distal. Typically, points for this condition are selected based on what side needs the most attention, so that would likely mean some points are only needled unilaterally. For example:

- N-UE-19 (Yāo Tòng Xué) is an extra point, which is actually four points – two points on each hand. This point is usually needled on the same side as the main area of concern in the lower back.[61] Therefore, if the patient was suffering from acute left-sided low back pain and tension with sciatica traveling down the left leg, then you would needle N-UE-19 (Yāo Tòng Xué) on the left hand only.

This local-and-distal combination is so effective because of the relationships of the points:

- BL 23 and BL 25 are local points that link well with the distal points of BL 40 and BL 60 because they are on the same channel. The same applies to GB 30 and GB 34.

- N-UE-19 (Yāo Tòng Xué) is the only distal point located on the arm, so it creates a nice whole-body treatment.

- GV 3 and GV 4 are local points used to consolidate BL 23, BL 25 and GB 30.

Tennis elbow (lateral epicondylitis)[62]

Local points – LI 10, LI 11, LI 12, LU 5, TE 10.

Distal points – LI 4, LI 5, TE 5, LR 3, SP 6, GB 34, ST 36.

Tennis elbow, or lateral epicondylitis, is usually diagnosed in Chinese medicine as Qì and Xuè Stagnation in the Large Intestine channel. It also typically only presents on one arm. Therefore, a large portion of the points above could be used unilaterally. If you did choose to needle them bilaterally, the treatment would total 24 needles: ten local and 14 distal. Personally, I would do a combination of both bilateral and unilateral. One possible combination is included in Case Study 5.1 below.

Tennis elbow tends to cause significant discomfort around the lateral epicondyle of the humerus bone. The closest channel to this area is the Large Intestine, which explains why there are so many local and distal points on the Large Intestine channel.

TE 10 acts as a further support, assisting with Vital Substance flow through the stagnation in the elbow.

LU 5 is the only other local point in this combination that isn't on the Large Intestine channel. It acts as a support by draining the Vital Substance stagnation down the arm, whereas the Large Intestine and Sān Jiāo channels attempt to drain the stagnation up the arm. This opposing flow potentially allows for more stagnation to leave the elbow, thereby speeding up the healing process.

The distal points also need some further discussion.

LI 4 and LI 5 are on the main channel of choice and provide some serious Vital Substance drive/push/force. As they are at a distance from the problem area, they can build up Vital Substance momentum, so that when it hits the stagnation in the elbow, it can force its way further into (and through) the blockage.

LI 4 clears painful obstruction with accompanying inflammation. It is also one of the best points on the body for pain relief.[63]

TE 5 acts in the same way with TE 10 as the Large Intestine channel local and distal points work. In addition, *The Great Compendium – Volume VIII* (*The Great Compendium of Acupuncture and Moxibustion*/Zhēn Jiǔ Dà Chéng/針灸大成. 第8卷) advises the use of TE 5 for elbow problems.[64]

TE 5 also clears heat and inflammation.

According to Sun (2011, pp.376–378), LR 3 and SP 6 are useful in a diagnosis of Xuè Stasis in the elbow. He says they are both good for moving stagnation of Qì (moving Qì will move the Xuè) and Xuè, as well as relieving the elbow pain.

LR 3 also makes its own point combination with LI 4 via 'opening the Four Gates' (see Chapter 6). In this instance, opening the Four Gates is effective to treat painful obstruction by activating the flow of Qì and Xuè.[65]

GB 34 and ST 36 are located near the knee and are distal mirrors or corresponding points for the elbow. The knee and elbow are mirrored joints on the body.

GB 34 acts as a distal mirror for the Sān Jiāo channel in the form of the Shào Yáng Six Division pairing. It is located in the knee region, which therefore makes it suitable to treat the elbow region. As Deadman *et al.* (2007, p.451) advise, '[GB 34] benefits the sinews and joints... In summary, Yanglingquan GB-34 can be used for pain, cramping, contraction, stiffness and sprain of the sinews and muscles in any part of the body.'

ST 36 acts as a distal mirror for the Large Intestine channel in the form of the Yáng Míng Six Division pairings. It is located in the knee region, which therefore makes it suitable to treat the elbow region.

CASE STUDY 5.1 A 35-YEAR-OLD MALE (AS) WITH PAIN/TENDERNESS IN HIS RIGHT ELBOW

AS was suffering from significant pain and tenderness at his right elbow near the lateral epicondyle of the humerus. He first noticed it five days prior after spending a weekend in the garden and it had not reduced in intensity at any stage in that five days.

AS commented that the pain was worse during and after use of the right arm, in particular when he was holding objects away from his body. He also found that typing on the computer keyboard was problematic. AS had full range of movement passively, but when I applied resistance, he complained of significant pain on wrist extension and pronation.

Upon Tuī Ná palpation, AS jumped and squealed when I pushed my thumbs into the region of LI 10, LI 11 and the common extensor tendon origin just distal to the lateral epicondyle. He also complained of discomfort when I ran my thumbs along the extensor digitorum communis muscle midway along the forearm. On further Tuī Ná, AS showed no discomfort at all on his left elbow/forearm and his neck was also fine.

My diagnosis for AS was Qì and Xuè stagnation of the Large Intestine and Sān Jiāo channels of the elbow and forearm of his right arm. The points I chose are listed in Table 5.1.

Table 5.1 Treatment for tennis elbow[66]

Points	Local/distal	Bilateral/unilateral
LI 4	Distal	Bilateral
LI 10	Local	Bilateral
LI 11	Local	Bilateral
LI 12	Local	Unilateral – right side only
LU 5	Local	Unilateral – right side only
TE 5	Distal	Bilateral
TE 10	Local	Unilateral – right side only
GB 34	Distal	Unilateral – left side only (swap sides for a mirror-image treatment)
ST 36	Distal	Unilateral – left side only (swap sides for a mirror-image treatment)
LR 3	Distal	Bilateral
Total points needled		15 needles used

The points chosen in Table 5.1 don't need additional explanation as they were discussed in detail earlier. I do want to add that, in the case of AS, I checked his signs and symptoms at every visit and made some changes to the points where necessary.

It took seven weekly treatments (my recommendation was twice a week but AS wouldn't come that often) for AS to notice any change at all. Then the benefits snowballed and he was virtually 100% better after nine treatments. He came for a tenth and then stopped coming.

I had advised AS to avoid using his arms as much as possible, but he didn't listen and continued to work long hours each day. He also continued to garden on the weekends as well as do his rock-and-roll dancing classes three nights a week. The fact that AS wasn't willing to make any changes to his weekly activities, combined with refusing to attend acupuncture treatments twice weekly, almost certainly lengthened his condition. In the end, however, we got there, and to date AS has not had any recurrence of his tennis elbow.

When might the local-and-distal point combination not be effective?

If there is too much Vital Substance stagnation between the points needled, then the local-and-distal method might not be the best choice, especially if the points are a great distance from one another. In this instance, you might be better off including more local and adjacent points and fewer distal points for the initial treatments. Then, as the local stagnation starts moving, you can include more distal points to speed up the Vital Substance flow in and out of the local area of concern.

The other consideration is that not every patient understands how acupuncture works. When this is the case, your patient typically expects needles to be inserted exclusively into the local area of complaint. Therefore, you will need to explain what you are doing before you put the distal points in.

4. Left and right[67]

The left-and-right method is also a fairly common point combination consideration in clinic. Its main specialty is that it can save needles by using only one of the bilateral points rather than both. For example, a patient is suffering from a right ankle sprain and so you needle GB 40 on the right side only.

This method is also useful to create a harmonious balance in the body by using a lot of different points, potentially on a lot of different channels.

The left-and-right method generally makes use of the following principle: the left side is Yáng/male and the right side is Yīn/female. This is stated in chapter 5 (Ni 1995, p.23) of *The Yellow Emperor's Classic* (*Inner Canon of the Yellow Emperor*/ Huáng Dì Nèi Jīng/黃帝內經): 'The east is the yang direction. The essence of yang circulates from the left… The western direction is considered yin, and the essence of yin descends down the right side.'[68]

However, what's interesting here is that we know east isn't to the left and west isn't to the right. In fact, it's the other way around, with east to the right and west to the left. But this statement is made because you are taking the eye view of the Emperor or a sage, and they face south. This is confirmed in chapter 6 (Ni 1995, p.27) of *The Yellow Emperor's Classic*: 'The sage stands facing south.'[69]

Therefore, if one was to view east and west in the eyes of the Emperor or sage, then east would be to the left and west would be to the right. So many rights and lefts!

In summary, if you plan to do unilateral needling, then you would typically use your Yáng channel points on the left side and the Yīn channel points on the right side.

There are, of course, exceptions to the rule. You may be treating a musculoskeletal complaint as in Case Study 5.1. In that instance, the unilateral points were purely based on the complaint and had nothing to do with the principle of putting Yáng channel points on the left and Yīn channel points on the right.

In the end, it's entirely up to you, as the practitioner, to decide what is best for your patient.

The left-and-right method can be used in a variety of different ways, including the following:

- It can be used as a bilateral method in certain circumstances where the patient is suffering from a one-sided complaint.

- Select a Yáng channel point on the left with a Yīn channel point on the right.

- Use dominant right-sided needling when a patient is suffering from Yīn Xū.

- Use dominant left-sided needling when a patient is suffering from Yáng Xū.

- Use unilateral needling on the same side as the patient complaint.

- Use unilateral needling on the opposite side to the patient complaint.

- Use unilateral needling on Yīn and Yáng partners (Wǔ Xíng).

- Use unilateral needling on Yīn/Yīn partners (Six Divisions).

- Use unilateral needling on Yáng/Yáng partners (Six Divisions).

- Use unilateral needling via the corresponding/mirror method.

As chapter 5 (Ni 1995, p.24) of *The Yellow Emperor's Classic* advises: 'When disease is on the right side, treat the left, and when it is on the left, treat the right.'

There really are a lot of different ways that the left-and-right method can be administered. Of the list above, I will only be discussing the first six, as the others listed have already been analyzed.

Bilateral needling for a unilateral complaint
Patient complaint is Bell's palsy – left-sided.[70]

Local points – ST 2, ST 4.

Distal points – LI 4, GB 20, LR 3.

The local points are selected based on the main areas that are affected with Bell's palsy. Therefore, the points chosen may vary somewhat with each patient.

LI 4 treats any disorder of the face and sense organs. As the four dominant points song goes: 'For mouth and face, Hegu's [LI 4] the ace' (Li 2007, p.75).

GB 20 and LR 3 are used to Clear the Wind, which is the typical cause of Bell's palsy when using the Zàng Fǔ pattern diagnostic tool.[71]

Yáng channel point on the left with a Yīn channel point on the right
Patient complaint is tiredness due to Qì Xū.[72]

Points – ST 36 and LU 9.

Needling ST 36 on the left and LU 9 on the right is a great combination for Qì production.[73]

ST 36 is an excellent point to tonify Qì as it can help nourish the organs that produce Qì. Deadman *et al.* (2007, p.159) state: 'Zusanli ST-36 is the single most important point in the body to stimulate the action of the Stomach and Spleen in generating qi and blood.'

LU 9 is the Yuán Source point of the Lungs. As such, it can be used for any disorder of the Lungs. It is also a great point to tonify Qì. Maciocia (2015, p.957) agrees: 'It [LU 9] is the main point to tonify Lung-Qi and Lung-Yin, especially in chronic conditions.'

Unilateral right-sided needling for Yīn Xū
Patient complaint is night sweats due to Yīn Xū.[74]

Points – KI 3, HT 6, SP 6, LU 9.

This combination works really well because it nourishes organs in the Upper Jiāo (Lungs and Heart), Middle Jiāo (Spleen) and Lower Jiāo (Kidneys). This creates a more harmonious and multifaceted approach to tonify Yīn. This is important, especially if the patient is quite deficient in Yīn; the more organs you can get involved, the better.

This combination is also good because it has needles in the arms and the legs, which is better than having all the points stacked in the one area.

It is worth noting that if the patient was very Yīn Xū, I would almost definitely needle the points bilaterally, and probably include additional points.

Unilateral left-sided needling for Yáng Xū

Patient complaint is edema and fatigue due to Yáng Xū.[75]

Points – BL 20, BL 22, BL 23, ST 36, TE 4.

This combination makes use of special point categories to enhance the overall benefits of the treatment. Included are the:

- Back Shù Transporting points (BL 20, BL 22, BL 23)
- Yuán Source points (TE 4)
- Lower Hé (Uniting) Sea points (ST 36)
- Horary points (ST 36).

BL 20 and BL 23 are Back Shù Transporting points of the Spleen and Kidneys respectively. Both of these points can be used to tonify Yáng.[76]

ST 36 is the Lower Hé (Uniting) Sea point of the Stomach channel. These points are useful to regulate/harmonize their associated organ. In this case, it will harmonize the Stomach, and aid in the tonification of Yáng. It's also the Horary point on the Stomach channel. In this case, it is the Earth point on an Earth channel. This feature makes it a tremendous point to balance the Stomach and Spleen organs. This will, in turn, tonify Qì and Yáng.[77]

This combination also takes advantage of the Sān Jiāo organ via the use of TE 4 and BL 22. The Sān Jiāo regulates Fire and Water, which makes it an effective organ to balance Yáng and Yīn.

TE 4 is the Yuán Source point, thereby making it an effective point to regulate the Sān Jiāo.[78]

BL 22 is the Back Shù Transporting point of the Sān Jiāo, and this can be used to regulate Yáng and Yīn.[79]

This combination is also good because it has needles in the trunk (back), arms and legs, which is better than having all the points stacked in the one area.

It is worth noting that if the patient was very Yáng Xū, I would almost definitely needle the points bilaterally, and probably include additional points.

Unilateral needling for same-sided unilateral complaint

Patient complaint is gout – right big toe.[80]

Local points – SP 1, SP 2, LR 1, LR 2.

Distal points – SP 6.

It is worth noting that if the patient is in significant pain and discomfort, you might be better off needling the opposite big toe because the use of local points will likely hurt quite a bit more on the affected side.

Having said that, if the patient can handle it, I have found clinically that you get faster results if you can needle the affected side.

SP 1, SP 2, LR 1 and LR 2 are all used as local points to activate the Vital Substances in the area and to help reduce the pain.

SP 6 is a very useful distal point because it connects the Spleen and Liver channels. This effectively makes it a distal point for both channels and helps to draw the Vital Substance stagnation out of the big toe.

If the gout is severe, I would almost certainly needle the points bilaterally – with the proviso that the patient will let me, of course.

Unilateral needling for opposite-sided unilateral complaint
Patient complaint is a temporal headache – left-sided.[81]

Points – GB 38, GB 41, TE 5, LI 4, BL 62.

This combination would be used on the right side only. If, however, the headache was on the right side, then the points would be needled on the left side only.

LI 4 is the best distal point on the body for any type of headache.[82]

BL 62 can similarly be used as a distal point for all types of headaches, in particular around the temple and ear regions.[83]

The Gall Bladder and Sān Jiāo channels travel around the ears and temple regions. Therefore, both channels have distal points that are excellent to use for temporal headaches. GB 38, GB 41 and TE 5 are probably the most commonly used, but there are other distal points that would also be effective.

If the headache is severe, I would almost certainly needle the points bilaterally.

When might the left-and-right point combination not be effective?

The left-and-right method won't work in all situations, and that applies for every point combination. As you know, I prefer to needle points bilaterally when I can as I consider this to be a more holistic method of needling. But everyone is entitled to their own view on this. If you get great results with unilateral needling, then I say: 'Keep up the good work!'

A few years ago, I had an interesting experience at Endeavour College of Natural Health (where I work as a lecturer and clinic supervisor), when I was partnered with another acupuncture lecturer in the student out-patient clinic. This is not an unusual situation and is dependent on student enrollment numbers.

The acupuncture lecturer I was teamed with was a big believer in unilateral needling, as well as using minimal needles where possible, so our views tended to clash, to say the least. But we got on really well and respected each other's Chinese medicine experience. As a result, even though the students got differing treatment views, the semester was a fascinating one for all of us, students included. Their end-of-semester feedback was positive, and their comments were appreciative towards the differences in their two lecturers' treatment styles.

5. Front and back[84]

As with the previous point combinations, the primary purpose of the front-and-back method is to create a harmonious balance. This equilibrium can be created across one treatment or multiple treatments. In one treatment, you can do some points on the front of the body and then halfway through the treatment take those needles out and flip the patient over and then needle some points on the back. This is all done in the one treatment.

The front-and-back method, however, also works well across multiple treatments. You could do an entire front treatment one session and an entire back treatment the next session.

In Chinese medicine, the front is considered a more Yīn aspect and the back a more Yáng aspect.[85] Therefore, you can use the front-and-back method to regulate the patient's Yīn and Yáng. Two of the best ways to do this are to choose:

- Rèn Mài and Dū Mài points

- Front Mù Collecting and Back Shù Transporting points.

Apart from that, the front-and-back method can be applied for points located in the regions of the:

- neck

- chest and upper thoracic

- upper abdomen and lower thoracic

- lower abdomen and lumbar

- groin and sacrum/coccyx.

There is also nothing to stop you from doing front-and-back treatments on the limbs, but this is certainly less common.

There are seven front-and-back point combinations discussed below using the Eight Extraordinary Vessels, special point categories and regions discussed above. This method will always treat the region that the points are located in as well as a variety of other signs, symptoms, disorders and Chinese medicine complaints.

Rèn Mài and Dū Mài

Rèn Mài point – CV 15.

Dū Mài point – GV 12.

CV 15 and GV 12 are an effective front-and-back combination for calming the Shén.[86]

I like calling CV 15 the unofficial Front Mù Collecting point of the Shén.[87] It sits between the Front Mù Collecting points of the Heart (CV 14) and Pericardium (CV 17). Both of these organs house the Shén and are also great points to calm the Shén.

GV 12 is located on the upper back, which governs the Upper Jiāo. Therefore, the point will regulate the function of the Lungs, Heart and Pericardium. Its specialty is to clear Excess conditions, and is an excellent point to calm down an overactive Shén.[88]

Front Mù Collecting and Back Shù Transporting points

Front Mù Collecting point – LU 1.

Back Shù Transporting point – BL 13.

LU 1 and BL 13 are an effective combination for bronchitis.[89]

LU 1 is the Front Mù Collecting point of the Lungs, and BL 13 is the Back Shù Transporting point of the Lungs. Both of these special point categories are effective at regulating the Lungs.[90] Therefore, the points can treat anything wrong with the Lungs, not just bronchitis. This could include asthma, wheezing, dyspnea, chest pain/fullness/obstruction, common colds, cough and shortness of breath. This combination can even treat pneumonia and emphysema.

Neck

Front point – CV 23.

Back point – GV 15.

As stated above, the front-and-back method will always treat the region in which the points are located – in this case, the neck. CV 23 and GV 15 will also benefit the tongue and speech.[91]

When CV 23 is needled towards the tongue, it treats the tongue and benefits the speech.

GV 15 treats the tongue and benefits the speech. It is also a Sea of Qì point.[92] According to the 33rd essay of *The Spiritual Pivot* (Líng Shū/靈樞), 'When the Sea of Qi is insufficient, it results in the qi being too sparse and insufficient to make speech' (Wu 1993, pp.132–133).

Chest and upper thoracic

Front point – CV 14.

Back point – BL 44.

CV 14 and BL 44 can treat the chest and upper thoracic regions as well as balance the Shén.[93]

CV 14 is the Front Mù Collecting point of the Heart. As such, it will treat anything wrong with the Heart. The Heart houses the Shén, and therefore CV 14 will calm the Shén.[94]

BL 44 is on the 'Outer Run' of the Urinary Bladder channel. This is the pathway that runs 3 cùn lateral to the spine. The Outer Run has five special points that will regulate the Wǔ Shén.[95] BL 44 is one of these and it regulates the Shén.[96]

This combination is particularly good for treating a range of Shén-based disorders, including:[97]

- depression, sadness, grief

- worry

- insomnia

- anxiety

- mental restlessness/agitation

- mania

- manic depression (Diān Kuáng)

- anger, rage, ranting and raving

- disorientation

- poor memory, lack of clarity

- improving intelligence.

CV 14 and BL 44 as a point combination also make the shape of a triangle. This is often termed the Triangle of Power method and will be discussed in Chapter 6.

The Triangle of Power method works as a set of three needles, inserted into the body, that make the shape of a triangle. They work together as a triumvirate to force big change in the body. None of the points is as powerful on its own. The triumvirate collective is what gives the Triangle its power.

Upper abdomen and lower thoracic

Front point – ST 21.

Back point – BL 21.

ST 21 and BL 21 can treat the upper abdomen and lower thoracic as well as nausea/vomiting and gastric/epigastric/abdominal distension and pain.[98]

ST 21 regulates the Middle Jiāo, in particular the Stomach and Spleen organs, which are heavily involved in treating nausea/vomiting as well as gastric/epigastric/abdominal distension and pain.[99]

BL 21 is the Back Shù Transporting point of the Stomach. As such, it will regulate the Stomach, thereby treating nausea/vomiting, gastric/epigastric/abdominal distension and pain.[100]

Lower abdomen and lumbar

Front point – CV 4.

Back point – BL 26.

CV 4 and BL 26 can treat the lower abdomen and lumbar as well as tonify Yuán Qì.[101]

This is a truly fascinating point combination and, from my experience, one that is rarely taught. At Endeavour College of Natural Health (ECNH), where I lecture, we teach the students all of the special point categories, including the Back Shù Transporting points. But we only discuss the twelve that relate specifically to the twelve Zàng Fǔ organs. We don't include any others and, in my opinion, there are Back Shù Transporting points all the way from BL 11 to BL 30.

BL 26 is, what I call, an unofficial Back Shù Transporting point. 'But of what?' I hear you ask. The answer is in the Pīn Yīn name, which is Guān Yuán Shū. It is the Back Shù Transporting point of CV 4, or Guān Yuán. What this means in clinical practice is that you have a CV 4 point on the front of the body as well as a CV 4 point on the back of the body with BL 26.

By using this combination, you are giving CV 4 a triple shot of energy across the three needles. You also create a nice harmonious balance by having a front point as well as a back point in the same treatment. This will enhance the overall benefits you are striving for when you use these points to tonify Yuán Qì.

As Ellis *et al.* (1989, p.307) advise: 'CV-4 is a "passageway of original qi", the "critical juncture of original yang and original yin", or the place where "original qi is stored [locked in]".'

CV 4 and BL 26 as a point combination also make the shape of a triangle, referred to as a Triangle of Power.

Groin and sacrum/coccyx

Front point – LR 11.

Back point – BL 32.

LR 11 and BL 32 can treat the groin and sacrum/coccyx as well as infertility and/or irregular menstruation.[102]

BL 32 is located in the second sacral foramen and is excellent to harmonize the Lower Jiāo organs. In doing so, BL 32 can be an effective point to treat infertility and/or irregular menstruation.[103]

LR 11 is also a good point to treat infertility and/or irregular menstruation. Deadman *et al.* (2007, p.487) state: 'Many classical texts recommend moxibustion at this point [LR 11] for the treatment of infertility.'

When might the front-and-back point combination not be effective?

This combination won't suit every treatment. The single biggest negative is the need to flip the patient over halfway through the treatment. But if this is something you do regularly, then it's not a negative at all. I'm still of the view that a selection of 8–16 needles retained for roughly 30 minutes achieves a better outcome than doing eight or so needles on the front for 10–15 minutes and then flipping them to do the same on the back.

I am, however, a big fan of the front-and-back treatment when it's done across two separate treatments, session one as a front treatment and then session two as a back treatment.

6. Whole body

The idea of the whole-body method is to create harmony and balance by ensuring there are points needled in all areas of the body – namely:

- head and/or face
- trunk – front and/or back
- arms and/or hands
- legs and/or feet.

The harmony/balance comes because the Qì is being charged at shorter intervals throughout the body, thereby ensuring that momentum is maintained during the treatment.

Patients' bodies are often quite stagnant. By ensuring that there are points scattered all over the body, there is less risk of Vital Substances backing up behind large stagnant areas. This is because Qì is coming at the stagnations from multiple directions.

This method can be used for many disorders but its specialty is maintaining health and wellbeing. I have had a lot of patients over the years seeing me purely to stay healthy, and I have used this combination on these patients regularly. By ensuring that the patient's Vital Substances are flowing, they are much less likely to develop disorders if they maintain a regular treatment protocol.

Of particular interest to me is treating Shén-based disorders, and the whole-body method is also very effective for that too. An example is shown in Table 5.2.

Table 5.2 Whole-body Shén-balancing treatment[104]

Location of point	Acupuncture point	
Head/face/neck	GV 20	M-HN-3 (Yìn Táng)
Trunk (front)	CV 15	CV 4
Arms/hands	SI 7	HT 7
Legs/feet	SP 6	BL 62
Total points needled	12 needles used bilaterally	

Further, the points are scattered all over the body, ensuring the whole-body method is adhered to. If you take a closer look at the points, you will also see that some are on channels that travel up the body (CV 4, CV 15, SI 7, SP 6) and some that travel down the body (HT 7, BL 62). GV 20 is located at the top of a channel that travels up and down the body, and M-HN-3 (Yìn Táng) is located on the head/face, where the Shén can be activated.

When might the whole-body point combination not be effective?

The whole-body method won't be effective all of the time, and if the patient has a lot of stagnation, you might be better off narrowing your focus and targeting a few key areas first. Once the Vital Substances are moving, the whole-body method will be significantly more effective.

Notes

1   Lau 2003, pp.61–63. The *Mencius* was originally written around 300 BCE. Mencius or Mèng Zǐ (371–289 BCE) is, quite possibly, the second most famous Chinese philosopher of all time. He became so popular in Europe in the Middle Ages that Western society decided to latinize his name so they could pronounce it better. His popularity came about because he never proclaimed himself to be a god, and nothing that he said went directly against Christian beliefs in Western countries, where Christianity was still the ruling power of thought. He also took Confucianism to a whole new level, which made it even more popular in China than it already was.

2   For an excellent discussion on chrono-acupuncture, or the ten heavenly stems and twelve earthly branches, see Lorraine Wilcox's amazing translation and commentary of *The Great Compendium – Volume V* (*The Great Compendium of Acupuncture and Moxibustion/ Zhēn Jiǔ Dà Chéng*) in 2010. The original text was written by Jizhou Yang in 1601 CE.

3   Deadman *et al.* 2007, pp.336–338, 552–554.

4   O'Connor and Bensky 1981, p.298.

5   Hartmann 2009, p.85.

6   Deadman *et al.* 2007, p.566.

7   Lade 1989, pp.329, 341.

8   Ross 1995, pp.277–279.

9   I have both been treated using these points and been a practitioner giving these points to my patients. From these two different perspectives, I have found this treatment to be very sedating. Therefore, I would encourage you to get your patient to take a walk for about ten minutes after the treatment to help get their minds back into their daily activities. It's best that they don't jump straight into their car and drive as their mental faculties may be dulled.

10   Deadman *et al.* 2007, p.570; O'Connor and Bensky 1981, p.163.

11   O'Connor and Bensky 1981, p.144.

12   I actually have all of these points (from the 'Head/face and arms/hands' and 'Head/face, legs/feet and arms/hands' sections) as my 'main acupoints' for insomnia of any cause in my *Acupoint Dictionary* (Hartmann 2009, p.85).

13   Hartmann 2009, p.79.

14   Maciocia 2015, p.1010. Treating the Heart means you are treating the Emperor organ. When you tonify Heart Yīn, it can help tonify Kidney Yīn.

15   Lade 1989, p.185.

16   Ibid., p.186.

17   Deadman *et al.* 2007, pp.501, 511, 518.

18   Ellis *et al.* 1989, pp.105, 237–238.

19   Lade 1989, pp.45, 72.

20   Ellis *et al.* 1989, pp.35, 100.

21   Ellis *et al.* 1991, pp.87, 148, 459.

22   Deadman *et al.* 2007, pp.90, 182.

23   Maciocia 2015, p.832.

24   Deadman *et al.* 2007, p.90.

25   Ibid., p.182.

26   Ibid., pp.90, 182.

27   Cheng 2010, pp.198, 213; Deadman *et al.* 2007, pp.393–394, 462; O'Connor and Bensky 1981, pp.238, 323.

28   Maciocia 2015, pp.1065–1066, 1090–1091.

29   Flaws 2004, pp.120–121. *The Classic of Difficulties* (*Canon of the Yellow Emperor's Eighty-One Difficult Issues*/Huáng Dì Bā Shí Yī Nán Jīng) was originally written between 0 and 200 CE.

30   Flaws (2004, p.121) translates the text as 'The triple burner [Sān Jiāo] is the special messenger of this original [Yuán] qi'. Unschuld (1986, p.561) translates the text as 'The Triple Burner is the special envoy that transmits the original influences'.

31   Maciocia 2015, pp.157–158.

32   Deadman *et al.* 2007, pp.165–167, 374–376.

33   O'Connor and Bensky 1981, pp.273–274.

34 Maciocia 2015, p.145.
35 Ibid., pp.224–226.
36 Ellis *et al.* 1989, p.225.
37 Ibid., p.297.
38 Deadman *et al.* 2007, pp.372, 485.
39 Ibid., p.372.
40 Ibid., p.485.
41 Ibid., pp.372, 485.
42 Kaatz 2005, pp.226, 404.
43 Ni 1995, p.16: 4th chapter. *The Yellow Emperor's Classic* (*Inner Canon of the Yellow Emperor/ Huáng Dì Nèi Jīng*) was written somewhere between 200 and 0 BCE.
44 Kaatz 2005, pp.226, 404.
45 Maciocia 2006, p.356.
46 Ibid., pp.180–182; Ross 1995, pp.50–51.
47 Hartmann 2009, p.60.
48 Kaptchuk 2000, p.439.
49 Deadman *et al.* 2007, p.43.
50 Ibid., p.40.
51 Ellis *et al.* 1989, p.283.
52 Ibid.
53 Deadman *et al.* (2007, p.104) reference *The Classic of the Jade Dragon* (*Bian Que's Spiritual Guide to Acupuncture and Moxibustion, Jade Dragon Classic*/Biǎn Què Shēn Yīng Zhēn Jiǔ Yù Lóng Jīng) written by Wang Guo Rui in 1329 CE. The quotation used is 'Hegu LI-4 treats all diseases of the head, face, ears, eyes, nose, cheeks, mouth and teeth'.
54 Hartmann 2009, p.108.
55 Maciocia 2015, p.26.
56 Deadman *et al.* (2007, p.104) reference *The Classic of the Jade Dragon*.
57 Deadman *et al.* 2007, pp.83–85; Hartmann 2009, p.108; Maciocia 2015, pp.954–956; Ross 1995, pp.297–299.
58 Li 2007, pp.43, 45.
59 Ellis *et al.* 1991, p.311; Quirico and Pedrali 2007, pp.62–63.
60 Hartmann 2009, pp.96, 138.
61 Deadman *et al.* 2007, p.580.
62 Hartmann 2009, p.57; Hecker *et al.* 2005, p.429; Legge 2011, p.209; Sun 2011, pp.374–378.
63 Deadman *et al.* 2007, pp.104–105.
64 Yang 2011, p.131.
65 Deadman *et al.* (2007, p.105) reference the *Ode to Elucidate Mysteries*/Biāo Yōu Fù, which was first recorded in the 'Guide to Acupuncture and Moxibustion' written in 1241 CE.
66 The point combination that I have suggested in Table 5.1 is just one of many possible treatment options for tennis elbow. I would treat each patient on their merits rather than always using the same points for tennis elbow. In doing so, this ensures I am always treating the person and not the disease. Therefore, I would decide on my actual points at the time my patient presents to me in clinic after taking a full case history and doing Tuī Ná (Chinese massage) on their arm/elbow/neck to gauge where the stagnation is lying.

67 Maciocia 2006, pp.194–205; Ross 1995, pp.54–55.
68 Ni 1995, p.23: 5th chapter.
69 Ibid., p.27: 6th chapter.
70 Sionneau and Gang 1996, pp.136–139. This reference applies to both the local and distal points.
71 Maciocia 2004, p.573; Sionneau and Gang 1996, p.135.
72 Hartmann 2009, p.129.
73 Maciocia 2006, pp.200–201.
74 Lade 1989, p.327.
75 Hartmann 2009, pp.5, 18, 173.
76 Deadman *et al.* 2007, p.43.
77 Maciocia 2015, pp.985–986.
78 Flaws 2004, pp.120–121.
79 All Back Shù Transporting points can regulate the organ they are associated with.
80 Hartmann 2009, p.69. This reference applies to both the local and distal points.
81 Ibid., p.74.
82 Deadman *et al.* 2007, p.104.
83 Ibid., pp.320–321.
84 Maciocia 2006, pp.191–194; Ross 1995, p.52.
85 Maciocia 2015, p.9.
86 Kaatz 2005, pp.48, 71; Maciocia 2009, pp.275–278.
87 Hicks *et al.* 2010, p.340.
88 Maciocia 2009, pp.277–278.
89 Ross 1995, p.52.
90 Deadman *et al.* 2007, pp.43–44.
91 Ellis *et al.* 1991, pp.364, 380.
92 There are typically four Sea of Qì points referred to in the literature. The 33rd essay of *The Spiritual Pivot* (Líng Shū) refers to the points as being CV 17, GV 14, GV 15 and ST 9.
93 Maciocia 2009, pp.258, 273–274.
94 Hicks *et al.* 2010, p.340.
95 The Wǔ Shén, or Five Spirit, special points on the Outer Run of the Urinary Bladder channel are: BL 42 (Pò Hù), which regulates the Pò (Corporeal/Grounded/Earthly Soul); BL 44 (Shén Táng), which regulates the Shén (Spirit); BL 47 (Hún Mén), which regulates the Hún (Ethereal/Heavenly Soul); BL 49 (Yì Shè), which regulates the Yì (Thought/Post-Heaven Intellect); and BL 52 (Zhì Shì), which regulates the Zhì (Willpower/Pre-Heaven Intellect).
96 Maciocia 2009, p.258.
97 Deadman *et al.* 2007, pp.514–515; Ellis *et al.* 1991, p.358; Lade 1989, pp.163, 266; Maciocia 2009, pp.258, 273–274.
98 Cheng 2010, pp.149–150, 176.
99 Ibid., pp.149–150; Ellis *et al.* 1991, p.125.
100 Cheng 2010, p.176; Ellis *et al.* 1991, pp.208–209.
101 Ellis *et al.* 1989, pp.162, 306–307.
102 Deadman *et al.* 2007, pp.293–294, 487.
103 Quirico and Pedrali 2007, pp.70–71.
104 Maciocia 2009, pp.251, 253, 255, 259, 272, 275, 278, 280–281.

I hope that posterity will judge me kindly, not only as to the things which I have explained, but also as to those which I have intentionally omitted so as to leave to others the pleasure of discovery.

René Descartes (1596–1650)[1]

With respect to man's appointment of fate, when his parents give forth their vital forces, he already gets his fortunes and misfortunes. Man's nature is different from his fate. There are people whose nature is good but whose fate is unlucky, and there are others whose nature is evil but whose fate is lucky. Whether one is good or evil in his conduct is due to his nature, but calamities and blessings, and fortunes and misfortunes, are due to fate.

Wáng Chōng/王充 (27–97 CE)[2]

6

Strategies/Types of Acupuncture Point Combinations – Small Combinations

1. Yuán (Original) Yīn and Yáng

Points – CV 4 and CV 6.

The Yuán (Original) Yīn and Yáng method is a simple yet powerful combination that employs the use of the Kidneys to ensure the patient gets a strong boost of Yīn and Yáng.[3]

The Kidneys are the site of our Yuán (Original) Qì, Jīng, Yīn and Yáng.[4] This is sometimes referred to as 'Pre-Heaven'. Other translations include 'Primary', 'Source', 'Origin', 'Basic', 'Fundamental' or 'First'.[5]

> What is called the single *Yuan* (Origin) is the great beginning… It is only the sage who is capable of relating the many to the one, and thus linking then to *Yuan*… This *Yuan* is like a source. Its significance is that it permeates Heaven and Earth from beginning to end… Therefore *Yuan* is the root of all things, and in it lies man's own origin. How does it exist? It exists before Heaven and Earth. (Dǒng Zhòng-shū/董仲舒, 179–104 BCE)[6]

The Kidneys are the first organs developed, or made, in us after conception. They are the site where our mother's and father's Qì, plus our ancestral Qì, is blended. This site is commonly referred to as our Dān Tián and is where our Yuán (Original) Yīn and Yáng is stored.[7] To stimulate this energy, you need to access the Kidneys. CV 4 and CV 6 are a two-point combination that is excellent to use for this purpose.

CV 4 and CV 6 are located in the vicinity of the Kidneys and are also considered to be directly over the top of the Dān Tián.[8]

Ellis *et al.* (1989, pp.307, 309) discuss these two points further:

> CV-4 is a 'passageway of original qi', the 'critical juncture of original yang and original yin', or the place where 'original qi is stored [locked in]'... This area [CV 6] serves as a reservoir of qi for the whole of the body. It is the place from which qi emanates and to which it returns and is thus the Sea of Qi.

The Yuán (Original) Yīn and Yáng method will therefore tonify the Yīn and Yáng of the patient. Further, it will also tonify the patient's Qì and Jīng and, by default, the Xuè and Jīn Yè.

When you treat a patient for Yīn and/or Yáng Xū, it is generally a good idea to use more than just CV 4 and CV 6. Although this is a great combination on its own, it is often considered to be part of a larger treatment that takes advantage of local and distal points on a variety of different channels. I have listed three different treatment options in Tables 6.1–6.3 that include the use of CV 4 and CV 6 as part of a holistic point combination for Yīn Xū, Yáng Xū as well as Yīn and Yáng Xū.

Table 6.1 General Yīn Xū treatment[9]

Location of points	Points	
Trunk (front)	CV 4	CV 6
Arms/hands	HT 6	LU 9
Legs/feet	KI 3 KI 6	SP 6
Total points needled	12 needles used bilaterally	

Table 6.2 General Yáng Xū treatment[10]

Location of points	Points	
Trunk (front)	CV 4 CV 6	CV 8 – moxibustion only CV 17
Trunk (back)	GV 4 GV 14	BL 23
Legs/feet	ST 36	SP 6
Total points	11 needles used bilaterally; one point with moxibustion only	

Table 6.3 General Yīn and Yáng Xū treatment[11]

Location of points	Points	
Trunk (front)	CV 4 CV 6	CV 17
Arms/hands	HT 6	LU 9
Legs/feet	KI 3 SP 6	ST 36
Total points needled	13 needles used bilaterally	

2. Crown and Third Eye

Points – GV 20 and M-HN-3 (Yìn Táng).

The Crown and Third Eye method is an excellent combination to calm the Shén.[12]

This is one of the rare combinations where you could use just these points. Personally, I use it regularly with Tuī Ná, by pressing both points at the same time. The patient visibly relaxes right before my eyes. Another option is to start the treatment by needling GV 20 and M-HN-3 (Yìn Táng), and then follow them up with the rest of the needles. This can be very effective to calm the patient down so that they relax into the treatment more easily.

GV 20 and M-HN-3 (Yìn Táng) are located on the head and face but they are still considered local points for the Shén. Even though the Heart houses the Shén, the brain is also a site for Shén.

> [T]here have been doctors who attributed mental functions [Shén] to the brain rather than the Heart: in particular, Sun Si Miao of the Tang dynasty, Zhao You Qin of the Yuan dynasty, Li Shi Zhen of the Ming dynasty and especially Wang Qing Ren of the Qing dynasty... For example, Li Shi Zhen said: 'The Brain is the Palace of the Original Shen.' (Maciocia 2015, p.241)

The Crown and Third Eye method is effective at calming the Shén in Shí/Excess patterns, Xū/Deficient patterns, Zhì/Stagnant patterns and Internal Wind patterns.[13]

The Crown and Third Eye combination won't be effective in every case of Shén calming. I have outlined three scenarios below where the Crown and Third Eye won't be the best point combination.

Only two needles in the entire treatment

This is rather unorthodox in a clinical setting. We all have our differing views on this, and if we get good results with our patients, then we can needle as many needles as we see fit to use. My range is typically 8–16 needles. Therefore, it's likely there will need to be some additional points used to supplement the Crown and Third Eye method.

The need for some distal anchors

You should also give serious consideration to using some distal points as anchors to GV 20 and M-HN-3 (Yìn Táng), which are in the head. This is because having all your points in just one area can be problematic. This is especially the case with head points. The neck region is often stagnant, which limits the effective flow of Vital Substances (Qì, Xuè, Jīn Yè and Jīng) into and out of the head. If this is the case with your patient, then having all the points in the head will create a frantic/ agitated mess and this can create quite a disturbance in the head and Shén.

Regardless of whether the neck is stagnant or not, you should seriously consider adding in some distal anchors to assist the Crown and Third Eye method with the flow of Vital Substances into, and out of, the head.

Patient may experience significant agitation with these needles in

Some patients just don't like GV 20 and/or M-HN-3 (Yìn Táng) being needled. If that is the case, your patient will tend to complain about some of the following: pain, hot flushes/flashes, increased pressure in the head, feeling hypertensive, the start of a headache (sometimes even migraines), localized electrical sensation, brain fogginess, brain quietness, increased noise in the brain, or that their brain won't switch off and in fact is getting more frantic.

If this is the case, for whatever reason, GV 20 and M-HN-3 (Yìn Táng) aren't performing their function of moving the Vital Substances in whatever direction the patient needs most. This is an unusual situation in clinic, but it can happen. If it does, then don't persist with the Crown and Third Eye combination to calm the Shén. There are plenty of other methods and point combinations available to calm the Shén. I have already outlined quite a few in the book, and there are more to follow.

3. Triangle of Power (Sān Jiāo Lì)

The Triangle of Power method works as a set of three needles, inserted into the body, that make the shape of a triangle. They work together as a triumvirate to force big change in the body. None of the points is as powerful on its own. The triumvirate collective is what gives the Triangle its power.

The Triangle of Power is incredibly potent, especially when you consider that the method uses only three needles. The power or force comes from the fact that the method doesn't just move Vital Substances along one dimension. The triangle shape generates Vital Substance flow across three dimensions, so in fact the method works more like a pyramid than a triangle. Therefore, the Triangle of Power method can move Vital Substances up/down, inside/outside, medial/ lateral and anterior/posterior.

The key feature of the Triangle of Power method is that it can move the Vital Substances with extreme force, but the Vital Substances need to be moving, at least a bit, for this method to shine.

Although this method is very powerful, it won't work all of the time. You see, its greatest strength is also its biggest weakness. That is, the Vital Substances need to be moving, at least a little bit, for this method to be effective. If there is stagnation, then the Triangle of Power will be severely limited in its potential force. This method needs flow to generate significantly better movement. Without flow, the Triangle of Power simply won't be powerful.

Let me give you an example. Your car needs petrol/gas to run. Without it, your car won't move. But your car also won't drive effectively/efficiently if there is a blockage in the fuel line.

The same applies with the Triangle of Power method. Without the flow of Vital Substances, or if they are partially blocked along the channels and collaterals, then this method will be inefficient. But if you can get the Vital Substances moving, then the Triangle of Power will be much more effective and efficient.

If your patient appears to have some level of Vital Substance stagnation, then you need to get it moving before using the Triangle of Power method. Your patient doesn't have to have perfect flow – it just needs to be moving a little bit. Then you can shift your point combination to the Triangle of Power and watch it go to work. This is because the method needs some movement as this is where it generates the extra power. The Triangle of Power can't create power and force if there is none to start with.

So please remember, don't use this method when the Vital Substances are stagnant. Choose a different method to get flow, then shift across to the Triangle of Power.

There are hundreds of different Triangle of Power combinations. I have included four examples below with explanations of which conditions these point combinations treat as well as how/why the points combine well together. As you can see, these examples also cover some of the other point combinations already discussed, such as the top-and-bottom and front-and-back methods.

Move Vital Substances up and down the body[14]

Top point – GV 20.

Bottom points – KI 1.

This combination can lift/raise energy, drop/descend energy, and even a bit of both in the same treatment. They are also the highest and lowest points and naturally make the largest triangular shape on the body.

When GV 20 and KI 1 are used together, they have the ability to help the body determine whether the Vital Substances need to move up or down. This combination has the capacity to do both in the same treatment, if required.

Qì/Yáng tonic[15]

Front point – CV 6.

Back points – BL 24.

Where the previous combination was a top-to-bottom triangle, this triumvirate travels across/through the body as a front-to-back combination. Its primary function is to produce Qì and Yáng.

CV 6 (Qì Hǎi) translates as Sea of Qì and is an excellent point to tonify Qì. The point is also located near the Kidneys, and is particularly good for nourishing Yuán/Original Yáng.[16] Ellis *et al.* (1989, p.309) advise us: 'This area [CV 6] serves as a reservoir of qi for the whole of the body. It is the place from which qi emanates and to which it returns and is thus the Sea of Qi.'

BL 24 is what I call the unofficial Back Shù Transporting point for CV 6. What this means in clinical practice is that you effectively have a CV 6 point on the front of the body as well as on the back of the body with BL 24 (acting as the transporter). This is clearly stated in Ellis *et al.* (1989, p.161): 'BL-24 is located directly opposite Sea of Qi (CV-6), and is named Sea-of-Qi Shu because of its location and for reasons that are similar to those that account for CV-6 being named Sea of Qi.'

By using this combination, you are giving CV 6 a triple shot of energy across the three needles. You also create a nice harmonious balance by having a front point as well as a back point in the same treatment. This will enhance the overall benefits you are striving for when you use these points to tonify Qì and Yáng.

I provided a similar example in Chapter 5 with the points CV 4 and BL 26.

Water (Shuǐ) Separation[17]

Trunk (Front) point – CV 9.

Leg points – SP 9.

This combination acts as a Jīn Yè resolver. Other terms that refer to this include 'Water Separation', 'Transforms and Transports Body Fluids', 'Disinhibits Water Damp', 'Transforms Damp', 'Resolves Dampness', 'Regulates the Waterways' and 'Regulates the Water Passages'.[18]

What's interesting about this triumvirate is the use of CV 9. Interesting because throughout history there has been commentary about whether you should needle the point or use moxibustion on the point or do both. In the end, my view is that it comes down to personal preference.

Some of the classics are very direct in their commentary and say acupuncture is contraindicated for use on CV 9 but moxibustion is fine. An example of this is from volume I (Wang 2014, pp.74–75) of *The Classic of Supporting Life (The Classic of Supporting Life with Acupuncture and Moxibustion*/Zhēn Jiǔ Zī Shēng Jīng/針灸資生經) which states: 'It is very good to apply seven cones of moxibustion [to CV 9], stopping at a hundred cones for water disease [edema]; needling is contraindicated. The patient will die of water overflowing [if needled].'

During my studies I was never told to avoid this needle when resolving Jīn Yè; in fact, I was advised the opposite. Therefore, I have needled CV 9 regularly for resolving the Jīn Yè for over two decades and not a single patient has died of water overflowing.

SP 9 is also a terrific point to resolve the Jīn Yè.[19] Combining SP 9 with CV 9 also makes use of different parts of the body when needling, with the trunk (front) and the legs being used in the combination, further enhancing the harmonious nature of this Triangle of Power combination.

Ellis *et al.* (1991, p.154) referenced the *Ode of a Hundred Patterns* (Bǎi Zhèng Fù/百症武) when they said: 'SP-9 and CV-9 treat water swelling in the umbilical region.'[20] Unfortunately, no mention is made of whether SP 9 and CV 9 are needled, if moxibustion is applied, or if both methods are employed. Obviously, this would be helpful to know, especially considering the needling contraindication associated with CV 9 in some classical texts.

Calm the Shén[21]

Head/face point – M-HN-3 (Yìn Táng).

Arm/hand points – HT 7.

This is a sensational triumvirate for calming the Shén.

HT 7 (Shén Mén) translates as Spirit Gate. The name says it all: HT 7 is the gateway to our Shén. I am of the view that it is the single best point on the body to calm the Shén. Deadman *et al.* (2007, p.220) agree when they say: 'Shenmen HE-7 (Spirit Gate) is the foremost acupuncture point to calm and regulate the spirit.'

M-HN-3 (Yìn Táng) is a great local point to calm the Shén. As previously mentioned in this chapter, even though the Heart houses the Shén, the brain is also a site for Shén.[22] Therefore, you technically have two local areas for calming the Shén: the head/face and the trunk over the Heart organ.

According to Wang Xue Tai, some of the eminent figures in Chinese medicine history attributed the Shén to the brain, including Sun Si Miao (581–682 CE), Li Shi Zhen (1518–1593 CE) and Wang Qing Ren (1768–1831 CE).[23]

Maciocia (2015, p.241) tells us: 'Li Shi Zhen said: "The Brain is the Palace of the Original Shen"… Wang Qing Ren said specifically: "Intelligence and memory reside not in the Heart but in the Brain."'

HT 7 and M-HN-3 (Yìn Táng) together form a wonderful Shén-calming triumvirate. The combination uses points on the arms and the face, which makes use of the local-and-distal method, and it is also a Triangle of Power combination.

4. Open the Four Gates (Sì Guān)

Points – LI 4 and LR 3.

The Four Gates method is one of the best-known point combinations in Chinese medicine.

The Four Gates were first mentioned in the *Ode to Elucidate Mysteries* (Biāo Yōu Fù/標幽賦) from *The Guide to Acupuncture and Moxibustion*/Zhēn Jiǔ Zhǐ Nán/針灸指南), which was written in 1241 CE. The ode said: '[F]or cold and heat with painful obstruction, open the Four Gates.'[24] Over subsequent centuries the actions and indications have increased so that now practitioners will consider opening the Four Gates for:[25]

- body pain and muscle spasms

- Bì/painful obstruction syndrome

- calming the Shén

- expelling Internal Wind

- clearing External Wind

- moving Qì and Xuè

- descending Rebellious Qì

- treating Liver Yáng Rising

- resetting the channels and collaterals/Jīng Luò

- tonifying Qì and Xuè.

The Four Gates are termed as such for the following reasons:

- LR 3 and LI 4, when needled bilaterally, make up four points.

- LR 3 is the gate of Xuè. Therefore, it can be used to move Xuè or to tonify Xuè. LI 4 is the gate of Qì. Therefore, it can be used to move Qì or to tonify Qì.[26]

- They are located in a similar place on each limb. LR 3 is located on the foot, between the first and second metatarsal bones in a valley. LI 4 is located on the hand, between the first and second metacarpal bones in a valley.

- LR 3 and LI 4 are both Yuán Source points on their respective channels.

Using the Yuán Source points on your patient allows you to treat anything wrong with their associated organ and channel.[27] In this instance, they will work together to regulate Qì and Xuè. This means that if Qì and Xuè need to be moved, then LR 3 and LI 4 can do that. If Qì and Xuè need to be tonified, the Four Gates can do that. If a mix of tonification and movement is needed, then this combination can also be used.

According to chapter 24 of *The Yellow Emperor's Classic* (*Inner Canon of the Yellow Emperor*/Huáng Dì Nèi Jīng/黃帝內經), the Yáng Míng channels (Large Intestine and Stomach) have more Qì and Xuè and the Jué Yīn channels (Liver and Pericardium) have more Xuè, but less Qì.[28]

This implies that by opening the Four Gates, you will achieve significant movement of Xuè, with less movement of Qì. Although this is the case, the combination still has the ability to move both Qì and Xuè.

Let's now look at how opening the Four Gates works on the actions and indications discussed earlier.

Body pain and muscle spasms[29]

The Four Gates are effective at treating pain anywhere in the body. This can include stationary pain, moving pain and pain in multiple locations.

This method is also good at treating muscle spasms, cramps, tics, twitches or contractions.

The primary method used to achieve this is via the strong movement of Qì and Xuè through the Jīng Luò channels and collaterals. This allows for the flushing of the muscles, joints, tendons and bones, both externally and internally. Good Qì and Xuè flow is a terrific method to ensure that blockages don't build up which are directly or indirectly responsible for toxic build-up. This toxic build-up is what can create pain, muscle spasms, cramps, tics, twitches and/or contractions.

Bì/painful obstruction syndrome[30]

Bì is a traditional Chinese term to describe what modern Western medicine would call rheumatic/arthritic complaints (in Chinese medicine, we tend to translate Bì as painful obstruction syndrome).[31]

It is typically caused by three different triggers – Wind, Cold or Damp. These triggers can also combine together to generate Wind Cold, Wind Damp or Cold Damp. They can also manifest into Heat (Cold and Damp are good examples) if they become chronic, stagnant and toxic.[32] Otherwise, Heat can combine with another trigger – Wind Heat or Damp Heat. Heat can also generate itself, although this is not always discussed in textbooks.[33]

> [Bì is] a disorder characterised by obstruction of the circulation of qi (primarily due to penetration of wind, cold and damp) that leads to pain. The pain most frequently occurs in the muscles, sinews, joints and bones, although any part of the body may be affected, including the internal organs. In terms of modern medicine it corresponds to rheumatic and arthritic disease. (Deadman *et al.* 2007, p.630)

The Four Gates method is a great combination to treat Bì syndrome. However, LR 3 and LI 4 are unlikely to treat each of the different Bì syndromes on their own, especially if it's a combined obstruction. Therefore, you would tend to look at combining the Four Gates with other points to enhance the benefits of the treatment.

It would also be a good idea to include some local points for the problem area.

Calming the Shén[34]

> [LR 3] is effective in calming very tense people who are prone to short temper or experience feelings of deep frustration and repressed anger… [I]t is also effective in general irritability and tendency to worry from emotional stress. Its [Shén's] calming action is enhanced when combined with L.I.-4 Hegu (the 'Four Gates'). (Maciocia 2015, p.1122)

When you plan to calm the Shén, you have to decide: are you going to raise the Vital Substances in cases of Xū/Deficiency? Or are you going to dump the Vital Substances in cases of Shí/Excess?[35] Or maybe you are unsure what's going on and so you just want to balance the Shén? In good news, the Four Gates can combine to treat Xū or Shí or to balance the Shén. But if you want to enhance the benefits of one of them specifically, you will want to add some extra points into the combination to make it more effective. The three possible point combinations are shown in Tables 6.4–6.6.

Table 6.4 Shén Xū treatment – raise the Vital Substances[36]

Location of points	Points	
Head/face/neck	GV 20	
Trunk (front)	CV 6	
Trunk (back)	BL 15	BL 44
Arms/hands	HT 7	LI 4
Legs/feet	ST 36 LR 3	SP 3
Total points needled	16 needles used bilaterally	

Table 6.5 Shén Shí treatment – decrease the Vital Substances[37]

Location of points	Points	
Head/face/neck	GB 15	
Trunk (front)	CV 15	
Arms/hands	LI 4 HT 8	HT 7
Legs/feet	SP 6 LR 3	KI 1
Total points needled	15 needles used bilaterally	

Table 6.6 Shén-balancing treatment[38]

Location of points	Points	
Head/face/neck	GV 20	M-HN-3 (Yìn Táng)
Trunk (front)	CV 15	

Trunk (back)	BL 15	BL 44
Arms/hands	LI 4 HT 3	HT 7
Legs/feet	LR 3	
Total points needled	15 needles used bilaterally	

Expelling Internal Wind[39]

LR 3 opens the gate of Xuè and belongs to the Jué Yīn pairing of the Liver and Pericardium. LI 4 opens the gate of Qì and belongs to the Yáng Míng pairing of the Large Intestine and Stomach. The Four Gates ensure that there is strong circulation of Qì and Xuè, thereby isolating the Internal Wind and forcefully removing it from the body.[40]

The Internal Wind signs and symptoms that LR 3 and LI 4 can treat include but are not limited to:[41]

- facial paralysis, including Bell's palsy

- tremors, tics, muscle spasms

- numbness

- dizziness

- convulsions

- paralysis

- body aches.

Internal Wind can be a very tricky pattern to treat, and therefore it's often a good idea to combine the Four Gates with other points to ensure that a much stronger treatment is employed. An example of such a treatment is shown in Table 6.7.

Table 6.7 Expelling Internal Wind treatment[42]

Location of points	Points	
Head/face/neck	GV 20 GV 16	GB 20
Trunk (front)	CV 17	
Trunk (back)	BL 13	BL 18
Arms/hands	LI 4	
Legs/feet	LR 3	
Total points needled	13 needles used bilaterally	

Clearing External Wind[43]

The Four Gates ensure that there is strong circulation of Qì and Xuè, thereby isolating the External Wind and forcefully removing it from the body.[44]

The External Wind signs and symptoms that LR 3 and LI 4 can treat include but are not limited to:[45]

- aversion to wind

- alternating chills and fever

- body aches and possible headache

- neck and shoulder tension

- foggy head

- sore throat or tickle in the throat

- cough

- runny or blocked nose depending on accompanying pathogen.

External Wind can be treated quickly and easily, and therefore it's a good idea to hit it hard and fast by combining other points with the Four Gates. An example of such a treatment is given in Table 6.8.

Table 6.8 Clearing External Wind treatment[46]

Location of points	Points	
Head/face/neck	GV 16	GB 20
Trunk (front)	LU 1	CV 17
Trunk (back)	BL 12	BL 13
Arms/hands	LU 7	LI 4
Legs/feet	LR 3	
Total points needled	16 needles used bilaterally	

Moving Qì and Xuè[47]

LR 3 is the gate of Xuè and is effective at moving the Xuè. LI 4 is the gate of Qì and is effective at moving the Qì. Further to that, LR 3 is also effective at moving the Qì. Together they can move Qì and Xuè in every direction – up, down, inside, outside, front, back, sideways, 'slantways and any other way you can think of'.[48]

As Wang and Robertson (2008, p.565) advise: '[The Four Gates] has a broad systemic effect derived from its ability to dredge the pathways of qi and blood throughout the body.'

Descending Rebellious Qì[49]

As the Four Gates can move Qì and Xuè in any direction, it logically makes sense that it can move Rebellious Qì downwards.

This would be effective for the following signs/symptoms among others:[50]

- acid reflux, heartburn, dyspepsia

- belching, burping

- hiccup

- nausea, vomiting

- bad breath

- gingivitis

- asthma, wheezing, cough, shortness of breath.

The main organs that are affected by Rebellious Qì are the Stomach and Lungs, although technically any organ can be affected by Rebellious Qì. This assumes that the term 'Rebellious' refers to the Qì going in the wrong direction to the preferred movement of the affected organ's Qì flow.

For example, Spleen Qì Sinking is not something you would generally refer to as being Rebellious. However, technically it is. This is because the Spleen sends Qì upwards in health. In ill-health the Qì sinks, and therefore it is Rebellious in nature because it is going in the opposite direction to the way the organ prefers to send Qì.

Typically, Rebellious Qì is only used as a term to describe Qì that has ascended, and therefore your treatment principle is to descend the Rebellious Qì. In the case of Spleen Qì Sinking, your treatment principle is to raise the Qì.

Regardless of the organ affected, and the subsequent signs and symptoms of the patient, you can use the Four Gates for Rebellious Qì. The more chronic the patient is, the more likely it is that you would combine additional points with the Four Gates to produce a stronger treatment effect.

Treating Liver Yáng Rising[51]

Liver Yáng Rising is an interesting Zàng Fǔ pattern because it refers to a patient who has some Shí signs and some Xū signs. The deficiency is usually Xuè Xū or Yīn Xū. The excess is usually Heat Rising.

Liver Yáng Rising therefore has some considerations when deciding on your treatment approach. These include whether you plan to:

- sedate the Shí first and then tonify the Xū later

- tonify the Xū first and then sedate the Shí later

- try to do both in the same treatment.

The good news is that, regardless of the treatment principle you plan to adopt, the Four Gates method can be used because it can flow with any style of treatment you employ. However, it does generally make sense to combine other points with the Four Gates to get a stronger effect with the treatment. Treatment approaches for the three considerations when treating Liver Yáng Rising are shown in Tables 6.9–6.11.

Table 6.9 Sedating Liver Heat treatment[52]

Location of points	Points	
Head/face/neck	GB 13	GB 20
Trunk (back)	GV 14	
Arms/hands	LI 4 LI 11	TE 5
Legs/feet	LR 2	LR 3
Total points needled	15 needles used bilaterally	

Table 6.10 Tonify Liver Xuè/Yīn treatment[53]

Location of points	Points	
Trunk (front)	CV 4	
Trunk (back)	BL 17	BL 18
Arms/hands	HT 6	LI 4
Legs/feet	SP 6 KI 6	LR 3
Total points needled	15 needles used bilaterally	

Table 6.11 Liver Yáng Rising treatment[54]

Location of points	Points	
Head/face/neck	GB 8	GB 20
Trunk (front)	CV 4	
Trunk (back)	BL 18	
Arms/hands	LI 4	
Legs/feet	GB 34 KI 3	LR 3
Total points needled	15 needles used bilaterally	

According to McDonald and Penner (1994, p.146), the typical signs and symptoms of Liver Yáng Rising are:

- irascibility (anger and irritability)
- throbbing headache with distended feeling

- dizziness

- flushed face

- blurred vision

- red, dry eyes, with feeling of grit in eye

- tinnitus

- dry mouth and throat with bitter taste in mouth

- insomnia

- palpitations

- tongue: red and dry, little or no coat

- pulse: thready and wiry, or wiry and rapid.

McDonald and Penner (1994, p.146) also attribute the following Western diseases to Liver Yáng Rising:

- hypertension

- neurasthenia: this is an obsolete term in modern times; some doctors refer to it as chronic fatigue syndrome[55]

- Ménière's disease (aural vertigo)

- hyperthyroidism

- problems associated with the menopause.

This combination [Four Gates] can therefore be used for hypertension with dizziness, headache and aggressive behavior. (Ross 1995, p.308)

Resetting the channels and collaterals/Jīng Luò[56]

This is a fascinating function of the Four Gates and goes something like this.

The needles for LR 3 and LI 4 are inserted into the body. After a few minutes the patient relaxes and winds down. As they continue to relax, the body goes into a deep state of sedation to the point where the body and mind effectively shut down. This allows for a body and mind reset (hard reset), at which point the body and mind wind back up again.

This is the crucial concept to grasp – that there is a winding down and then a winding back up again. This is why I am happy enough to use the Four Gates on a patient that is Shí or Xū. If they are Shí, they will benefit from the wind-down; if they are Xū, they will benefit from the wind-up.

The body and mind reset that occurs is almost like a hard reset that you might do on your mobile/cell phone from time to time because it's not operating as effectively as it was a week or two earlier. Our bodies need that hard reset sometimes too. It allows for everything to go back to what I call 'factory settings' and helps to bring organs that are Xū back into balance with the nourished organs. It also helps to reduce organs that are Shí and bring them back into balance too.

If your patient's body and mind are too wired and always on the go, then this hard reset allows for them to relax and slow down. It allows for vacancy in the mind and total relaxation in the muscles of the body. Pure bliss!

Alternatively, if your patient's body and mind are too empty and weak, then this hard reset allows for them to wind back up again. It allows for a mental and muscular recharge – a bit like accidentally touching an exposed electrical socket. They are flying!

This also explains why so many patients who receive the Four Gates are so sedated and dopey when they get off the table after the treatment has finished: their bodies are still adjusting to the hard reset. This is why I always tell my patients to take a walk around the block after a Four Gates treatment. This encourages the winding back up of the hard reset and they are almost always firing and ready for anything within five or ten minutes.

Wang and Robertson (2008, pp.564–565) use this function of the Four Gates in cases where a patient hasn't responded successfully to treatment when, in their minds, they should have. They call this 'channel exhaustion' or 'channel confusion': 'In these cases, the four gates can be helpful to reset the patient's channel qi transformation' (Wang and Robertson 2008, p.565).

Tonifying Qì and Xuè[57]

LR 3 is the gate of Xuè and is effective at building/tonifying the Xuè. LI 4 is the gate of Qì and is effective at building/tonifying the Qì.

There are two theories here with regard to this function of the Four Gates:

- They can tonify Qì and Xuè in general.[58]

- They can tonify Qì and Xuè in the channels.[59]

In my view, the Four Gates can be used for both, but more so for the tonification in the channels. But let's look at each theory a little more closely before we move on.

THEY CAN TONIFY QÌ AND XUÈ IN GENERAL

There is little doubt that LR 3 can tonify and move the Xuè as well as move the Qì. This is one of the main functions of the point. Using LI 4 as a Qì tonic is the main sticking point in this function for the Four Gates. Maciocia (2015, pp.963–964) states that LI 4 does tonify Qì, but I have struggled to find many other references that support Maciocia in this view.

Deadman *et al.* (2007, p.104) suggest that some authorities recommend the use of LI 4 for the tonification of Wèi Qì, but that's only one form of Qì, and not Qì in general.

Li (2007, p.76) supports the idea that LI 4 can tonify Qì. The argument used is that the Lungs are an important organ to make Qì and the Large Intestine is the Yáng partner for the Lungs. By using a tonifying method of needling on LI 4, it should, because it's the Yuán Source point on the Large Intestine channel, be able to tonify Lung Qì. This, by default, would then provide strong Qì to other parts of the body.

THEY CAN TONIFY QÌ AND XUÈ IN THE CHANNELS

LR 3 is the Yuán Source point of the Liver. As such, it can tonify, sedate and/or move Qì and Xuè in the body. This includes flushing the extremities in cases of stagnation, but also to draw Qì and Xuè into the extremities for nourishment in cases of Xū.

LI 4 can do likewise for Qì and Xuè. According to chapter 24 of *The Yellow Emperor's Classic*, the Yáng Míng channels (Large Intestine and Stomach) have more Qì and Xuè. This indicates that LI 4, because it is part of the Large Intestine channel, can move Qì and Xuè, in this case into the channels.[60]

> [T]he abundance of qi and blood in the arm and foot yangming channels [which includes LI 4] means that their points are not only important to dispel stagnation, but also to tonify qi and blood in the channels and thus bring nourishment to the limbs. (Deadman *et al.* 2007, p.105)

When might the Four Gates point combination not be effective?

Opening the Four Gates won't be effective every single time you use the method. It also won't always treat everything that is listed above. The main sticking point with this combination is its small number of points. It would be two needles if done unilaterally or four needles if done bilaterally. Sometimes it's just not quite strong enough to get the effect you were after. Obviously, acupuncturists have different views on the number of needles needed in a treatment to get amazing results.

For example, I have a friend in Israel who uses only one needle on his patients and gets great results. I know of quite a few practitioners in Australia that use in excess of 50 needles and also get great results. Who is right? Well, the debate that would follow that question is for another time. Suffice to say that if your treatments are successful, then stick with whatever number of needles you use because it clearly works for you.

You would also want to be careful with patients who have significant deficiency/Xū. The Four Gates method is designed more as an active treatment which ultimately uses up the Vital Substances during its attempts to correct the imbalance. In patients with minor deficiencies/Xū, it's not such a big deal, but in severe deficiencies/Xū the Four Gates would not be the best point combination choice.

When using the Four Gates method, it's also beneficial to make the treatment target-specific. This is important because it can do so many different things in so many different parts of the body. Therefore, the Four Gates typically need additional points to help target a condition and/or area that needs special attention. This helps make it target-specific and is why I have included multiple treatment tables above. Those tables are designed to show you how to direct the Four Gates towards a particular purpose. As I said – make the treatment target-specific.

5. The Three Regions/Powers – Heaven, Earth, Human (Tiān Dì Rén)[61]

The Three Regions, or Three Powers, refers to the Chinese medicine triumvirate of Heaven, Earth, Human (Tiān Dì Rén). As the 75th essay in *The Spiritual Pivot* (Líng Shū/靈樞) states: 'Man [Human] is a triad with heaven and earth' (Wu 1993, p.244).

Deadman *et al.* (2007, p.194) refer to Tiān Dì Rén as the Three Regions. But Bertschinger (2013, p.102) prefers the term Three Powers. This is interesting because the Three Regions and the Three Powers are referred to in *The Great Compendium* (*The Great Compendium of Acupuncture and Moxibustion*/Zhēn Jiǔ Dà Chéng/針灸大成) with separate point combinations offered for each.[62] Let's look at these point combinations separately.

As stated in the previous paragraph, the Three Regions point combination was referred to in *The Great Compendium*, which was written by Yang Jizhou in 1601 CE. Having said that, expert commentary suggests it was taken from a much earlier book called *The Guide to Acupuncture and Moxibustion* (Zhēn Jiǔ Zhǐ Nán/針灸指南), where the 'Ode to Elucidate Mysteries' (Biāo Yōu Fù/標幽賦) was written in 1241 CE. The ode says: 'Above, Middle and Below are the Three Regions, The Great Enveloping [SP 21], Heavenly Pivot [ST 25] and Earth Motivator [SP 8]' (Bertschinger 2013, p.102).

In Bertschinger's (2013, p.102) translation, there is another ode which refers to the Three Powers. It says: 'One Hundred Meetings [GV 20] is a point on the head, it echoes the sky [Heaven] above. Jade Pearl [CV 21] is a point on the breast, it echoes man himself. The Bubbling Spring [KI 1] comes through two points on the sole of the foot, echoing the earth. These are the Three Powers.'

The acupuncture point combinations for the Three Regions and Three Powers are summarized in Table 6.12.

Table 6.12 The Three Regions/Powers

Location of point	The Three Regions	The Three Powers
Head/face/neck	N/A	GV 20 (Heaven/Tiān)
Trunk (front)	SP 21 (Heaven/Tiān) ST 25 (Human/Rén)	CV 21 (Human/Rén)
Legs/feet	SP 8 (Earth/Dì)	KI 1 (Earth/Dì)
Total points needled	6 needles used bilaterally	4 needles used bilaterally

As you can see in Table 6.12, each of the point combinations treats Heaven, Earth and Human. I have used both combinations over the years and found them to be excellent for balancing out Tiān Dì Rén.

Having said that, I am definitely more inclined to use the point combination of the Three Powers (GV 20, CV 21 and KI 1) as I find it to be more specific to the purpose of the combination. After all, GV 20 is the highest point on the body, thereby having direct access to Heaven/Tiān. KI 1 is the lowest point on the body, thereby having direct access to Earth/Dì. That just leaves CV 21 to act as the middle ground, or Human/Rén level.

I have also experimented with the points in the different combinations and have decided that my current favorite is using GV 20 for Heaven/Tiān, SP 21 for Human/Rén and KI 1 for Earth/Dì.[63]

What is Heaven, Earth and Human/Tiān Dì Rén?

Using the simplest explanation, they are the three inherent aspects of ourselves that make up our microcosm – Heaven, Earth and Human. This is also replicated in the macrocosm, which is classic Chinese medicine! Before we move on, let's look at each of the three parts individually.

Heaven/Tiān

Tiān = Heaven, celestial, sky, divine, God.[64]

This is where we have access to our greatest/grandest dreams. It's where our inspiration resides. It's also where we can access our destiny (why we are really here). Up here anything is possible! The Hún also resides up here.[65]

Earth/Dì

Dì = Earth, land, place, territory.[66]

This is where we take our dreams and make them reality. The Earth is where we get stuff done, where we perform/act/work. The Pò also resides down here.[67]

Human/Rén

Rén = Human being, humankind, person, man.[68]

This is the part of us that takes our dreams from Heaven (Tiān) and filters them through our Shén, Yì and Zhì to decide what to move down on to the Earth (Dì) for action.

It's also the part of us that includes our self-esteem, which includes our view/sense of self as well as our perception of other people's views of us.

What do the Three Regions/Powers treat?

This point combination works on regulating/balancing Heaven, Earth and Human (Tiān Dì Rén). I often get my patients to visualize the Three Regions/Powers and to give each of these parts a big hug. Embrace your regions/powers and love and respect them for what they are because they are *you*! And if your microcosmic self is more balanced, then it will resonate so much more effectively with the macrocosm.

The Three Regions/Powers will also work on regulating/re-balancing your Five Element guardian archetype (see Chapter 14). After all, your Heaven, Earth and Human (Tiān Dì Rén) is every part of you. It's what makes you *you*!

That being the case, the Three Regions/Powers point combination is incredibly important for overall mental/spiritual/emotional health. One could even argue that they have the capacity to tweak our personality, particularly if it's not in a balanced state.

Therefore, I have decided to construct a Three Regions/Powers point combination for each of the Five Element guardian archetypes. I will explain why I have selected each of the points. In the end, there are many point combinations available to you, with these five being just one example for each.

The Three Regions/Powers point combination
Wood archetype

As we are working on a Wood archetype, the points will be predominantly on the Liver and Gall Bladder channels, which are the organs associated with the Wood element. Aside from that, the Front Mù Collecting points for the Liver and Gall Bladder are necessary choices because they work on the more Yáng aspect of our being,[69] and the Wood archetype is a Yáng archetype. Finally, the Urinary Bladder channel point for the Wǔ Shén of the Wood element, which is the Hún, has been included. Table 6.13 shows the point combination listed with a reason provided for why each point was chosen.

Table 6.13 Wood archetype point combination

Location of point	Point	Tiān Dì Rén	Reasoning
Head/face/neck	GB 9 GB 18	Tiān/Heaven Tiān/Heaven	Translates as 'Heavenly Rushing'[70] 'Cover of the celestial spirit'[71]
Trunk (front)	LR 14 GB 24	Rén/Human Rén/Human	Front Mù Collecting point of the Liver Front Mù Collecting point of the Gall Bladder
Trunk (back)	BL 47	Rén/Human	Regulates the Hún (Wǔ Shén spirit of the Wood archetype)
Legs/feet	LR 3 GB 42	Dì/Earth Dì/Earth	Yuán Source point of the Liver Translates as 'Earth Five Meetings'[72]
Total points needled		14 needles used bilaterally	

If you wanted to stick to just one point for each of the Three Regions/Powers, that would certainly be possible. Any of the points listed would be suitable (as would plenty of other points not included in Table 6.13), but one example could look like this:

- GB 18 – Heaven/Tiān.
- LR 14 – Human/Rén.
- GB 42 – Earth/Dì.
- Total of six needles used bilaterally.

Fire archetype

As we are working on a Fire archetype, the points will predominantly be targeting the Heart, Pericardium, Small Intestine and Sān Jiāo organs because they are the organs associated with the Fire element. The Front Mù Collecting points are necessary choices because they work on the more Yáng aspect of our being,[73] and the Fire archetype is a Yáng archetype. Finally, the Urinary Bladder channel point for the Wǔ Shén of the Fire element, which is the Shén, has also been included. Table 6.14 shows the point combination listed with a reason provided for why each point was chosen.

Table 6.14 Fire archetype point combination

Location of point	Point	Tiān Dì Rén	Reasoning
Head/face/neck	SI 17 TE 16	Tiān/Heaven Tiān/Heaven	Translates as 'Heaven's Contents'[74] Translates as 'Heaven's Window'[75]
Trunk (front)	CV 4 CV 5 CV 14 CV 17	Rén/Human Rén/Human Rén/Human Rén/Human	Front Mù Collecting point of the Small Intestine Front Mù Collecting point of the Sān Jiāo Front Mù Collecting point of the Heart Front Mù Collecting point of the Pericardium
Trunk (back)	BL 44	Rén/Human	Regulates the Shén (Wǔ Shén spirit of the Fire archetype)
Legs/feet	ST 39 BL 39	Dì/Earth Dì/Earth	Lower Hé (Uniting) Sea point of the Small Intestine Lower Hé (Uniting) Sea point of the Sān Jiāo
Total points needled		14 needles used bilaterally	

If you wanted to stick to just one point for each of the Three Regions/Powers, that would certainly be possible. Any of the points listed would be suitable (as would plenty of other points not included in Table 6.14), but one example could look like this:

- TE 16 – Heaven/Tiān.
- CV 14 – Human/Rén.

- ST 39 – Earth/Dì.

- Total of five needles used bilaterally.

Earth archetype

As we are working on an Earth archetype, the points will be predominantly on the Spleen and Stomach channels, which are the organs associated with the Earth element. Aside from that, the Front Mù Collecting and Back Shù Transporting points for the Spleen and Stomach are necessary choices because they work equally on the Yīn and Yáng aspect of our being,[76] and the Earth archetype is a Yīn and Yáng archetype. Finally, the Urinary Bladder channel point for the Wǔ Shén of the Earth element, which is the Yì, has been included. Table 6.15 shows the point combination with a reason provided for why each point was chosen.

Table 6.15 Earth archetype point combination

Location of point	Point	Tiān Dì Rén	Reasoning
Head/face/neck	ST 8	Tiān/Heaven	Highest Stomach channel point; closest to Tiān/Heaven
	ST 9[77]	Tiān/Heaven, Rén/Human	Regulates both Tiān/Heaven and Rén/Human[78]
Trunk (front)	LR 13	Rén/Human	Front Mù Collecting point of the Spleen
	CV 12	Rén/Human	Front Mù Collecting point of the Stomach
Trunk (back)	BL 20	Rén/Human	Back Shù Transporting point of the Spleen
	BL 21	Rén/Human	Back Shù Transporting point of the Stomach
	BL 49	Rén/Human	Regulates the Yì (Wǔ Shén spirit of the Earth archetype)
Legs/feet	SP 3	Dì/Earth	Horary point (Earth of Earth)
	ST 36	Dì/Earth	Horary point (Earth of Earth)
Total points needled	17 needles used bilaterally		

If you wanted to stick to just one point for each of the Three Regions/Powers, that would certainly be possible. Any of the points listed would be suitable (as would plenty of other points not included in Table 6.15), but one example could look like this:

- ST 9 – Heaven/Tiān.

- CV 12 – Human/Rén.

- SP 3 – Earth/Dì.

- Total of five needles used bilaterally.

Metal archetype

As we are working on a Metal archetype, the points will be predominantly on the Lung and Large Intestine channels, which are the organs associated with the Metal element. Aside from that, the Back Shù Transporting points for the Lungs and Large Intestine are necessary choices because they work on the more Yīn aspect of our being,[79] and the Metal archetype is a Yīn archetype. Finally, the Urinary Bladder channel point for the Wǔ Shén of the Metal element, which is the Pò, has been included. Table 6.16 shows the point combination with a reason provided for why each point was chosen.

Table 6.16 Metal archetype point combination

Location of point	Point	Tiān Dì Rén	Reasoning
Head/face/neck	LI 17 LI 18	Tiān/Heaven Tiān/Heaven	Translates as 'Heaven's Tripod'[80] Window of the Sky/Window of Heaven
Trunk (back)	BL 13 BL 25 BL 42	Rén/Human Rén/Human Rén/Human	Back Shù Transporting point of the Lungs Back Shù Transporting point of the Large Intestine Regulates the Pò (Wǔ Shén spirit of the Metal archetype)
Legs/feet	ST 37	Dì/Earth	Lower Hé (Uniting) Sea point of the Large Intestine
Total points needled			12 needles used bilaterally

If you wanted to stick to just one point for each of the Three Regions/Powers, that would certainly be possible. Any of the points listed would be suitable (as would plenty of other points not included in Table 6.16), but one example could look like this:

- LI 17 – Heaven/Tiān.

- BL 13 – Human/Rén.

- ST 37 – Earth/Dì.

- Total of six needles used bilaterally.

Water archetype

As we are working on a Water archetype, the points will be predominantly on the Kidney and Urinary Bladder channels, which are the organs associated with the Water element. Aside from that, the Back Shù Transporting points for the Kidneys and Urinary Bladder are necessary choices because they work on the more Yīn aspect of our being,[81] and the Water archetype is a Yīn archetype. Finally, the Urinary Bladder channel point for the Wǔ Shén of the Water element, which is the Zhì, has been included. Table 6.17 shows the point combination listed with a reason provided for why each point was chosen.

Table 6.17 Water archetype point combination

Location of point	Point	Tiān Dì Rén	Reasoning
Head/face/neck	BL 8 BL 10	Tiān/Heaven Tiān/Heaven	'Cover of the celestial spirit'[82] Translates as 'Heaven's Pillar'[83]
Trunk (back)	BL 23 BL 28 BL 52	Rén/Human Rén/Human Rén/Human	Back Shù Transporting point of the Kidneys Back Shù Transporting point of the Urinary Bladder Regulates the Zhì (Wǔ Shén spirit of the Water archetype)
Legs/feet	KI 1 BL 67	Dì/Earth Dì/Earth	Lowest point on the body; has direct access to Earth Translates as 'Reaching Yīn'[84]
Total points needled			14 needles used bilaterally

If you wanted to stick to just one point for each of the Three Regions/Powers, that would certainly be possible. Any of the points listed would be suitable (as would plenty of other points not included in Table 6.17), but one example could look like this:

- BL 10 – Heaven/Tiān.

- BL 23 – Human/Rén.

- KI 1 – Earth/Dì.

- Total of six needles used bilaterally.

When might the Tiān Dì Rén point combination not be effective?

This depends on which of the point combinations you plan to use. The combinations mentioned in Table 6.12 are safe to use in most situations. They were those referenced from *The Great Compendium* (*The Great Compendium of Acupuncture and Moxibustion*/Zhēn Jiǔ Dà Chéng/針灸大成) and are a great regulator of the triumvirate of Heaven, Earth and Human/Tiān Dì Rén.

If you plan to target one of the Five Element archetypes, then you need to be 100% sure that you have diagnosed the correct guardian archetype before using that specific point combination. If you are even slightly hesitant, then don't use it – wait until you are completely sure, as these point combinations are designed to specifically target a guardian archetype.[85]

6. Three Yīn sixes[86]

Points – HT 6, SP 6 and KI 6.

The three Yīn sixes method is a special point combination to tonify Yīn.

The three Yīn sixes name comes about because:

- there are three points

- they are all Yīn channel points and all of them tonify Yīn

- they are all the sixth point on their associated channel.

One of my lecturers mentioned this combination to our class back in the mid-1990s and I have been using it ever since. Having said that, I am yet to see the combination referred to as the three Yīn sixes in any textbooks. The three points are mentioned in textbooks for Yīn Xū but are mixed in with other points. Regardless, I have no doubts as to its effectiveness as I have used the three Yīn sixes method for more than 20 years now.

Interestingly, some of the lecturers at Endeavour College of Natural Health, where I work, also use the three Yīn sixes method, but substitute HT 6 for PC 6. Personally, I prefer using PC 6 for moving Qì Stagnation, calming the Shén or for nausea/vomiting.

I like the three Yīn sixes combination because it has points on the arms and the legs, which provides a more balanced treatment. I also use the method bilaterally and either use the points as the only needles in the treatment or add a few extra points to consolidate the treatment. If I do choose to do additional points, these are selected based on the overriding Zàng Fǔ patterns. I have listed five examples in Tables 6.18–6.22.

Table 6.18 Heart Yīn Xū treatment[87]

Location of points	Points	
Trunk (front)	CV 4	CV 14
Trunk (back)	BL 15	
Arms/hands	HT 6 HT 7	PC 6
Legs/feet	SP 6	KI 6
Total points needled	14 needles used bilaterally	

Table 6.19 Kidney Yīn Xū treatment[88]

Location of points	Points	
Trunk (front)	CV 4	CV 6
Trunk (back)	BL 23	
Arms/hands	HT 6	
Legs/feet	SP 6 KI 3	KI 6
Total points needled	12 needles used bilaterally	

Table 6.20 Liver Yīn Xū treatment[89]

Location of points	Points	
Trunk (front)	CV 4	
Trunk (back)	BL 18	BL 23
Arms/hands	HT 6	
Legs/feet	SP 6 KI 6	LR 8
Total points needled	13 needles used bilaterally	

Table 6.21 Lung Yīn Xū treatment[90]

Location of points	Points	
Trunk (front)	CV 4	CV 12
Trunk (back)	BL 13	BL 43
Arms/hands	HT 6	LU 9
Legs/feet	SP 6	KI 6
Total points needled	14 needles used bilaterally	

Table 6.22 Stomach Yīn Xū treatment[91]

Location of points	Points	
Trunk (front)	CV 4	CV 12
Trunk (back)	BL 20	BL 21
Arms/hands	HT 6	
Legs/feet	SP 6 KI 6	ST 36
Total points needled	14 needles used bilaterally	

When might the three Yīn sixes point combination not be effective?

The three Yīn sixes combination won't be effective in every single patient. For starters, Yīn Xū is typically a chronic condition, and three points isn't often enough to generate strong and distinct change.

You will have noticed from Tables 6.18–6.22 that there are a lot of other points to consider when treating the various Yīn Xū patterns. Sometimes these treatment combinations work more effectively if one of the three Yīn sixes points is left out and replaced with another point.

7. The Great Five

The Great Five is a point combination mentioned in *The Great Compendium* (*The Great Compendium of Acupuncture and Moxibustion*/Zhēn Jiǔ Dà Chéng/針灸大成),

which was written by Yang Jizhou in 1601 CE. It refers to the five extremities – arms, legs and head:

> The two Mounds, two Qiao points and two Crossings connect and tie up the Great Five [arms, legs and head]. The two Mounds are the Yin Mound Spring [SP 9] and the Yang Mound Spring [GB 34]. The two Qiao points are the Yin-Qiao (meaning the Illuminated Sea) [KI 6] and Yang-Qiao (meaning the Extended Meridian) [BL 62]. The two Crossings are Yin Crossing [SP 6] and Yang Crossing [GB 35]. They connect, meaning they join and connect onto. The Great Five are the five 'limbs' of the body. These six points present a connection to both arms, both legs and the head. (Bertschinger 2013, pp.103–104)

To understand how this point combination works, let's dissect the six points (yes, six, not five) and see what each is doing in the combination. For starters, there are three separate point combinations within the larger grouping of the Great Five. SP 9 and GB 34 have their own personal connection within the combination, as do KI 6 and BL 62. This is anchored by the final pairing of SP 6 and GB 35. So, the Great Five works as a collective but could also be separated into three separate groups. I give three examples in Tables 6.23–6.25.

Further, each of the three individual combinations send Vital Substances in different directions, thereby ensuring better flow throughout the body.

They are all very powerful points in their own right and have the capacity to stimulate Vital Substance flow throughout the entire body and not just to the extremities. Let's look at each of the points in a little more detail.

The Great Five points

Although the point combination name refers to the number five, there are actually six points, which is very confusing. The Great Five refers to the extremities of the legs, arms and head and not to the number of points used.

SP 6

The Spleen channel travels up the legs, with one of its internal pathways finishing at the head. SP 6 (Sān Yīn Jiāo) translates as 'Three Yīn Intersection'.[92] This means the point accesses three channels to move the Vital Substances, namely the Spleen, Liver and Kidney channels. Apart from the significant list of conditions that SP 6 can treat on the legs, it is also a good point for the other three extremities by treating heaviness of the body and limbs as well as cold hands and feet. It can also calm the Shén and assist with sense organ disorders.[93]

SP 9

The Spleen channel, as previously mentioned, travels up the legs, with one of its internal pathways finishing at the head. The channel can treat three of the Great Five (extremities), but there is no connection to the arms that I could find during my research. SP 9 also doesn't treat any signs/symptoms on the arms.

GB 34

The Gall Bladder channel travels down the body and on to the legs, with its origin at the head. Therefore, it has a direct connection to three of the Great Five (extremities). GB 34 is also an excellent point for any muscle, tendon, ligament or joint in the body, including the arms. According to Deadman *et al.* (2007, p.451): 'Yanglingquan GB-34 may be used for pain, cramping, contraction, stiffness and sprain of the sinews and muscles in any part of the body.'

GB 35

As mentioned, the Gall Bladder channel travels down the body and on to the legs, with its origin at the head. Therefore, it has a direct connection to three of the Great Five (extremities).

GB 35 is also the Xì Cleft point of the Yáng Wéi Mài, which moves Vital Substances up the body, where it connects to the Large Intestine, Sān Jiāo and Small Intestine channels on the shoulder before finishing on the head. This connection allows for all of the Great Five (extremities) to be linked.

KI 6

The Kidney channel travels up the legs, with one of its internal pathways finishing at the head.

KI 6 is also the opening point of the Yīn Qiāo Mài, which moves Vital Substances up the body, finishing at the head. Apart from the significant list of conditions that KI 6 can treat on the legs, it is also a good point for the other three extremities by treating 'pain and weakness of the limbs...heat vexation in the five hearts[94]... cramp in the hands and feet preventing movement...swelling of the face and limbs; hemiplegia. [It also] clears the spirit [Shén]-disposition [and] disinhibits the throat' (Ellis *et al.* 1991, pp.250–251).

BL 62

The Urinary Bladder channel travels down the body and on to the legs, with its origin at the head. Therefore, it has a direct connection to three of the Great Five (extremities).

BL 62 is also the opening point of the Yáng Qiāo Mài, which moves Vital Substances up the body, where it connects to the Large Intestine and Small Intestine channels on the shoulder before finishing on the head. This connection allows for all of the Great Five (extremities) to be linked.

The Great Five is a terrific point combination in its own right. If you are like me and are concerned about all the points being stacked in one area, and would prefer to change it up, I have listed three alternative point combinations for the Great Five. I have kept the three point combination connections together; that of SP 9 and GB 34, KI 6 and BL 62, and SP 6 and GB 35. These point combinations are in Tables 6.23–6.25.

The Great Five point combinations

The Great Five point combination 1

This point combination focuses on the Great Five combination of SP 9 and GB 34.

Table 6.23 The Great Five point combination 1

Location of point	Point	Reasoning
Head/face/neck	ST 8 GB 20	I sometimes use these two points to regulate Vital Substance flow into/out of the head
Trunk (front)	SP 21	Treats pain and/or flaccidity of the whole body[95]
Arms/hands	LI 10 PC 6	A big Vital Substance mover through the extremities A big Vital Substance mover through the extremities
Legs/feet	SP 9 GB 34	See description above See description above
Total points needled		14 needles used bilaterally

The Great Five point combination 2

This point combination focuses on the Great Five combination of KI 6 and BL 62.

Table 6.24 The Great Five point combination 2

Location of point	Point	Reasoning
Head/face/neck	BL 7 BL 10	I sometimes use these two points to regulate Vital Substance flow into/out of the head
Arms/hands	LU 7 SI 3	Assists KI 6 in stimulating the Yīn Qiāo Mài. Also opens the Rèn Mài Assists BL 62 in stimulating the Yáng Qiāo Mài. Also opens the Dū Mài
Legs/feet	KI 6 BL 62	See description above See description above
Total points needled		12 needles used bilaterally

The Great Five point combination 3

This point combination focuses on the Great Five combination of SP 6 and GB 35.

Table 6.25 The Great Five point combination 3

Location of point	Point	Reasoning
Head/face/neck	GV 20 GB 20	I sometimes use these two points to regulate Vital Substance flow into/out of the head
Trunk (front)	SP 21	Treats pain and/or flaccidity of the whole body[96]
Arms/hands	TE 8 LU 5	A big Vital Substance mover through the extremities A big Vital Substance mover through the extremities[97]
Legs/feet	SP 6 GB 35	See description above See description above
Total points needled		13 needles used bilaterally

When might the Great Five point combination not be effective?

The Great Five combination is a massive extremity flush, so it would be inappropriate for patients who were deficient/Xū. This is because it moves Vital Substances and will therefore also deplete Vital Substances.

From a purely personal perspective, I have concerns about this point combination, and that's no disrespect to one of the greatest classical books ever written. It comes down to point location preferences. For me, the combination is too leg-heavy/dominant. I much prefer points sensibly scattered throughout the body, and this personal belief isn't changed by the Great Five point combination.

8. Host-Guest combination (Yuán Source and Luò Connecting)[98]

The Host-Guest point combination is a particularly famous one that was promoted in *The Great Compendium – Volume V* (*The Great Compendium of Acupuncture and Moxibustion*/Zhēn Jiǔ Dà Chéng/針灸大成. 第5 卷). It targets the Yuán Source and Luò Connecting points on the interiorly–exteriorly related Yīn and Yáng channel partners.[99]

The term Host is given to the chief organ/channel that is diseased. The term Guest is given to the Yīn or Yáng partner of the injured organ/channel. For example, your patient is suffering from Lung Qì Xū. The Host organ is the Lungs, and the Guest organ is the Large Intestine.

The organ that is the Host makes use of its Yuán Source point. The organ that is the Guest makes use of its Luò Connecting point. In the previous example, that would mean we used LU 9 (Yuán Source point on the Lung channel) and LI 6 (Luò Connecting point on the Large Intestine channel).

Table 6.26 lists the interiorly–exteriorly related Yīn and Yáng organs/channels.

Table 6.26 Interiorly–exteriorly related Yīn and Yáng organs/channel partners[100]

Yīn organ/channel	Yáng organ/channel
Lungs	Large Intestine
Heart	Small Intestine
Pericardium	Sān Jiāo
Spleen	Stomach
Kidneys	Urinary Bladder
Liver	Gall Bladder

Tables 6.27 and 6.28 list the Host/Guest points for the Yīn and Yáng organs/channels.[101]

Table 6.27 Host as Yīn and Guest as Yáng

Yīn organs/channels	Host as Yīn	Guest as Yáng
Lungs	LU 9	LI 6
Heart	HT 7	SI 7
Pericardium	PC 7	TE 5
Spleen	SP 3	ST 40
Kidney	KI 3	BL 58
Liver	LR 3	GB 37

Table 6.28 Host as Yáng and Guest as Yīn

Yáng organs/channels	Host as Yáng	Guest as Yīn
Large Intestine	LI 4	LU 7
Small Intestine	SI 4	HT 5
Sān Jiāo	TE 4	PC 6
Stomach	ST 42	SP 4
Urinary Bladder	BL 64	KI 4
Gall Bladder	GB 40	LR 5

Let me finish by giving a couple of acupuncture point combinations that make use of the Host–Guest relationship.

Liver Qì Stagnation

Host point for Liver = LR 3.

Guest point for Gall Bladder = GB 37.

In this fairly straightforward example, your patient has been diagnosed with Liver Qì Stagnation. You choose the Host and Guest points and then decide if you want to do any additional needling. If you don't (and the theory suggests you don't have to), then you would use two needles unilaterally or four needles bilaterally.

However, if you are like me, some additional points to help move Liver Qì wouldn't go astray. If you also considered a sensible scattering of points, then you might end up with this point combination:[102]

- Head/face/neck – GV 20.

- Trunk (front) – LR 13, LR 14.

- Arms/hands – PC 6, LI 4.

- Legs/feet – LR 3 (Host point), GB 37 (Guest point).

- Total of 13 needles used bilaterally.

Spleen and Kidney Yáng Xū

Host point for Spleen = SP 3.

Guest point for Stomach = ST 40.

Host point for Kidneys = KI 3.

Guest point for Urinary Bladder = BL 58.

In this example, the patient has two main organs that are diseased. Therefore, you will have two Host points and two Guest points. In this situation, you already have eight needles if you were to do them all bilaterally (or four unilaterally). If you are happy with that number of needles, then go for it.

I just have one issue with this point combination: they are all in the legs/feet. I would personally like to see at least two or three more points used elsewhere in the body to provide a better spread of needles. Some other options could include:[103]

- Trunk (front) – CV 4, CV 6, CV 9, CV 12, ST 28, GB 25.

- Trunk (back) – BL 20, BL 22, BL 23, BL 52, GV 4, GV 14.

- Arms/hands – TE 4, TE 6.

When might the Host-Guest point combination not be effective?

There are two main reasons why this combination might not be effective: a lack of points used in the treatment and the fact that the points are always going to be on only one area of the body.

A lack of points

As a general rule, I would consider two or four points needled in a treatment as not being enough to help heal the patient.

Stacked in one area only

I prefer to have my point combinations with needles sensibly scattered across a wide area of the body. This combination will only ever have points in the arms/hands or legs/feet.

Notes

1   Descartes 1954, p.240. René Descartes (1596–1650) was an extraordinary Western philosopher; what he gave the world cannot be underestimated. He took advantage of the new wave of free thinking that occurred through the late 1500s onwards in a way that few other people were able to do at that time.

2   Mou 2009, p.297. Wáng Chōng (27–97 CE) was a fascinating philosopher because he merged this love of wisdom with his love for astronomy and meteorology. This triumvirate led him to decide that there was no higher being that governed the Universe. Instead, life came about 'through the spontaneous interaction of cosmic forces such as yin and yang' (Liang 1996, p.263).

3   Maciocia 2015, pp.163–164.

4   Ibid., p.164.

5   Ellis *et al.* 1989, pp.306, 409.

6   Mou 2009, p.287. Dǒng Zhòng-shū (179–104 BCE) was a Confucian official who played a major role in ensuring that the newly implanted Han dynasty took Confucianism as its official ideology after the collapse of the Legalist-driven Qin dynasty.

7   Hicks *et al.* 2010, pp.163–164; Maciocia 2015, pp.162–165.

8   Deadman *et al.* 2007, p.502.

9   Hartmann 2009, p.174.

10   Ibid., p.173.

11   Ibid., pp.173–174.

12   O'Connor and Bensky 1981, pp.141, 144.

13   Deadman *et al.* 2007, pp.552–554, 565–566; Ellis *et al.* 1991, pp.383, 399; Lade 1989, pp.288–289, 293; Maciocia 2015, pp.1155–1156, 1159–1160.

14   Deadman *et al.* 2007, pp.336–338, 552–554.

15   Ellis *et al.* 1989, pp.161, 309.

16   Shi 2007, p.328.

17   Deadman *et al.* 2007, pp.194–195, 508–509; Ellis *et al.* 1991, pp.153–154, 354.

18   Shi 2007, pp.139, 330.

19   O'Connor and Bensky 1981, pp.285–286.

20   Ellis *et al.* 1991 (pp.154, 466–467) mention a classical Chinese medical text, *The Glorious Anthology of Acupuncture and Moxibustion*/Zhēn Jiǔ Jù Yīng, written by Gao Wu in 1529 CE. In the text there is a section titled *Ode of a Hundred Patterns*/Bǎi Zhèng Fù, and this is where the quotation came from.

21   Ellis *et al.* 1991, pp.169, 399.

22   Maciocia (2015, p.241) advises as such when he references chapter 17 of *The Yellow Emperor's Classic* (*Inner Canon of the Yellow Emperor*/Huáng Dì Nèi Jīng). Maciocia also refers to Wang Xue Tai's text *Great Treatise of Chinese Acupuncture*/Zhōng Guó Zhēn Jiǔ Dà Quán.

23   Maciocia 2015, p.241.

24   Deadman *et al.* 2007, p.105.

25   Ibid.; Maciocia 2015, p.964; Ross 1985, pp.249, 308; Wang and Robertson 2008, pp.563–565.

26   Maciocia 2015, p.964; Wang and Robertson 2008, pp.563–565. It is important to note that both texts promote the use of the Four Gates for moving Qì and Xuè. They do, however, differ in their view on tonification. Maciocia (2015) says that LR 3 can tonify Xuè and LI 4 can be used to tonify Qì. Wang and Robertson (2008, p.564) says that the Four Gates 'are not used for tonification'. My 20-plus years of clinical experience have shown me that the Four Gates can be used to tonify Qì and Xuè.

27   Deadman *et al.* 2007, p.40.

28   Ni 1995, p.98; Wang 1997, p.132. *The Yellow Emperor's Classic* (*Inner Canon of the Yellow Emperor*/Huáng Dì Nèi Jīng) was written somewhere between 200 and 0 BCE.

29   Deadman *et al.* 2007, p.105.

30   Ibid.

31   Ibid., p.630.

32   Maclean and Lyttleton 2010, p.640.

33   Maclean and Lyttleton (2010, pp.638–640) do consider Heat to be an important trigger for painful obstruction syndrome (Bì).

34   Ross 1995, p.308.

35   Ibid.

36   Maciocia 2009, p.228. Note that LR 3 and LI 4 are not in his treatment protocol, but they can be used to calm the Shén, when combined with the points listed in the table.

37   Maciocia 2009, pp.221–222. Note that LR 3 and LI 4 are not in his treatment protocol, but they can be used to calm the Shén when used with the other points listed in the table.

38   Hartmann 2009, p.139. Note that LR 3 and LI 4 are not in my treatment protocol, but they can be used to calm the Shén, when combined with the points listed in the table.

39   Wang and Robertson 2008, p.564.

40   Ibid.

41   Ibid.

42   Hartmann 2009, p.9.

43   Wang and Robertson 2008, p.564.

44   Ibid.

45   Deadman *et al.* 2007, pp.104, 477.

46   Hartmann 2009, p.171. LR 3 isn't included in the list of points used to treat Wind. However, LR 3 is excellent for moving Qì and Xuè, thereby ensuring that Wind is more effectively eliminated from the body.

47   Deadman *et al.* 2007, p.105.

48   An appropriate quotation from the 1971 movie *Willy Wonka and the Chocolate Factory*.

49   Maciocia 2015, p.1122.

50   Deadman *et al.* 2007, pp.104, 477.

51   Ross 1995, p.308.

52   Hartmann 2009, p.9. LR 3 and LI 4 are not part of the treatment in the reference used. Having said that, they can both be used to bring down Liver Heat/Fire.

53   Hartmann 2009, p.9. LI 4 is not included in the referenced treatment. It isn't a typical point choice to tonify Xuè or Yīn.

54   Hartmann 2009, p.9. LI 4 isn't included in the referenced treatment. However, it is a good point to treat Liver Yáng Rising, particularly to bring down the Liver Heat/Fire.

55   www.psychnet-uk.com/x_new_site/DSM_IV/neurasthenia.html.

56   Wang and Robertson 2008, pp.564–565.

57   Maciocia 2015, pp.963–964, 1121–1122.

58   Ibid.

59   Deadman et al. 2007, pp.105, 478.

60   Ni 1995, p.98; Wang 1997, p.132.

61   Tiān Dì Rén is typically translated as Heaven, Earth, Human. However, they are also referred to as the Three Powers and the Three Regions; just to make it confusing.

62   Bertschinger 2013, p.102.

63   In this instance I am using SP 21 as a point for Human/Rén rather than for Heaven/Tiān. It is worth noting that SP 21 can actually embrace Heaven/Tiān, Earth/Dì and Human/Rén. This is why SP 21 (Dà Bāo) translates as 'Great Embrace'.

64   Ellis et al. 1989, p.396.

65   Dechar 2006, p.136.

66   Ellis et al. 1989, p.360.

67   Dechar 2006, p.136.

68   Ellis et al. 1989, p.389.

69   Deadman et al. 2007, pp.42–43. This is an interesting dichotomy in Chinese medicine. The front of the body is considered Yīn, with the back of the body being Yáng. But then it gets interesting because the Front Mù Collecting points are more for Yáng and the Back Shù Transporting points are more for Yīn. As I said: interesting!

70   Deadman et al. 2007, p.428. GB 9 (Tiān Chōng) Tiān = Heavenly/Celestial; Chōng = Rushing.

71   Ellis et al. 1989, p.267. GB 18 is in the vicinity of 'the place the ancient Chinese termed the "cover of the celestial spirit"'.

72   Ellis et al. 1989, p.287.

73   Deadman et al. 2007, pp.42–43.

74   O'Connor and Bensky 1981, p.163.

75   Ibid., p.164. Interestingly, both SI 17 and TE 16 are Windows of the Sky/Windows of Heaven points.

76   Deadman et al. 2007, pp.42–43.

77   I don't personally needle ST 9. Therefore, I would leave it out and use ST 8. Having said that, if you do needle ST 9, it would be an excellent point for this combination.

78   First, ST 9 (Rén Yíng): Rén = Human/person/man; Yíng = predict, welcome, receive. With Rén in the name, it can be used to regulate the Human region/power. Second, Ellis et al. (1989, p.64) say 'to receive the days and predict events' when describing what ST 9 can treat. Third, ST 9 (Rén Yíng) has an alternative Pīn

Yīn name – Tiān Wǔ Huì, which translates as 'Heaven's Five Meetings'. This matches with the fact that it's also a Window of the Sky/Window of Heaven point.

79   Deadman et al. 2007, pp.42–43.

80   Ibid., p.118.

81   Ibid., pp.42–43.

82   BL 8 is in the vicinity of 'the place the ancient Chinese termed the "cover of the celestial spirit"' (Ellis et al. 1989, p.267).

83   Lade 1989, p.129. BL 10 also happens to be a Window of the Sky/Window of Heaven point.

84   Ellis et al. 1989, p.195. BL 67 (Zhì Yīn): Zhì = reach; Yīn = Yīn. Reaching Yīn is referring to the fact that BL 67 is the last point on the Urinary Bladder channel, before the Qì travels to the Kidney channel at KI 1. Therefore, BL 67 has a direct connection to the ground/Earth.

85   Franglen 2014, pp.73–82.

86   Maciocia 2015, pp.1000–1001, 1010, 1067; Ross 1995, pp.171–172, 214–215, 277.

87   Hartmann 2009, p.4. It is worth noting that KI 6 isn't in the referenced point prescription, but is still an effective point to use for Heart Yīn Xū. This is because KI 6 can tonify Original Yīn, which is responsible for all of the Yīn in the body, including Heart Yīn.

88   Hartmann 2009, p.5.

89   Ibid., p.9.

90   Ibid., p.11. SP 6 isn't in the referenced point prescription, but is still a good point for Lung Yīn Xū. SP 6 is the intersecting point of the Three Leg Yīn channels of the Spleen, Liver and Kidneys. As such it can strengthen the Kidneys' tonification of Original Yīn, which is responsible for all of the Yīn in the body, including Lung Yīn.

91   Hartmann 2009, p.20. HT 6 isn't in the referenced point prescription, but can still be used for Stomach Yīn Xū. Having said that, HT 6 isn't one of the more commonly used points for Stomach Yīn Xū.

92   Ellis et al. 1989, p.105.

93   Deadman et al. 2007, pp.189–191.

94   Heat vexation in the five hearts is also known as 'Five Hearts Hot' or 'Five Palms Heat'. It's a disorder that is categorized by five areas being hot at the same time. This is typically the two palms, both soles of the feet and the face. Sometimes the chest is hot and not the face, and sometimes it's both the chest and the face. This is a common condition in patients with Yīn Xū.

95   The Spiritual Pivot (Líng Shū), chapter 10, says: 'A solid [Shí] disease causes pain in the whole body. A hollow [Xū] disease causes all of the hundred joints to loosen… These can be treated by using the point of the great luo linking channel of the spleen [SP 21]' (Wu 1993, p.65).

96   See previous note.

97   Deadman et al. 2007, pp.81–82.

98   Yang 2010, pp.12, 97–108. *The Great Compendium - Volume V (The Great Compendium of Acupuncture and Moxibustion/ Zhēn Jiǔ Dà Chéng)* was originally published in 1601 CE.

99   Yang 2010, p.12.

100 Maciocia 2015, p.104.

101 It is worth noting that the Host–Guest point combination doesn't use the three extra Luò Connecting points of CV 15, GV 1 and SP 21; only the 12 standard Luò Connecting points.

102 Hartmann 2009, p.9. Bear in mind that GB 37 isn't included in the reference; neither are a lot of other points that could work for a patient with Liver Qì Stagnation.

103 Hartmann 2009, pp.5, 18.

Do not think that you know. Be aware of all that is and dwell in the infinite. Wander where there is no path. Be all that heaven gave you, but act as though you have received nothing. Be empty, that is all.

Zhuāng Zǐ/莊子 (369–286 BCE)[1]

You can't teach anybody anything, only make them realize the answers are already inside them.

Galileo Galilei (1564–1642 CE)[2]

7

Strategies/Types of Acupuncture Point Combinations – Larger Combinations

1. Figure Eight

I do need to include an author disclaimer on this Figure Eight method. To date, I have yet to read anything that discusses this method exactly as it has been written here. This method is my own design and has been developed over decades of researching, reading, writing and treating patients.

During this time, I have gathered interesting treatment methods from many different sources, tinkered with these methods and combined treatment suggestions from different authors to determine what works. Some have and some have not. The Figure Eight method is an accumulation of all this work and is a recent, but brilliant, addition to my clinical practice.

The Figure Eight method is a point combination designed specifically to rebalance the Wǔ Shén/Five Spirits (see Chapter 13). The Wǔ Shén are:[3]

- Hún = Ethereal/Heavenly/Dream-Big Soul.

- Shén = Spirit.

- Yì = Thought/Post-Heaven Intellect.

- Pò = Corporeal/Grounded/Earthly/Do-Big-Be-Big Soul.

- Zhì = Willpower/Pre-Heaven Intellect.

The idea with the Figure Eight method is to reset a patient's Wǔ Shén, thereby bringing all five of our spirits back into alignment. This is a crucial concept to grasp – that is because we *all* tend to have an imbalance in our Wǔ Shén. This occurs as a result of how we live our life and how that gears in with Universal Qì.

What I mean is this: as we live our daily lives, we tend to get pushed and pulled in different directions, and it's how we react to these factors that defines who we are. The way that we live will invariably drive some of our Wǔ Shén into Excess/Shí and some into Deficiency/Xū.

The Figure Eight point combination has shown itself to be the second most amazing point combination that I have ever come across (behind only the Eight Extraordinary Vessels). I have included a patient case study (7.1) at the end of this section to provide an example of how good this method is.

For the Figure Eight method to work best, I would advise getting the patient ready by ensuring they are in a good/balanced state before you start. For me, this requires a number of treatments geared towards strong Vital Substance (Qì, Xuè, Jīn Yè and Jīng) production as well as balancing out any problematic Zàng Fǔ patterns. You don't have to get them to perfect health; just start them on the journey!

For me the Figure Eight method represents the following:

- There is no beginning or end. Just like the figure 8, or infinity standing on its end if you like.

- There are peaks and troughs as you run along the figure 8. This means you will have ups and downs in life, but this creates the balance needed.

- If I were to lay the 8 down flat, I would see a total of eight eights piled on top of one another. Essentially, this suggests that we have the ability to live out eight different lifetimes within the one life.

- Life and death are in a constant state of cycles – some high and some low, but within the flow of the eight eights.

- This is who we are, and these eights are where we sit in response to Universal Qì.

- Quite a number of Chinese, and Western, philosophies believe that we are born with our life already laid out for us, essentially suggesting that we have no free will. This can also be called our destiny. Some of these philosophical systems also believe that you can alter, to some degree, how you live that pre-planned life. This is our free will, which can also be called our desires.

The eight eights allow us to accept both. The eight locks us into a life we were always meant to lead (no free will; our destiny). But with the eights laid on top of one another, it tells us that we have some room to move up and down these eights. This movement is our free will/desires and allows us to choose the way our day-to-day activities unfold.

In a most basic sense it shows that, although our lives are predetermined, we have the capacity, within certain limits, to live our desires. These yearnings, via their limitations, will ensure that we meet similar people that will set us on the correct path.

We will all have significant relationships with people that can give us the same basic fulfilment and assistance. The variables remain within the Figure Eight.

- Our Wǔ Shén can be rebalanced within these eights.

- Not one single Chinese philosophical system that I have read has ever suggested that life was easy and was actually even meant to be easy. Life is hard, but that's for a very good reason! Without the tough times, we can't appreciate the good times!

- Can you imagine only ever knowing anger? And all other emotions didn't exist. It's not possible, is it? Then what about joy? It's the same thing; because if all you knew was joy, then happiness becomes meaningless because it's the standard. Regardless, it's not possible in Chinese medicine/philosophy anyway.

- The Chinese have known this for thousands of years, but the West is only just beginning to appreciate this very fact. Why? Because they have only been allowed free thought for the last 500-plus years. And this is a small moment in time in the context of the world.

- And, yes, we can fit the Wǔ Shén/Five Spirits into eight. Classic TCM! But first you need to see Diagram 7.1 for the Wǔ Xíng/Five Elements and the Wǔ Shén. This diagram is important because it sets the stage for how you can fit five into eight.

To start to get a better understanding of what we are dealing with in the Figure Eight combination, I will provide a series of diagrams to aid with the visualization. Diagram 7.1 shows the Wǔ Xíng/Wǔ Shén in the shape of a 'plus' sign rather than the traditional 'pentagon' sign.

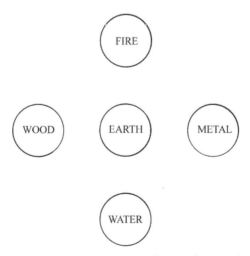

Diagram 7.1 Wǔ Xíng/Wǔ Shén Earth Central

The Wǔ Xíng/Wǔ Shén Earth Central diagram (7.1) represents:[4]

- Fire and Shén at the top

- Water and Zhì at the bottom

- Earth and Yì in the middle

- Metal and Pò on the right

- Wood and Hún on the left.

Diagram 7.2 looks at how the Wǔ Xíng/Wǔ Shén fit into the Figure Eight symbol.

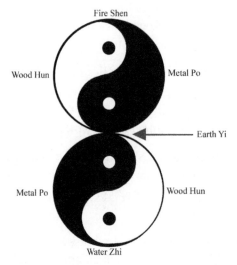

Diagram 7.2 Wǔ Xíng/Wǔ Shén and the Figure Eight

The Wǔ Xíng/Wǔ Shén and the Figure Eight diagram (7.2) is imagining the Supreme Ultimate Yīn Yáng symbol in a slightly different way. Rather than having the symbol as a singular, I have placed one on top of the other so that it represents an eight. In this way the Figure Eight image is represented as follows:

- Fire is at the top. The Heart is a Fire element organ and houses our Shén.

- Water is at the bottom. The Kidneys are a Water element organ and house our Zhì.

- Earth is in the middle. The Spleen is an Earth element organ and houses our Yì.

- Metal is Yīn (Black) and is represented here as top right and bottom left. The Lungs are a Metal element organ and house our Pò.

- Wood is Yáng (White) and is represented here as top left and bottom right. The Liver is a Wood element organ and houses our Hún.

- In addition, more balance can be created using links between each of the Wǔ Shén.

Now that we have managed to fit five into eight we need to construct a point combination to support this Figure Eight method. I have experimented with a number of different points over the past few years, and the combination that seems to work the best is shown in Table 7.1.

Table 7.1 Figure Eight point combination[5]

Location of point	Points	Effective to treat
Head/face/neck	GV 20	Fire Shén
Trunk (front)	SP 21 CV 17 CV 12 CV 5	Uplifting point – pivot between all of the Wǔ Shén Balances the Fire Shén which, by default, will positively affect the rest of the Wǔ Shén Earth Yì Water Zhì, but also provides a link on the Rèn Mài with the Yì, Pò and Shén
Arms/hands	LU 3 LI 4	Metal Pò Metal Pò and Wood Hún – via the Four Gates (in combination with LR 3)
Legs/feet	GB 40 LR 3 KI 1	Wood Hún Wood Hún and Metal Pò – via the Four Gates (in combination with LI 4) Water Zhì
Total points needled		16 needles used bilaterally

Diagram 7.3 builds on Diagram 7.2 by inserting the Figure Eight acupuncture point combination on to it.

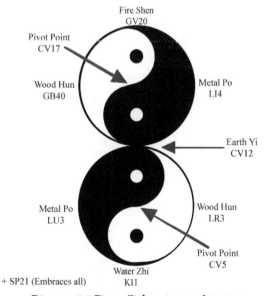

Diagram 7.3 Figure Eight point combination

As you can see from the treatment in Table 7.1 and Diagram 7.3, there is a good scattering of points over the whole body for the Figure Eight combination. There are also connections between points which allows for a stronger balance with the treatment.

These don't have to be the points you use for every patient. Sometimes it would make sense to adjust the points slightly based on the original diagnosis and the patient's personality. I have stuck with this combination almost every time. Of the few occasions I haven't, it has been to focus on a Zàng Fǔ pattern, while at the same time using the Figure Eight method.

Assuming that the patient is ready for positive change, then the Figure Eight method will reset the Wǔ Shén. This is partly done at the time of the treatment, but typically the rest is done the next time the patient has a proper sleep. As I stated above, the idea here is to get each of the Wǔ Shén on an equal playing field where each is operating on a level footing. This allows for much better balance in our day-to-day lives.

For a more in-depth discussion on the Wǔ Shén, see Chapter 13.

Important considerations

This combination won't be effective for everyone. For starters, your patient needs to be 100% committed to the treatment process. You need to explain the entire procedure and what they could expect.

All patients will react in different ways, and sometimes the changes they exhibit are unusual, unexpected and unwanted. For example, a patient who is normally calm may show signs of anger for a day or two after the treatment. This is the body resetting itself, and sometimes unexpected reactions appear briefly. These are not usually a bad sign – in fact, they are a good sign, because they are allowing the body to remove some locked-in and unwanted emotional baggage.

Therefore, the patient needs to know that they may experience some strange emotional output. There may also be some distinct changes to your patient's personality. This is to be expected because that is why you are doing the Figure Eight method in the first place.

Let your patient know that you are with them all the way. Allow them to contact you if they need to chat about something unexpected, unusual and/or exciting. Try to be flexible with your treatment program, thereby allowing for increased or decreased appointments as the patient adapts to their new self.

Ensure that the patient's immediate family (and perhaps close friends?) are aware of potential changes to their emotions and personality. That way they are involved in the process and won't be as surprised if some big changes occur in the short term. What are some possible changes you can expect based on each of the Wǔ Shén? That will depend on whether they are Excess/Shí or Deficient/Xū.

Tables 7.2 and 7.3 illustrate each of the Wǔ Shén in the context of whether they are Deficient/Xū or Excess/Shí. I don't mean that all of the Wǔ Shén will be Xū at the same time or all Shí at the same time. From experience, I tend to see only one or two Xū or Shí at the same time. For each diagnosed patient you will typically only be targeting one or two rows (from one or both of Tables 7.2 and 7.3). When you use the Figure Eight method, you will move the Xū or Shí back into balance, thereby ensuring that all of the Wǔ Shén are stable and healthy.

Tables 7.2 and 7.3 can't possibly include all the changes that may be exhibited by your patient. Every patient is unique and you can't know exactly how they will react. You also can't know how unbalanced their Wǔ Shén might be. You will probably have a fair idea but you may not have diagnosed everything. Some of the Wǔ Shén could be Shí; some could be Xū; some might be Shí at the same time as some are Xū. Therefore, Tables 7.2 and 7.3 are simply a guide to what you might expect.

These changes will typically only be present for a day or two – a week at the most. To date I have never had a patient who hasn't had some short-term upheaval, but this has never lasted longer than a week. If you have a patient who is still exhibiting change around the week mark, then treat them again, moving back to your typical diagnostic method. For me, that would be diagnosing them with a Zàng Fǔ pattern and treating accordingly. You don't need to do the Figure Eight method again as it has performed its function.

Table 7.2 Wǔ Shén Xū potential emotional/personality changes[6]

Wǔ Shén	Emotional/personality changes
Hún Xū	• Compromises, submits, passive, timid, ineffectual, ambivalent, powerless, frustrated, stressed, resentful, suspicious, self-punishing. • Feeling down/low/flat (unlikely to use the word 'depression' but that's what it is). • May feel a vague sense of unease. • Feeling as if the day hasn't gone the way they had hoped/dreamed. • Poor decision making and planning due to inability to actually decide: 'It's all too hard!' Blames others if they fail. • Obsessed with ensuring that everything in their lives is planned down to the minutest detail. Habit bound. • Too rigid and no longer open to change because change is scary.
Pò Xū	• Disillusioned, dispirited, pessimistic, indifferent, conservative, worried, sad, grief-stricken, depressed. • Makes hasty decisions as a result of inadequate planning/not thinking things through. • All talk and no action – they come up with heaps of ideas but never finish what they start. • Off with the fairies. • Will 'dream big', but won't 'do big' or 'be big'.[7]
Zhì Xū	• Soft, spineless, dishonest, dull, forgetful, frugal. • Will lock themselves away from the world. • Poor willpower, drive, determination, initiative, enthusiasm. • Easily discouraged; gives up – never completes anything. • Can have significant fears/phobias. • Suspicious of everyone and everything. • May have non-specific feelings of dread and foreboding.

cont.

Wǔ Shén	Emotional/personality changes
Yì Xū	• Unmotivated, feels stuck, vague; sloppy, conforming, melancholic, broody, lethargic, tired, submissive, obsequious. • Worried about everyone and everything. Further, they worry so much about the past that they become obsessed with it; therefore, they live in the past. • Pensive but with a poor memory and is a slow learner. Also, can't concentrate, procrastinates and is too tired to think.
Shén Xū	• Quiet, withdrawn, depressed, disheartened, easily startled, anxious, gullible, naïve, dazed, confused, lost, panicky, apathetic, lethargic, stressed. • Memory problems – short-term, long-term or when trying to study. • Suffers from shock. • Suffers from insomnia.

Table 7.3 Wǔ Shén Shí potential emotional/personality changes[8]

Wǔ Shén	Emotional/personality changes
Hún Shí	• Angry, frustrated, feels overwhelmed, stressed, intolerant, arrogant, impulsive, aggressive, reckless, pretentious, impatient and/or confrontational. • Makes hasty decisions as a result of inadequate planning/not thinking things through and then blames others if they fail. • All talk and no action – they come up with heaps of ideas but never finish what they start. • Off with the fairies. • Will 'dream big', but won't 'do big' or 'be big'. • Subject to uncontrollable impulses.
Pò Shí	• Overly strict, dogmatic, self-righteous, indifferent, hypocritical, worried. Over-analyzes everything. • Poor decision making and planning due to inability to actually decide: 'It's all too hard!' • Obsessed with ensuring that everything in their lives is planned down to the minutest detail. • Too rigid and no longer open to change because change is scary.
Zhì Shí	• Critical, cynical, blunt, unforgiving, dishonest, anxious, forgetful, fussy. • Suspicious of everyone and everything. • Can show false confidence. • Poor willpower, drive, determination, initiative, enthusiasm. • Can have significant fears/phobias. • Constantly getting distracted from a task because of a fear of failure and anxiety. • May have non-specific feelings of dread and foreboding.
Yì Shí	• Overprotective, overbearing, meddlesome, obsessive. • Worried about everyone and everything. Further, they worry so much about the future that they become obsessed with it; therefore, they live in the future. • Pensive but with a poor memory and is a slow learner.
Shén Shí	• Over-excited, hypersensitive, manic, manic depressive, psychotic, aggressive, anxious, confused, selfish, agitated, stressed. • Memory problems – short-term, long-term or when trying to study. • Addicted to stimulants. • Suffers from shock. • Suffers from insomnia but then has nightmares (when they do sleep).

Finally, I would also never treat a patient with the Figure Eight method if they were unaware I was planning to do it. I also wouldn't do it if the patient was only having the treatment because someone else told them they should. Both of these instances are loaded with problems, ethically and otherwise.

This method is only for patients 100% committed to the process once they have been informed about its benefits and potential short-term pitfalls.

CASE STUDY 7.1 A 33-YEAR-OLD FEMALE (MG) WITH LOW BACK AND HIP PAIN

MG was a patient of mine a few years ago. She originally came to see me because of a sore lower back and hips. She was quite overweight and worked at a sedentary job. As I took her case history, I found out that MG had recently had a bad relationship break-up with her partner. To make matters worse, she was not told why he broke it off with her. This left her in quite a deal of distress and she was unable to move forward with her life as a result.

She worked extremely long hours (typically 4am–8pm, six days a week – roughly 100 hours per week) and disliked her job immensely. When enquiring about her long hours, she told me it was primarily because she had to supervise her fellow staff members to ensure they got their work done. This meant she didn't even start her own work until 12pm, once the other staff had signed off for the day.

MG suffered from mild depression and anxiety, neither of which were medicated. She also advised me that since her break-up she couldn't stop her brain from analyzing every small detail about her relationship to see what could have been the cause of it ending so suddenly.

She had recently started doing mindfulness meditation three evenings a week after she got home from work and found it to be quite helpful, but it didn't keep the analyzing brain at bay for long. When I told her that acupuncture could be a good adjunct to her mindfulness meditation, she jumped at the chance.

Once her low back pain was under control, I started to balance out her Zàng Fǔ patterns, which at the time was Spleen and Heart Qì Xū with Liver Qì Stagnation. I did seven weekly treatments for those patterns and felt I had reached the stage where she was ready for the Figure Eight method.

There was a slight delay because MG had booked herself into surgery for a gastric sleeve. This resulted in me doing three more treatments over a ten-day period to help her body recover post-surgery. MG was not working at her job during this time.

So although it took me nearly three weeks longer to use the Figure Eight method, it was necessary in MG's case.

I did the Figure Eight point combination on her and we chatted on several occasions before her next scheduled weekly appointment. She observed feeling really content and at peace in her mind, which she said started almost as soon as the treatment commenced. The analyzing brain had simply ceased to exist and it stayed away for almost five days. Even when it returned, the brain was significantly less analytical, and instead became more processed in its thinking. This allowed MG to deal with stuff to help her move through the relationship issues, rather than falling back into the continual rehashing of relationship dramas.

MG came to the conclusion shortly thereafter that although she may never find out why her partner had ended the relationship so suddenly and surprisingly, this was out of her control. She started focusing on what she could control about herself and her current relationships with family, acquaintances and work colleagues. This also dramatically reduced her levels of depression and anxiety.

She went back to work for the first time since her surgery, five days after the Figure Eight point combination. Then the most incredible thing happened.

MG sat down at her desk at 4am and started working. Around about 6am a work colleague walked up to her desk to see if MG was feeling okay. She said she was feeling wonderful and asked her, 'Why?' The colleague declined to comment but did tell her she was pleased to hear she was well. At around about 8am another staff member enquired as to her health and received the same answer from MG. Before the end of the day she was asked twice more about whether she was ill and gave the same answer. Then she signed off from work at 12pm with everyone else and went home.

Did you work out what was so amazing? MG certainly didn't until shortly before she came for her acupuncture appointment two days later. She had instantly stopped caring about what her fellow staff members were doing, and instead was simply focusing on her job. After all, MG wasn't the employer at the company; she was a staff member, just like everyone else. So she shouldn't have been worrying so much about what everyone else was doing – especially when it meant working double the hours each day as well as making her unpopular in the workplace.

This revelation that she was a very controlling person shed new light on her entire life, both past and present. She proposed that this was the reason her partner had left her and why she didn't have any close friends. And although this was quite a confronting revelation, it was one that gave her new-found strength and resolve.

She quit the job she hated. She joined a couple of sporting groups, as well as a yoga group, which she had been unable to do before because of her long work hours and obesity. And although her weight loss took time, her head was in the best place it had been her entire life.

I put the Figure Eight method down as being a critical part of the massive change in MG's headspace. I accept that the previous acupuncture treatments played their part, as did her mindfulness meditation. I also accept that MG was in a space where she was ready for big change, and this is a crucial element for potential success.

At the time of writing, MG is not currently coming for acupuncture treatments. But she is a friend on social media and I have therefore had the pleasure of seeing her blossom into an extraordinary human being. She is almost at goal weight. She is in a new relationship (he just proposed to her!) and has close friends for the first time since she was at school.

2. Zàng Fǔ/Sān Jiāo balance

This combination acts in a similar manner to the whole-body method discussed in Chapter 5. However, the Zàng Fǔ/Sān Jiāo balance is designed specifically to give all the organs in the body a Vital Substance boost.

This method places more emphasis on the trunk when needling, with a lesser focus on the extremities. In that way we still get a whole-body balance but with the Sān Jiāo as the key. One of the best ways to access the organs is to needle them locally. The entire trunk should be needled at intervals, with some needles in the Upper Jiāo, some in the Middle Jiāo and some in the Lower Jiāo for best results.

Tables 7.4 and 7.5 offer two acupuncture point combination examples for the Zàng Fǔ/Sān Jiāo balance, with explanations on what the points treat as well as how/why the points combine well together.

Table 7.4 Front-of-body Zàng Fǔ/Sān Jiāo treatment[9]

Session 1 – face up		
Location of point	**Points**	**Points treat**
Trunk (front)	CV 4 CV 6 CV 12 CV 14 CV 17 CV 21	Lower Jiāo and Xuè/Yīn Lower/Middle Jiāo and Qì/Yáng Middle Jiāo and Qì/Yáng Middle/Upper Jiāo and Qì/Xuè Upper Jiāo and Qì Descends into the entire Sān Jiāo
Arms/hands	TE 4 LU 7	Balances the entire Sān Jiāo Opens the Rèn Mài
Legs/feet	ST 36 SP 6 KI 6	Balances the entire Sān Jiāo Lower/Middle Jiāo and Qì/Xuè Coupled point to open the Rèn Mài
Total points needled		16 needles used bilaterally

As you can see from Table 7.4, the Zàng Fǔ/Sān Jiāo combination is anchored with six Rèn Mài points on the trunk. These six points have the ability to treat every organ in the body, with the points at regular intervals along the trunk. The points have multiple jobs, with some working on one of the Jiāos, and some working on multiple.

Some of the Rèn Mài points work on Yīn and Xuè, whereas others work on Yáng and Qì. This provides additional balance for the treatment.

CV 4 and CV 6 regulate all the organs in the Lower Jiāo as well as balancing Yīn, Xuè, Yáng and Qì. CV 6 also acts as a connection between the Lower Jiāo and Middle Jiāo.

CV 12 and CV 14 regulate all the organs in the Middle Jiāo as well as balancing Xuè, Yáng and Qì. CV 14 also acts as a connection between the Middle Jiāo and Upper Jiāo.

CV 17 and CV 21 regulate all the organs in the Upper Jiāo as well as balancing Qì. CV 21 also acts as a connection for all of the Sān Jiāo.

This combination also accesses the arms with TE 4 and LU 7 as well as the legs by using ST 36, SP 6 and KI 6. These points further aid the Rèn Mài points and ensure that Vital Substance flow is both leaving and returning to the trunk as well as assisting the production and movement of Vital Substances.

Finally, the points are scattered sensibly all over the body, ensuring a solid whole-body treatment.

Table 7.5 Back-of-body Zàng Fǔ/Sān Jiāo treatment[10]

Session 2 – face down		
Location of point	**Points**	**Points treat**
Trunk (back)	BL 13 – right side only BL 15 – left side only BL 18 – left side only BL 20 – right side only BL 22 BL 23	Upper Jiāo and Qì/Yīn Upper Jiāo and Qì/Xuè/Yīn/Yáng Middle Jiāo; Xuè tonic; Qì mover Middle Jiāo and Qì/Xuè/Yáng Balances the entire Sān Jiāo Lower Jiāo and Qì/Xuè/Yīn/Yáng
Arms/hands	HT 7 LU 9	Upper Jiāo and Qì/Xuè/Yīn/Yáng Upper Jiāo and Qì/Yīn
Legs/feet	BL 39 KI 3	Balances the entire Sān Jiāo Lower Jiāo and Qì/Yīn/Yáng
Total points needled		16 needles used bilaterally

The face-down treatment is designed to act in the same way as the face-up treatment. Both Zàng Fǔ/Sān Jiāo combinations are anchored on the trunk, with the face-down treatment using six Urinary Bladder channel points. These six points have the ability to treat every organ in the body, with the points at regular intervals along the trunk. The points have multiple jobs, with some working on one of the Jiāos and some working on multiple.

You will see alongside the six Urinary Bladder channel points that some are needled unilaterally and some bilaterally. This ensures that the entire treatment stays within my 8–16 needle range. Feel free to needle those points however you wish. If you did do them all bilaterally, the treatment would use 20 needles.

BL 13 and BL 15 regulate all the organs in the Upper Jiāo as well as balancing Yīn, Xuè, Yáng and Qì.

BL 18 and BL 20 regulate all the organs in the Middle Jiāo as well as balancing Xuè, Yáng and Qì.

BL 22 and BL 23 regulate all the organs in the Lower Jiāo as well as balancing Yīn, Xuè, Yáng and Qì. BL 22 also acts as a connection for all of the Sān Jiāo.

This combination also accesses the arms with HT 7 and LU 9 as well as the legs by using BL 39 and KI 3. These points further aid the Urinary Bladder channel points and ensure that Vital Substance flow is both leaving and returning to the trunk as well as assisting the production and movement of Vital Substances.

Finally, the points are scattered sensibly all over the body, ensuring a solid whole-body treatment.

When might the Zàng Fǔ/Sān Jiāo point combination not be effective?

As with the whole-body method discussed earlier, the Zàng Fǔ/Sān Jiāo method won't be effective all of the time. This is particularly the case if the patient has a lot of stagnation, in which case you might be better off narrowing your focus down and targeting a few key areas first. Once the Vital Substances are moving, the Zàng Fǔ/Sān Jiāo method will be significantly more effective.

3. Chain and lock[11]

And now finally in longstanding suffering or partial paralysis,
The rule is to connect the qi all through the channels…
Suppose you clear out a waterway by letting through water
Do you not at once see results?
And why does catastrophe not then set in?…
If the climate is fairly adjusted then the waterways are clear and working,
The people at peace and all things flourish. (Bertschinger 2013, pp.153–154)[12]

The chain-and-lock method is a treatment combination that employs points on the one channel – some local, some distal and some adjacent to the main site of complaint for the patient. The idea here is to be target-specific, and if you know which channel is most affected, then putting a series of points along this stagnant channel can be very effective.

The word 'chain' refers to the selected points being all on one channel, thereby ensuring they are linked together like the links in a chain.

The 'lock' has three different meanings. First, it refers to the links in the chain being connected or locked together. Second, it refers to the points selected as being locked, unique and separate to any other treatment you may be employing in that session. Third, it refers to the technique the practitioner employs as the last step in the chain-and-lock method, which is to stimulate the two furthest needles in the chain, thereby ensuring the technique has been securely locked in.

This doesn't mean that the chain-and-lock method isolates the Vital Substances – far from it. The final locking technique is used to 'fire up' the Vital Substances so that they surge through the chain before being unleashed into the main body circulation. The power that is generated is one of the great strengths of the chain-and-lock technique.

Chain-and-lock treatment approaches

There are a few different approaches that can be employed when using the chain-and-lock point combination.

Needle the points bilaterally for a unilateral complaint

This is a consideration if you believe that the patient has bilateral imbalances, even though their signs and symptoms are only presenting as one-sided. The best way to determine that is via questioning and Tuī Ná (Chinese massage).

You might also consider needling bilaterally if you believe that the opposite side will still come to the aid of the injured side. This is something I am a big believer in, and I will discuss my implementation of bilateral points in the two examples I give below. Briefly, however, I would typically select a few key points along joints and needle them bilaterally, and use the other points unilaterally.

Needle the points unilaterally on the affected side only

The emphasis here is to target the affected area only. This gives the patient's body very specific information, thereby allowing it to go to work knowing exactly what's required, without any other points confusing or diluting the treatment.

Needle the points unilaterally on the unaffected side only

There are two reasons why you would consider this option. The first is that you simply can't get to the affected side. For example, this might apply if your patient has a broken tibia and the affected side is in a cast or splint. It may therefore be impossible to employ the chain-and-lock method along your chosen Spleen channel (or whichever channel you chose). As a result, you use the method on the opposite leg because it is the mirror image. Alternatively, you use the opposite forearm as a corresponding/mirror image.

The second reason is that the affected side is just too sore, and as much as you may wish to needle the affected side, the patient won't let you. A perfect example of that is gout:

- You could employ the chain-and-lock method on the Liver channel in the treatment of gout. In this example you would needle the unaffected side with a range of points including, but not limited to, LR 1, LR 2, LR 4, LR 6, LR 8 and LR 11. This point selection ensures that the joints of the metatarsophalangeal, ankle, knee and hip are employed. The Xì Cleft point on the Liver channel has also been used (LR 6), the benefits of which will be discussed shortly. This treatment allows for a tremendous Vital Substance flush of the Liver channel and its associated joints.

I discussed a separate treatment for gout in Chapter 5.

Use the method as the only form of acupuncture treatment in the designated session

The chain-and-lock method can be a very strong treatment during and often afterwards. Patients will often describe the affected area as having a deep, dull ache, throb, pain, discomfort, tightness, burning and even a partial cramp/spasm. The entire area needled will be active and may remain active for days after the treatment.

From my experience, the patient will feel the needles during the treatment and perhaps for an hour or so after the needles have been removed. Then there tends to be a sense of lightness – as if the affected joints have relaxed/loosened. This can generate quite a euphoric sense of being, particularly if they have had the complaint for a long time.

However, they will commonly notice the affected joints again a day or two after the treatment. This may present as a deep ache/discomfort/pain/tightness. Usually, acute disorders remain localized but chronic complaints are often different. This is because the longer the disorder has been present, the longer the area has had to stagnate. This stagnation often becomes toxic, and when it's moved, additional signs and symptoms may present to the patient. Some of the more common include generalized body aches/pain, headaches, nausea, fatigue, greasy sweat and/or unusual bowel movements/bladder discharge.

These are the reasons why you have to consider whether to use the chain-and-lock method exclusively in the designated treatment.

Use other points on different channels to supplement the method

In both acute and chronic cases, there needs to be some consideration about whether to supplement the chain-and-lock technique with additional points on different channels.

In acute cases you may really want to rip in and give a super-strong treatment, the idea being that the more recent the complaint, the faster it will heal.

In chronic cases you're conscious of the fact that there may be side effects which, for the patient, could appear out of the blue a day or two after the treatment. This was discussed above, so I don't need to go into detail again; suffice to say, if you think it's possible there will be side effects, then you choose points in the treatment to try to stop those side effects occurring, or at least to minimize the impact to the patient. For example, add in PC 6 and LI 4 for pain relief, as stated by O'Connor and Bensky (1981, p.233): '[Use LI 4] with P-6 (Neiguan) for various anesthetic purposes.' PC 6 will aid with any nausea.[13]

Use other points on different channels to treat a separate patient complaint

You might be of the view that treating the patient for multiple complaints is perfectly okay in a clinic setting. I am certainly of this belief in many instances. But the chain-and-lock method is not your standard treatment, so I would recommend caution in this instance. I would only consider this if my patient was very robust and an otherwise healthy individual.

The chain-and-lock technique is already strong enough. Other than considering some additional points on other channels to consolidate, and perhaps a few of the points in the method used bilaterally, I would be unlikely to consider this option. In the end, it is entirely up to you and your own views on patient treatments.

Always use a Xì Cleft point on the affected channel, as long as it's in the vicinity

Xì Cleft points are a special point category that treat acute-stage disorders, especially when there is pain.[14] They're excellent at moving Vital Substances, which makes them a great category to consider when using the chain-and-lock method.

Chain-and-lock needling techniques/options

You also need to consider how you will needle the points. The following options should be considered.

Needle with the flow of the channel

For example, for severe muscle fatigue and wasting/atrophy along the Spleen channel, you would start needling in the ankle and progressively work your way up the channel to the hips.

This method is employed if the patient is suffering from a Deficiency/Xū complaint. This is because moving the Vital Substances towards the trunk (where they are made) is a more nourishing/tonifying technique.[15] This is further enhanced by needling with the flow of Qì of the channel, which is typically a tonifying technique.[16]

Needle against the flow of the channel

For example, your patient has adductor muscle groin pain (along the Liver channel) that is radiating down the leg *and* up into the lower abdomen. You would start needling in the lower abdomen and progressively work your way counterflow down the channel.

This method is employed if the patient is suffering from an Excess/Shí complaint. This is because moving the Vital Substances away from the trunk (where they are made) is a more draining/dispersing/sedating technique.[17] This is further enhanced by needling against the flow of Qì of the channel, which is typically a draining technique.[18]

Insert the needles with minimal stimulation

This is definitely not standard needling for the chain-and-lock method. The patient is supposed to feel the Vital Substances surging through the affected channel. Using minimal stimulation is unlikely to give your patient that sensation.

There are instances, of course, where you might employ this needling technique. The most obvious are patients that are severely needle-phobic, elderly patients and/or patients who are quite unwell. My view is that something is still better than nothing, and if this is the needling technique needed in your patient's current state, then only apply minimal needle stimulation. Otherwise, stick with the following needling method which employs strong stimulation.

Insert the needles with strong stimulation

The chain-and-lock method is supposed to be strong and this is therefore the preferred needling technique. There are two ways you can go about this. The first is to insert each needle (in your pre-planned direction) and then stimulate them before moving on to the next one. The other option is to insert all of the needles (in your pre-planned direction) first and then come back to the first one and stimulate them one after the other.

I prefer the second option because once all of the needles are in, your patient tends to physically and visibly relax. I imagine this is because they think the worst is over. With the chain-and-lock method, they couldn't be more wrong, but they don't know that yet. You will have told them you plan to stimulate each needle beforehand, but most patients think this is less painful than the actual needle penetrating the skin.

Further, I like the second option because each needle will already be stimulating Vital Substance flow even before you get to each one and give them further stimulation. This means you have gained a few minutes of extra benefit from the treatment.

Stimulate two needles at once

Once the needles have been inserted and then stimulated individually, start stimulating the two closest needles to try to get the Vital Substances flowing between the two needles. If the patient can feel a distinct sensation between each of the needles, then you will have enhanced the benefits of the treatment.

If there is a decent distance between the two needles, or if you have tried but failed to get a sensation between the two needles, give the following a try. In a line along the channel, scrape a fingernail between the two needles. This provides a motivating force for the Vital Substances, plus gives the patient's body (and mind) a clear instruction of what you are trying to achieve. Then grip the two needles and visualize the Vital Substances flowing between the points. This visualization could be an energy or vibration; for me, it's the color white.

Repeat for all needles that are beside one another.

Finish with the 'lock'

The 'lock' is stimulating the two furthest needles in the chain, thereby ensuring the technique has been securely locked in. This final act is used to 'fire up' the Vital Substances so that they surge through the chain/channel before being unleashed into the main body circulation. The power that is generated is one of the great strengths of the chain-and-lock method.

Use an electro-acupuncture machine on some/all of the needles

It is worth noting that you can employ one further technique after you have finished stimulating the needles with the lock method. If you feel that it's necessary, you can apply electro-acupuncture to some or all of the needles used in the chain-and-lock point combination. At the very least, they could be applied to the main problem area along the chain or used only on the needles at either end of the chain.

Obviously, this has the potential to enhance the benefits of the treatment. However, it can also increase the possibility of any initial side effects of the treatment. As the chain-and-lock method is already incredibly powerful, I am usually reluctant to apply electro-acupuncture, but I would consider it for a patient who is very robust and an otherwise healthy individual.

Chain-and-lock treatment examples

I have provided three examples of the chain-and-lock method below (Tables 7.6–7.8). Please be aware that you can alter the point selections somewhat. You should, however, always remember to have a point at each joint, a point between joints and the Xì Cleft point.

Table 7.6 Lateral leg chain-and-lock treatment (Gall Bladder channel)

Points	Bilateral/ unilateral	Reasoning
GB 30	Bilateral or unilateral	Local hip point – this will activate the highest joint in the leg, which is important to allow for free flow of Vital Substances back into general body circulation.
GB 31	Unilateral	Used as a stop-gap to ensure Vital Substances are moving effectively between the hip and knee.
GB 33	Unilateral	Local knee point – this will activate the middle joint in the leg. This will ensure there is minimal disruption of Vital Substance flow down, and up, the leg.
GB 34	Bilateral or unilateral	Local knee point for reasons already stated in GB 33 above. Also an excellent point to treat all muscles, tendons, ligaments and joints.[19]
GB 36	Unilateral	Used as a stop-gap to ensure Vital Substances are moving effectively between the knee and ankle. Xì Cleft point on the Gall Bladder channel.[20]

GB 40	Bilateral or unilateral	Local ankle point – this will activate the lower joint in the leg. As one of the most distal joints in the legs, it is an important area to have strong Vital Substance flow.
Total points needled	6 needles used if done unilaterally only 9 needles used if doing three bilateral and three unilateral	

The chain-and-lock combination in Table 7.6 uses six needles unilaterally on the affected leg only. As you can see from the points chosen, the emphasis is squarely on the Gall Bladder channel, which makes sense when the patient complaint is a lateral leg disorder.

The method takes advantage of three main joints along the entire leg – the hip (GB 30), knee (GB 33 and GB 34) and ankle (GB 40). There are also some consolidating points between the hip and knee joints (GB 31) and between the knee and ankle joints (GB 36).

The joints are sites where Vital Substance flow can be compromised. This is because the joints have space for stagnation to occur, in the same way that blood will often pool in joints after a muscle or tendon tear. Therefore, it is very important to treat the joints when using the chain-and-lock method.

Looking at the points chosen, I would personally consider doing three of the points bilaterally in order to target the three joints. In this example, I would likely choose GB 30, GB 34 and GB 40 as my bilateral points of choice. These will provide a double-shot of energy to the hip, knee and ankles.

Table 7.7 Anterior leg chain-and-lock treatment (Stomach channel)

Points	Bilateral/ unilateral	Reasoning
ST 31	Bilateral or unilateral	Local hip point – this will activate the highest joint in the leg, which is important to allow for free flow of Vital Substances back into general body circulation.
ST 32	Unilateral	Used as a stop-gap to ensure Vital Substances are moving effectively between the hip and knee.
ST 34	Unilateral	Local knee point – this will activate the middle joint in the leg. This will ensure there is minimal disruption of Vital Substance flow down, and up, the leg. Xì Cleft point on the Stomach channel.[21]
ST 36	Bilateral or unilateral	Local knee point for reasons already stated in ST 34 above.
ST 40	Unilateral	Used as a stop-gap to ensure Vital Substances are moving effectively between the knee and ankle.
ST 41	Bilateral or unilateral	Local ankle point – this will activate the lower joint in the leg. As one of the most distal joints in the legs, it is an important area to have strong Vital Substance flow.
Total points needled	6 needles used if done unilaterally only 9 needles used if doing three bilateral and three unilateral	

The chain-and-lock combination in Table 7.7 uses six needles unilaterally on the affected leg only. As you can see from the points chosen, the emphasis is squarely on the Stomach channel, which makes sense when the patient complaint is an anterior leg disorder.

The method takes advantage of three main joints along the entire leg – the hip (ST 31), knee (ST 34 and ST 36) and ankle (ST 41). There are also some consolidating points between the hip and knee joints (ST 32) and between the knee and ankle joints (ST 40).

Looking at the points chosen, I would personally consider doing three of the points bilaterally in order to target the three joints. In this example, I would likely choose ST 31, ST 36 and ST 41 as my bilateral points of choice. These will provide a double-shot of energy to the hip, knee and ankles.

Table 7.8 Lateral arm chain-and-lock treatment (Large Intestine channel)

Points	Bilateral/ unilateral	Reasoning
LI 4	Bilateral or unilateral	Local wrist/hand point – this will activate the lower joint in the arm. As one of the most distal joints in the arms, it is an important area to have strong Vital Substance flow. Also an excellent point for pain relief.[22]
LI 7	Unilateral	Used as a stop-gap to ensure Vital Substances are moving effectively between the wrist/hand and elbow. Xì Cleft point on the Large Intestine channel.[23]
LI 10	Unilateral	Used as a stop-gap to ensure Vital Substances are moving effectively between the wrist/hand and elbow. Also translates as 'Arm/Hand Three Miles', which indicates the power that this point has at its disposal in order to keep moving.[24]
LI 11	Bilateral or unilateral	Local elbow point – this will activate the middle joint in the arm. This will ensure there is minimal disruption of Vital Substance flow down, and up, the arm.
LI 14	Unilateral	Used as a stop-gap to ensure Vital Substances are moving effectively between the elbow and shoulder.
LI 15	Bilateral or unilateral	Local shoulder point – this will activate the highest joint in the arm, which is important to allow for free flow of Vital Substances back into general body circulation.
Total points needled	6 needles used if done unilaterally only 9 needles used if doing three bilateral and three unilateral	

The chain-and-lock combination in Table 7.8 uses six needles unilaterally on the affected arm only. The emphasis is squarely on the Large Intestine channel, which plays a major role in the treatment of lateral arm disorders.

The method takes advantage of three main joints along the entire arm – the wrist/hand (LI 4), elbow (LI 11) and shoulder (LI 15). There are also some consolidating points between the wrist/hand and elbow joints (LI 7 and LI 10) as well as the elbow and shoulder joints (LI 14).

Looking at the points chosen, I would personally consider doing three of the points bilaterally in order to target the three joints. In this example, I would likely choose LI 4, LI 11 and LI 15 as my bilateral points of choice. These will provide a double-shot of energy to the wrist/hand, elbow and shoulder.

When might the chain-and-lock point combination not be effective?

Obviously, the chain-and-lock method is very specific and that's where its greatest strength and biggest weakness lie. Its strength is using large numbers of points on a channel to force rapid change, which is typically better than using just one or two points on the affected channel.

Its weakness is that it's very specific and doesn't allow for points on other channels to aid the treatment. Another negative to consider is that there might be stagnation on more than one channel, which is very common in a lot of sports injuries or repetitive strain injuries.

For example, you get a patient in clinic with shin splints. They describe the stabbing pain as being on the medial and lateral aspect of the tibia. This would therefore likely involve the Spleen, Liver and Stomach channels. It might even involve the Kidney and Gall Bladder channels. In this example, the chain-and-lock method may not be the best combination to choose.

Finally, as already mentioned, the treatment can be quite painful and can generate some side effects a day or two after the treatment (see above for additional discussion).

CASE STUDY 7.2 A 38-YEAR-OLD MALE (CJ) WITH NECK PAIN/STIFFNESS AND HEADACHES/MIGRAINES

CJ was a patient of mine 15 years ago when I lived and worked on the Gold Coast, Australia. I had been in practice for a number of years at that point and was working with a chiropractor (PP) in his clinic. Three days a week I did massage on his patients prior to their adjustments, and the other two days I worked as an acupuncturist, with PP referring many patients to me. It was a wonderful relationship that did wonders for my massage and acupuncture skills.

One day CJ came in to see PP as a new patient. As he walked into the clinic, you could see straight away that something wasn't right. CJ had a very funny gait and he looked as if he could fall over every step he took. His left arm was hanging useless at his side and his right arm was used to grab on to anything for support. Upon questioning CJ, his main complaint was neck pain/stiffness and headaches/migraines. His history revealed that he had had spinal surgery on his neck for a tumor. CJ had decompression surgery where they excised the entire tumor. This surgery had complications attached to it, especially two decades ago when CJ had his operation. He also had to have spinal stabilization surgery.

As was the rule with new patients, CJ was required to get a spinal X-ray so that PP could better establish what was going on inside the body. This was even more necessary in CJ's case for obvious reasons. The X-ray showed PP that there was no way he could treat CJ with chiropractic adjustments, so he recommended acupuncture with me. CJ agreed.

I went a little deeper with my questioning than PP had done because it was apparent to me that CJ was depressed. My approach was to get additional information about his musculoskeletal complaints as well as explore the sadness that was evident in him.

I discovered the following about his musculoskeletal complaints:

- CJ had been diagnosed with an aggressive and malignant spinal tumor two years earlier. His specialist was blunt and told him he had two choices. The first was he could have the operation to remove the tumor, but there was a very high risk that he would end up a quadriplegic. The second option was not to do the surgery and die. CJ chose option one.

- The outcome of the operation was more successful than the doctors expected and CJ only had one limb (left arm and non-dominant hand) that was completely paralyzed.

- Both his legs were inconsistent in their functioning and so he walked the best he could manage, but he did fall over regularly. He refused to use a walking stick or a mobility walker. His reasoning was that he was still young and didn't want to use an 'old person's device'. Plus he hadn't broken any bones when he did fall, so he figured he was okay to keep walking. In addition, the recovery nurses had recommended that he get used to walking without support.

- His left arm didn't work at all and he had zero feeling in it.

- His right arm did work quite well but he lacked fine motor skills, so it was pretty much impossible for him to write, type, pick up small things or grip anything such as a teacup handle. He also struggled to press the correct buttons on the television remote. He also couldn't do any buttons up on shirts, and zippers were a nightmare. He also couldn't tie shoelaces.

- CJ considered his neck pain/stiffness to be a direct result of the tumor growing as he had never suffered from neck pain/stiffness until about six months before the tumor was discovered. The subsequent spinal surgery wouldn't have helped the neck pain/stiffness either, I imagine.

- CJ also placed the blame for his headaches and migraines on the tumor as he had never suffered from them until about six months before the tumor was discovered. His headaches were managed semi-successfully with paracetamol. They were typically located at the base of the skull near GB 20 or behind/above one eye. They were almost always left-sided.

- His migraines always started at the left GB 20. As they progressed, they resulted in the headache traveling across to the right-sided GB 20. Before long, it felt as if it was slicing through his head, coming out at GB 14. This rapid shift also resulted in photophobia, nausea and an unbalanced feeling as if he was 'standing on a rocking boat out at sea'. This was obviously an issue as he already had problems with his balance. His treatment of choice for these migraines was codeine and rest.

This is what I found out about his sadness/depression:

- After the surgery CJ was initially ecstatic about the outcome. He worked hard in rehab and enjoyed life for about six months. But by then CJ was starting to tire of the continual neck pain/stiffness and headaches/ migraines. He also had reduced functioning/sensation for his bowel and bladder movements. His poor erectile function was also a big concern for him.

- These factors resulted in his initial positive mood becoming more somber and depressing. A gradual but continual decline of his mental health had his wife at her wits' end. He had reached a point where he would stay in bed all day and not engage with his young kids or his wife.

- It reached an explosive climax when his wife kicked him out and said that she couldn't understand why he was so unhappy. He was alive, the tumor hadn't returned and he wasn't a quadriplegic. He was alive but he might as well have been dead, she reported bluntly.

- In spite of all of this, CJ was not suicidal. He was just sad and lacked motivation to do anything. He wasn't on any medications from a doctor for depression.

So, CJ moved to the Gold Coast (he had been living in Adelaide, South Australia) to live with his sister and that is how he met me. I told him that I was confident I could help with his neck pain/stiffness and headaches/migraines. I also said I could probably help with his depression/sadness and see if we could improve the feeling/function in his bowels, bladder and penis. What I was also keen to try on CJ was the chain-and-lock method on his four limbs.

CJ was happy for me to try to treat any of those areas. After explaining that I would prefer to focus on only two of those four options to start with (so that my treatment wasn't too diluted), CJ chose the neck/headaches and limbs as his priorities. If/when they improved, he was keen on working the emotions and bowel/bladder/penis functioning.

CJ was a robust and healthy individual apart from his obvious complaints. He was not a deficient patient, and therefore I was happy to work more aggressively on him than I might otherwise have done.

PP advised me against working locally on the neck, other than on the lateral edge. But this still meant I could use GB 20 and GB 12. After explaining to CJ that I could only do minimal work on his neck, I said that we could still treat his neck/headaches distally and work the chain-and-lock method at the same time. I asked which limbs he preferred me to start with and he chose the arms.

I also advised him that the process could take quite some time. CJ didn't care as long as he saw some small results on a fairly regular basis. This made sense as he had never had acupuncture before and didn't know me at all. CJ was unable to afford more than one treatment a week.

First of all I recommended six treatments for the arms – one chain and lock every week for six weeks on each of the six arm channels. I did the following.

CJ TREATMENT 1: CHAIN AND LOCK ON THE LARGE INTESTINE CHANNEL PLUS NECK/HEADACHE POINTS

The treatment is outlined in Table 7.9.

Table 7.9 CJ treatment 1

Location of points	Points	Reasoning
Head/face/neck	GB 14 GB 20[25]	Headaches Neck pain and headaches
Arms/hands	LI 4 LI 7 LI 10 LI 11 LI 14 LI 15 LU 7	Chain and lock, headaches Chain and lock Chain and lock Chain and lock Chain and lock Chain and lock Neck pain and headaches
Legs/feet	BL 60	Neck pain and headaches
Total points needled	20 needles used bilaterally	

I was able to stick with my whole-body style of treatment with points on the face, neck, arms and legs. I also used more needles than I normally would, but in this instance I was perfectly happy to do so.[26]

CJ TREATMENT 2: CHAIN AND LOCK ON THE SĀN JIĀO CHANNEL PLUS NECK/HEADACHE POINTS

Before I needled CJ, I asked him how the week had been. He advised me that he didn't get a single migraine but did suffer two headaches which were quickly alleviated by paracetamol. His neck stiffness had lessened, as had the pain. There was no change to his left arm; however, his right arm/hand were noticeably more 'buzzy, but in a good way'. There was, however, no change to his fine motor skills.

The treatment is outlined in Table 7.10.

Table 7.10 CJ treatment 2

Location of points	Points	Reasoning
Head/face/neck	M-HN-3 (Yìn Táng) GB 12[27]	Headaches Neck pain and headaches
Arms/hands	TE 4 TE 7 TE 9 TE 10 TE 12 TE 14 SI 3	Chain and lock Chain and lock Chain and lock Chain and lock Chain and lock Chain and lock Neck pain and headaches
Legs/feet	BL 60	Neck pain and headaches
Total points needled	19 needles used bilaterally	

CJ TREATMENT 3: CHAIN AND LOCK ON THE SMALL INTESTINE CHANNEL PLUS NECK/HEADACHE POINTS

Before I needled CJ, I asked him how the week had been. He advised me that he did get one migraine later on the same day as treatment 2. He said it was a 'whopper' and took nearly 16 hours to subside, during which time he took 12 codeine tablets. Other than that, he didn't suffer any migraines or headaches. His neck pain and stiffness had reduced by about 30%. There was no change to his left arm; however, his right arm/hand had improved. He felt there was a distinct change in his grip and proceeded to show me by picking up a pen on my desk. His arm also felt stronger and more alive.

The treatment is outlined in Table 7.11.

Table 7.11 CJ treatment 3

Location of points	Points	Reasoning
Head/face/neck	GB 14 GB 20	Headaches Neck pain and headaches
Arms/hands	SI 3 SI 6 SI 7 SI 8 Ā Shì point on Small Intestine channel midway between SI 8 and SI 10 SI 10 LI 4	Chain and lock, neck, headaches Chain and lock Chain and lock Chain and lock Chain and lock Chain and lock Headaches
Legs/feet	BL 62	Neck pain and headaches
Total points needled	20 needles used bilaterally	

Interestingly, SI 3 and BL 62 are also opening and coupled points for the Dū Mài and the Yáng Qiāo Mài. This aided CJ's spine and the lateral aspect of his whole body.

It is also worth noting that I did choose the Yáng channels on the arm first on purpose. They are typically more dynamic than their Yīn counterparts for obvious reasons, and I was looking for some sort of reaction fast for CJ so that he could believe in the treatment more.

CJ TREATMENT 4: CHAIN AND LOCK ON THE PERICARDIUM CHANNEL PLUS NECK/HEADACHE POINTS

Before I needled CJ, I asked him how the week had been. He advised me that he did get one headache but it was so minor he didn't even bother with any painkilling medication. His neck pain and stiffness had reduced by about 50%. There was no change to his left arm; however, his right arm/hand had improved further still. His grip had improved even more and he was now able to pick most things up (apart from tea cups). His fine motor skills had also improved. To prove the point, he wrote his name on the patient file; although it was messy, he told me it was a massive improvement on what he had been able to do since the operation. He was now hogging the television remote from his sister because he could push the correct buttons. His right arm also felt stronger and more alive.

The treatment is outlined in Table 7.12.

Table 7.12 CJ treatment 4

Location of points	Points	Reasoning
Head/face/neck	M-HN-3 (Yìn Táng) GB 12	Headaches Neck pain and headaches
Arms/hands	PC 2 PC 3 PC 4 PC 6 PC 7 LU 7	Chain and lock Chain and lock Chain and lock Chain and lock Chain and lock Neck pain and headaches
Legs/feet	BL 60 KI 6	Neck pain and headaches Combines with LU 7
Total points needled	19 needles used bilaterally	

Interestingly, LU 7 and KI 6 were also used as opening and coupled points for the Rèn Mài and the Yīn Qiāo Mài. This aided CJ's anterior trunk and medial aspect of his whole body.

It is also worth noting that quite a few of the points used in this treatment also worked on CJ's Shén, but this was not intentional as the chain-and-lock method was the priority.

CJ TREATMENT 5: CHAIN AND LOCK ON THE HEART
CHANNEL PLUS NECK/HEADACHE POINTS

Before I needled CJ, I asked him how the week had been. He advised me that he did get a migraine late on the same day of the fourth treatment. It wasn't as severe as the previous migraine and didn't last as long either (he took six codeine tablets).[28] His neck pain and stiffness had reduced by about 75%. There was no change to his left arm; however, his right arm/hand had improved further still. To prove his point, he gestured to his feet: he was wearing closed-in shoes with shoelaces. Every time I had seen CJ, he was wearing thongs/flip-flops. He undid a shoelace and then tied it up again. I noticed that it was far from fluid but he did it successfully.

How did he tie his shoes up with only one arm? For starters, he tied up the laces in two knots, rather than a knot and bow. He also used his opposite foot as a stabilizer for the laces. Trust me when I say it was fascinating to watch how CJ was adapting to his disorder.

The treatment is outlined in Table 7.13.

Table 7.13 CJ treatment 5

Location of points	Points	Reasoning
Head/face/neck	GB 14 GB 20	Headaches Neck pain and headaches
Arms/hands	HT 1 HT 2 HT 3 Ā Shì point on the Heart channel midway between HT 3 and HT 6 HT 6 SI 3	Chain and lock Chain and lock Chain and lock Chain and lock Chain and lock Neck pain and headaches
Legs/feet	BL 62	Neck pain and headaches
Total points needled	18 needles used bilaterally	

Interestingly, SI 3 and BL 62 were also used as opening and coupled points for the Dū Mài and the Yáng Qiāo Mài. This aided CJ's spine and the lateral aspect of his whole body.

It is also worth noting that quite a few of the points used in this treatment also worked on CJ's Shén, but this was not intentional as the chain-and-lock method was the priority.

CJ TREATMENT 6: CHAIN AND LOCK ON THE LUNG
CHANNEL PLUS NECK/HEADACHE POINTS

Before I needled CJ, I asked him how the week had been. He advised me that he hadn't had a single headache or migraine. His neck pain and stiffness had reduced by about 80%. There was no change to his left arm; however, his right arm/hand had improved further still. He was now able to hold a tea cup in his hand and his fine motor skills were also better than they had been since the surgery.

CJ also pointed out that he was feeling more at peace with himself and his situation. He was talking about wanting to go back to Adelaide and try to get his marriage back on track.

The treatment is outlined in Table 7.14.

Table 7.14 CJ treatment 6

Location of points	Points	Reasoning
Head/face/neck	GB 14 GB 20	Headaches Neck pain and headaches
Arms/hands	LU 1 LU 4 LU 5 LU 6 LU 7 LU 9 LI 4	Chain and lock Chain and lock Chain and lock Chain and lock Chain and lock, neck, headaches Chain and lock Headaches
Legs/feet	BL 60	Neck pain and headaches
Total points needled	20 needles used bilaterally	

CJ TREATMENTS 7–12

Before I needled CJ, I asked him how the week had been. He advised me that he hadn't had a single headache or migraine. His neck pain and stiffness had reduced by about 90%. There was no change to his left arm; however, his right arm/hand had improved further still. CJ was feeling the best he had felt in ages. He was looking forward to his legs being treated.

CJ treatment 7: chain and lock on the Stomach channel plus neck/headache points

The chain-and-lock method included ST 31, ST 32, ST 34, ST 36, ST 40 and ST 41.

CJ treatment 8: chain and lock on the Gall Bladder channel plus neck/headache points

The chain-and-lock method included GB 29, GB 31, GB 33, GB 34, GB 36 and GB 40.

CJ treatment 9: chain and lock on the Urinary Bladder channel plus neck/headache points

The chain-and-lock method included BL 36, BL 37, BL 40, BL 57, BL 60 and BL 63.

CJ treatment 10: chain and lock on the Spleen channel plus neck/headache points

The chain-and-lock method included SP 5, SP 6, SP 8, SP 10, SP 11 and SP 13.

CJ treatment 11: chain and lock on the Liver channel plus neck/headache points

The chain-and-lock method included LR 4, LR 6, LR 8, LR 9, Ā Shì on the Liver channel between LR 9 and LR 11, and LR 11.

CJ treatment 12: chain and lock on the Kidney channel plus neck/headache points

The chain-and-lock method included KI 3, KI 5, KI 9, KI 10, Ā Shì point on the Kidney channel between KI 10 and KI 11, and KI 11.

CJ treatments 7–12: additional information

Bilateral needling was performed.

The left arm was continually needled with the chain-and-lock combination but with no recognizable improvement.

His neck pain/stiffness and headaches/migraines were continually needled locally and distally.

The right arm continued to stay strong and so I did one more treatment on it in session 13. I chose the Large Intestine channel for pure Yáng power.

After the ninth treatment, CJ was virtually pain-free in his neck and only had stiffness associated with the surgery. He had only had one headache in three weeks and no migraines.

There was no change to his left arm; however, his right arm/hand continued to stay strong. CJ continued to feel better in himself emotionally. He had started a dialogue with his wife about moving back to Adelaide. The initial signs showed promise.

His legs had improved. There was more flexibility in the muscles but not much change in his hip, knee and ankle joints. But he definitely felt that his muscles were working harder. 'They have certainly gotten sorer but in a good way. Like after exercise,' he stated.

What was also interesting is that CJ's low functioning/sensation of the bowels and bladder had changed. He was now aware of some sensation in that area. This also included his erectile function. Even though we weren't treating this directly, CJ was still seeing benefit from the chain-and-lock method and other distal points.

CJ also relayed a funny event that happened to him after the ninth treatment. He was wearing shoes all the time to clinic now, and after he got off the table he felt like his legs were 'on fire, but in a good way'. He paid for his appointment, and instead of walking back to the train station to travel home he decided to walk to the local park which was beside a river. He was walking along and feeling so happy and fired up in the legs that he made an impromptu decision to run. CJ hadn't run in over two years (since before the operation) but he made that snap decision and he was running.

He made it about 50 meters before his awkward gait resulted in him tripping and he slammed face-first into the grass. His right hand had cushioned the blow somewhat. What happened next was priceless! He started laughing and laughing. He said he laughed so much, tears were running down his cheeks. He was laughing and rolling around in the grass. Some of the people in the park had seen him take a tumble, and when he didn't rise immediately, they went over to check he was okay. When they saw him laughing/crying, they were confused as to what was going on. One person said he was going to call an ambulance because he must have hit his head and was delirious. CJ was able to assure them all that he was okay and that he wasn't injured. Luckily, they believed him, and after a few more minutes he got up and walked back to my clinic to tell me what happened.

CJ POST-TREATMENT 12

By the end of the twelfth treatment CJ was a changed man. Other than the odd headache that didn't require medication, he only had the neck stiffness associated with the surgery. He had not had a single migraine in over two months.

There was no change to his left arm; however, his right arm/hand continued to stay strong. CJ was feeling fantastic in himself emotionally. He had booked a flight back to Adelaide to see his wife and kids for the first time in nearly six months. He was going to sleep in the spare bedroom initially and see if the marriage could work.

His legs had also improved. There was more flexibility in the muscles, and his joints were also more flexible. His awkward gait was virtually non-existent.

CJ's low functioning/sensation in the bowels and bladder had also completely changed. He was now aware of sensation in most of the area. His erectile function also seemed to be nearly back to normal. 'The only way to know for sure is to give it a proper test-out,' he laughed.

What I find amazing about this case is that CJ didn't get any direct treatment for his Shén, his bowels/bladder or for his erectile dysfunction. But the chain-and-lock points from the different channels worked on those aspects anyway. Therefore his treatment program, which initially looked as if it could be more than 20 treatments, ended up only being 13.

To date, CJ is still one of the more remarkable treatment results I have ever had in my acupuncture career over more than 20 years, and I must place a huge chunk of that success on the chain-and-lock method.

4. Bright Foyer, Watch Tower, Court, Fence and Shield

Huang Di said, 'The Bright Foyer is the nose. The Watch Tower is between the eyebrows. The Court is the forehead. The Fence is the cheek. The Shield refers to the area around the Ear Door [TE 21]. For these places and in between one would desire that they be correct and large, so that from ten paces all the externals can be seen. If they are like this it means long life and one must hit a hundred years.' (Wu 1993, p.172)

That quotation is from the 49th essay of *The Spiritual Pivot* (Líng Shū/靈樞) and it poses two interesting questions:

- Is the quotation referring to the areas of the face needing to look 'correct'?

- Does the quotation refer to an acupuncture point combination?

Let's look at each question a little more closely.

Is the quotation referring to the areas of the face needing to look 'correct'?

In all likelihood the answer to this question is yes. But in order for the Bright Foyer, Watch Tower, Court, Fence and Shield to look correct, doesn't that mean there should be an emphasis on that person's health? If so, we know that acupuncture can aid a person's health and wellbeing, so why not treat a patient using a point combination that can target those areas of the face? And, further, use points that can treat the organs that are representative of those areas of the face. Finally, if you have a healthy internal environment, then your external environment will shine bright; this includes your face.

When deciding on which channels to access, you can consider the following options:

- Use points on channels that travel to, or from, the face.

- Use points that regulate the Zàng Fǔ organs that open into the related sense organs.

- Use points that regulate the Zàng Fǔ organs that are mirrored on those areas of the face.

Each of these options needs to be discussed in a little more detail.

CHANNELS THAT TRAVEL TO/FROM THE FACE

The Three Arm Yáng channels of the Large Intestine, Small Intestine and Sān Jiāo travel up to the face before ending somewhere near a sense organ. The Three Leg Yáng channels of the Stomach, Gall Bladder and Urinary Bladder start near a sense organ and then travel away from the face.

It would make sense to target any of these six channels to treat the Bright Foyer, Watch Tower, Court, Fence and Shield.

Zàng Fǔ organs and their related sense organs[29]

The eyes are nourished by the Wood element organs of Liver and Gall Bladder. The tongue is nourished by the Fire element organs of Heart, Pericardium, Small Intestine and Sān Jiāo. The mouth is nourished by the Earth element organs of Spleen and Stomach. The nose and throat are nourished by the Metal element organs of Lung and Large Intestine. The ears are nourished by the Water element organs of Kidney and Urinary Bladder.

This discussion shows that potentially any of the main organs' channels could treat the Bright Foyer, Watch Tower, Court, Fence and Shield.

Zàng Fǔ organs and their mirrored areas on the face

This is not as straightforward as the previous two discussions. Different theories have been around over the past 2000-plus years as to what areas of the face are the mirror of the Zàng Fǔ organs. So, I have made an executive decision to use *The Spiritual Pivot*, which makes sense to me, especially as this point combination has been inspired by this very classic.

> The Central Watchtower is the lungs. The Lower Pivot which is between the eyes relates to the heart. Straight below, the bridge of the nose relates to the liver. To the left of the liver location is the gallbladder. Lower on the nose is the spleen. Squared and above [both sides of nostril] is the stomach. Right in the middle below the cheekbones is the large intestine. Clasping the large intestine position on the face from the sides are the kidneys... Above the King of the Face, the tip of the nose, on the cheekbones is the small intestine. Below the King of the Face, on a level with the philtrum, on the sides, are the locations of the bladder and reproductive organs. (Wu 1993, p.174)

As you can see from the discussion above, any of the Zàng Fǔ organs can be used for treating the Bright Foyer, Watch Tower, Court, Fence and Shield. But before we discuss a possible point combination, let's look at the other question posed earlier.

Does the quotation refer to an acupuncture point combination?

In all likelihood the answer to this question is 'No', especially considering there is no point combination provided for the Bright Foyer, Watch Tower, Court, Fence and Shield.

But what if the answer is actually yes? This would mean that the reader gets the name of the point combination, along with what it treats, but then isn't given the points for the combination. What a fascinating possibility!

Why do you think that might be? Most Chinese medicine classical experts suggest that *The Spiritual Pivot* wasn't written by just one person, and was in fact probably written by quite a few different people.[30] But that doesn't account for the fact that a point combination is labeled in name/title but no points are actually given.

Could it be that the points were a secret and only handed down to a particular practitioner's disciples? And that this same practitioner was also one of the authors of *The Spiritual Pivot* but didn't want to reveal his special point prescription to anyone who read the book? I haven't seen any commentary to suggest that this hypothesis is correct, so we shall have to just consider it a possibility.

Regardless of which question is correct, I have taken it upon myself to attempt two different point combinations for the Bright Foyer, Watch Tower, Court, Fence and Shield. Before I do so, I need to confirm with *The Spiritual Pivot* which areas of the head/face I need to target:[31]

- Bright Foyer – nose

- Watch Tower – between eyebrows, upper head, face and throat

- Court – forehead, upper head and face

- Fence – cheeks and mouth

- Shield – ears.

The original quotation (Wu 1993, p.172) also states: 'For these places and in between.' Therefore, we can comfortably say that the Bright Foyer, Watch Tower, Court, Fence and Shield point combination is attempting to treat the eyes, ears, nose, mouth, throat, face, head and any extra areas this entails.

What would the points be?

After giving it some thought, I have come up with two separate point combinations. These are hardly set in stone and could be edited somewhat to include some of your favorite points for those areas needing treatment. These two treatments are provided in Tables 7.15 and 7.16.

Table 7.15 Bright Foyer, Watch Tower, Court, Fence and Shield point combination example 1

Location of point	Point	Target
Head/face/neck	LI 20 M-HN-3 (Yìn Táng) GB 14 ST 6 TE 21	Bright Foyer Watch Tower and Bright Foyer Court Fence Shield
Arms/hands	LI 4 SI 4 TE 3	Bright Foyer, Watch Tower, Court, Fence and Shield Fence Shield
Legs/feet	LR 3 GB 41	Watch Tower Watch Tower and Court
Total points needled		19 needles used bilaterally[32]

Table 7.16 Bright Foyer, Watch Tower, Court, Fence and Shield point combination example 2

Location of point	Point	Reasoning
Head/face/neck	M-HN-14 (Bí Tōng) BL 2 ST 4 ST 8 GB 2	Bright Foyer Watch Tower and Bright Foyer Fence Court Shield
Arms/hands	LI 5 SI 3	Bright Foyer and Court Fence and Shield
Legs/feet	GB 37 GB 42 ST 36	Watch Tower Shield Court
Total points needled		20 needles used bilaterally[33]

Can we call the point combinations the Bright Foyer, Watch Tower, Court, Fence and Shield?

Why not? If we have gone to the trouble of constructing a point prescription for the Bright Foyer, Watch Tower, Court, Fence and Shield, then we should be able to call it that if we want – especially when the combination didn't come with a prescription to begin with.

Even if *The Spiritual Pivot* had provided a point prescription, you have seen enough examples throughout this book (with plenty more to follow) where alternative point combinations have been provided. Which, in my opinion, is perfectly okay because it's free thinking, and that is what this book is all about.

Notes

1 Feng and English 2008, p.159. Zhuāng Zǐ (369–286 BCE) is quite possibly the second most famous ancient Daoist, behind only Lǎo Zǐ. This is primarily because of the book he wrote that was named after him. In my opinion his book was a lot easier to follow than the Lǎo Zǐ text, the *Dào Dé Jīng*, which was full of riddles.

2 Galileo Galilei (1564–1642 CE), or Galileo, as he is generally referred to, is considered to be the father of modern science. But he was also interested in astronomy, cosmology, mathematics and philosophy. The quotation was obtained from www.azquotes.com/author/5284-Galileo_Galilei.

3 Ni 1995, p.19: 5th chapter. *The Yellow Emperor's Classic (Inner Canon of the Yellow Emperor/Huáng Dì Nèi Jīng)* was written somewhere between 200 and 0 BCE.

4 Maciocia 2015, p.23.

5 Hartmann 2009, pp.45, 56, 59, 64, 102, 139, 156, 170–172; Hicks *et al.* 2010, pp.311, 339.

6 Beinfield and Korngold 1991; Dechar 2006; Franglen 2014, pp.19–23, 28–46, 150–162; Hicks *et al.* 2010; Maciocia 2009, pp.1–113; Rossi 2007, pp.47–69.

7 The Hún is directly responsible for our inspiration and dreaming. In the Hún we have access to unlimited dreaming; therefore, we can 'dream big'. The Pò is directly responsible for taking our dreams and actioning them, and this action is virtually limitless; therefore, we can 'do big'. But the Pò also needs to rest sometimes so that it can recharge. This is where we can simply be, and this is why it's also called 'be big'. This could also be termed as Wú Wèi.

8 Beinfield and Korngold 1991; Dechar 2006; Franglen 2014, pp.19–23, 28–46, 150–162; Hicks *et al.* 2010; Maciocia 2009, pp.1–113; Rossi 2007, pp.47–69.

9 Deadman *et al.* 2007, pp.83, 158–161, 189–191, 501, 505, 511, 514, 517–518, 521; Maciocia

2015, pp.897, 954, 985–987, 1000–1001, 1090–1091, 1132, 1134, 1139, 1141, 1143.

10 Deadman *et al.* 2007, pp.87, 219–220, 267, 270, 275–276, 278–280, 282–285, 298, 339–341; Maciocia 2015, pp.956–957, 1010–1012, 1034–1035, 1037–1043, 1047, 1065.

11 Bertschinger 2013, pp.153–154; Deadman *et al.* 2007, pp.60, 105; Ross 1995, p.51.

12 This quotation is from *The Great Compendium – Volumes II and III* (*The Great Compendium of Acupuncture and Moxibustion*/Zhēn Jiǔ Dà Chéng).

13 O'Connor and Bensky 1981, pp.233–234, 249–250.

14 Ross 1995, p.64.

15 There are opposing views on this, so if you have an alternative view and it's working for you, then stick with what you know.

16 Phillips 2017, pp.55–70.

17 There are opposing views on this, so if you have an alternative view and it's working for you, then stick with what you know.

18 Phillips 2017, pp.55–70.

19 Deadman *et al.* (2007, pp.450–452) reference the *Ode to Elucidate Mysteries*/Biāo Yōu Fù, which was first recorded in *The Guide to Acupuncture and Moxibustion*/Zhēn Jiǔ Zhǐ Nán and was written in 1241 CE.

20 Ellis *et al.* 1991, p.321.

21 Ibid., p.131.

22 O'Connor and Bensky 1981, p.233.

23 Ellis *et al.* 1991, pp.97–98.

24 Ellis *et al.* (1989, pp.45–46, 90–91) say: 'The name of this point [LI 10] is closely related to that of ST-36, Leg Three Li… An oral tradition has it that in ancient times, when the primary means of travel was on foot, stimulation of ST-36 was thought to relieve fatigue sufficient to allow one to journey another three li.' Therefore, if we were to take the first statement that says LI 10 (Shǒu Sān Lǐ) has a similar name to ST 36 (Zú Sān Lǐ), and we merge that with the second statement, it could suggest that arm fatigue would be reduced enough to allow for extra work to be carried out. The amount of extra time this point could generate would be dictated by how long it takes to walk three Lǐ. This could be as much as two or more hours of reduced arm fatigue.

25 GB 20 can be needled with the patient laying face up. With them lying down, you turn their head to one side and needle the point obliquely, ensuring the needle handle lies flat against the pillow when they turn their head back to the center position. Repeat for the other side. These needles will now be hidden from view, so don't forget to take them out at the end of the appointment.

26 Every treatment on CJ ended up being a higher needle count than I would normally use on a patient. This was a conscious decision on my part as I felt CJ could handle it. That decision turned out to be the right one.

27 GB 12 can be needled with the patient laying face up. With them lying down, you turn their head to one side and needle the point obliquely, ensuring the needle handle lies flat against the pillow when they turn their head back to the center position. Repeat for the other side. These needles will now be hidden from view, so don't forget to take them out at the end of the appointment.

28 This has happened before and since my treatments with CJ, and M-HN-3 (Yìn Táng) seems to be the culprit when a migraine appears the same day as the treatment. If this scenario occurs in my clinic these days I tend to avoid using M-HN-3 (Yìn Táng) on those patients. This is, however, rare and I love using M-HN-3 (Yìn Táng) for problems in the local area and for Shén-based disorders.

29 Kaptchuk 2000, p.439; Maciocia 2015, p.26.

30 Wu 1993, pp.xi–xii. *The Spiritual Pivot* (Líng Shū) was written somewhere between 200 and 0 BCE.

31 Wu 1993, pp.172–174: 49th chapter.

32 This point combination uses 19 needles, which is possibly at the high end of what you might use in a treatment. If that is the case, then consider splitting the treatment into two separate treatments a few days apart.

33 This point combination uses 20 needles, which is possibly at the high end of what you might use in a treatment. If that is the case, then consider splitting the treatment into two separate treatments a few days apart.

Part 3

Wǔ Xíng/Five Elements Point Category and Acupuncture Point Combinations

The task of the humane is surely to seek to promote the benefit of all the world and eliminate harm to all the world, and to take this as a standard (fa) in the world. Does something benefit people? Then do it. Does it not benefit people? Then stop.

Mò Zǐ/墨子 (470–391 BCE)[1]

Welcome to Part 3 of *The Principles and Practical Application of Acupuncture Point Combinations*. Over the next three chapters I will be taking you on a journey through the Wǔ Xíng/Five Elements. We will start with a quick overview outlining the way the Wǔ Xíng operate in health, which is similar to the quotation above.

The goal of the Wǔ Xíng is to ensure the health of the world by the elimination of harm (within a person's microcosmic world) and to keep this as a standard which, in the Wǔ Xíng, is the proper operation of the Shēng/Generating and Kè/Controlling cycles.

Throughout the three chapters we will work our way through a range of acupuncture point combinations, finishing with the more advanced content.

Note

1   Mou 2009, p.148. Mò Zǐ (470–391 BCE) was the founder of the Mohist school of philosophy which thrived during the Warring States Period (475–221 BCE) in China. He was all about Universal love, which juxtaposed beautifully with the massive civil war that was occurring in China at the time. Fǎ (法) is typically translated as model or standard.

Each of the Five Elements circulates according to its sequence; each of them exercises its own capacities in the performance of its official duties.

Dǒng Zhòng-shū/董仲舒 (179–104 BCE)[1]

The world had that from which it began
And this is taken as the mother of the world.
After you have got the mother
You can in turn know the son.
After you have known the son
Go back to abiding by the mother,
And to the end of your days you will not meet with danger.

Lǎo Zǐ/老子 (6th century BCE)[2]

8

Wǔ Xíng/Five Elements Point Category – Introductory Concepts

The next three chapters take a look at the Wǔ Xíng or Five Elements,[3] and how you can use them to construct acupuncture point combinations. I have split it into three chapters partly because of the size, but also because of the fact that the Wǔ Xíng has so many different aspects that can be discussed. Therefore, I have split the chapters up into concepts that are introductory (Chapter 8), intermediate (Chapter 9) and advanced (Chapter 10).

1. Introduction to the Wǔ Xíng/Five Elements

> The Chinese world view permits the simultaneous existence of seemingly conflicting theories, thus allowing for the selection of the particular theory that is best suited to cope with specific conditions. In point selection, this leaves practitioners free to choose five-phase correspondences when it seems appropriate to do so, and to ignore them when it seems to conflict with their clinical experience. (Ellis *et al.* 1991, p.438)

Using the Wǔ Xíng/Five Elements in clinical practice is another fascinating look into a varied and often conflicting Chinese medicine system. We aren't just talking about the Wǔ Xíng conflicting with other special point categories or other systems. We are also talking about the Wǔ Xíng conflicting with itself.

This might suggest that the Wǔ Xíng can't work in all of the varied ways people use them, because if one way is right, then the other ways must be wrong. But here's the kicker: in Wǔ Xíng theory and practice, more than one answer can be correct.

Should we really be surprised to hear that, though? After all, Wǔ Xíng theory has been around for more than 2500 years, originating as a philosophical school founded during the Warring States Period (472–221 BCE).[4] Several hundred years after the philosophical school was formed, the first book on Chinese medicine was written. It was called *The Yellow Emperor's Classic* (*Inner Canon of the Yellow Emperor*/Huáng Dì Nèi Jīng/黃帝內經) and it discussed the Wǔ Xíng consistently throughout.

Wǔ Xíng theory has remained prominent in Chinese medicine ever since. Therefore, we have more than 2000 years of Chinese medical theory to sift through, and not all of this theory complements the rest. One of the reasons for this would be the evolution of Wǔ Xíng theory during that time.

Another possible explanation would be the millions of Chinese medicine practitioners who have been practicing/mentoring/writing about the medicine. During the treatments of patients, they would have formulated their own unique treatment style that worked for them.

Yet another explanation is the different areas in China where the practitioners lived and practiced. The differing geographical and climactic locations would have required very different treatment styles. For example, diseases were different in northern China compared with southern China. Therefore, the treatment methods would have been vastly different.[5]

So which theory is correct? Is there only one answer or can there be multiple answers to the one question? When we decide to use one particular type of Wǔ Xíng treatment, we are focusing on one aspect of that theory to the detriment of another. This doesn't necessarily mean we wouldn't consider a different Wǔ Xíng approach next time. It just means we didn't this time!

Before we get to the various special point categories for the Wǔ Xíng, we need to discuss briefly the basics of the Five Elements. Of particular interest are:

- the Shēng/Generating cycle
- the Kè/Controlling cycle
- the Chéng/Overacting cycle
- the Wǔ/Insulting cycle.

Shēng/Generating cycle

In the Shēng cycle, each element generates another but is also generated by one, which looks like this: Fire generates Earth, Earth generates Metal, Metal generates Water, Water generates Wood and Wood generates Fire.[6] In that manner, each of the Wǔ Xíng will aid the next element, but will also be aided by the previous one. For example, Fire generates Earth, but Fire is generated by Wood. See Diagram 8.1.

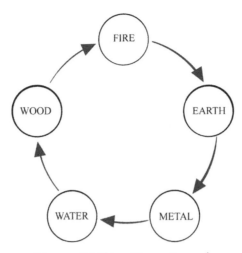

Diagram 8.1 Shēng/Generating cycle

Mother and Child (originally translated as 'Mother and Son') theory aligns with the Shēng cycle. Just like animals in nature, the term refers to the Mother element feeding/nourishing/generating its Child element. In its most basic form, we use this term to describe the close relationship between the elements that are beside each other.

If we use the same example we just applied, Fire is the Mother of Earth because Fire generates Earth; but Fire is the Child of Wood because Fire is generated by Wood.

The Shēng cycle is often used in clinical practice for patients with chronic and gradually forming disorders. See Chapter 9 for a more detailed discussion on this.

This is a somewhat generalized statement because there are alternative views on this, but for the sake of the special point categories to be discussed shortly, this is the theory we will apply to the Shēng cycle.

Kè/Controlling cycle

In the Kè cycle, each element controls another but is also controlled by one, which looks like this: Fire controls Metal, Metal controls Wood, Wood controls Earth, Earth controls Water and Water controls Fire.[7] In that manner, each of the Wǔ Xíng will regulate the next element, but will also be regulated by the previous one. For example, Fire controls Metal, but Fire is controlled by Water. See Diagram 8.2.

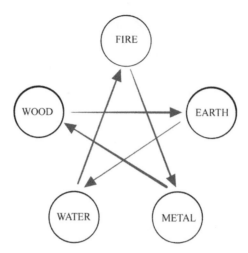

Diagram 8.2 Kè/Controlling cycle

Mother and Child theory can be applied to the Kè cycle, as it is in the Shēng cycle.

If we use the same example we just applied, Fire is the Mother of Metal because Fire controls Metal; Fire is the Child of Water because Fire is controlled by Water.

The Kè cycle is often used in clinical practice for patients with acute disorders. See Chapter 9 for a more detailed discussion on this.

This is a somewhat generalized statement because there are alternative views on this, but for the sake of the special point categories discussed below, this is the theory we will apply to the Kè cycle.

Chéng/Overacting cycle

The Chéng cycle tracks along the same pathway as the Kè cycle. But rather than control/regulate the next element, the Chéng over-controls or overacts on the next element. This will cause the next element to become deficient/Xū, because it isn't being regulated by its Mother.

That would look like this: Fire overacts on Metal, Metal overacts on Wood, Wood overacts on Earth, Earth overacts on Water and Water overacts on Fire.[8] In that manner, each of the Wǔ Xíng can overact on the next element, but can also be overacted on by the previous one. For example, Fire overacts on Metal, but Fire can be overacted on by Water. See Diagram 8.3.

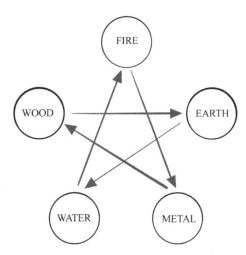

Diagram 8.3 Chéng/Overacting cycle

Mother and Child theory can also be applied to the Chéng cycle, as it is in the Shēng cycle.

If we use the same example we just applied, Fire is the Mother of Metal because Fire controls Metal. In this instance, however, the Mother (Fire) won't feed the Child (Metal) because they are keeping what they have for themselves, resulting in the Child (Metal) becoming Xū.

Also, don't forget that Fire is the Child of Water because Fire is controlled by Water. In this instance the Child (Fire) won't be fed by the Mother (Water) and this will lead to Xū in the Child (Fire).

The Chéng cycle is often used in clinical practice to describe an imbalance between two or more organs/elements.[9] Again, this is a somewhat generalized statement because there are alternative views on this. See Chapter 10 for a more thorough analysis of the Chéng cycle and acupuncture point combinations.

Wǔ/Insulting cycle

The Wǔ cycle tracks along the same pathway as the Kè cycle but in the opposite direction. Therefore, rather than the Kè cycle controlling/regulating the next element, the Wǔ insults the previous element. This will cause the previous element to become Deficient/Xū, because it is being insulted by its Child.

That would look like this: Fire insults Water, Water insults Earth, Earth insults Wood, Wood insults Metal and Metal insults Fire.[10] In that manner, each of the Wǔ Xíng can insult the previous element, but can also be insulted by the next one. For example, Fire insults Water, but Fire can be insulted by Metal. See Diagram 8.4.

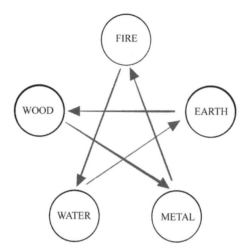

Diagram 8.4 Wŭ/Insulting cycle

If we use the same example we just applied, Fire is the Mother of Metal because Fire controls Metal. In this instance, however, the Mother (Fire) is being continually harassed by the Child (Metal) because the Child wants more than they already have. This will result in the Mother (Fire) becoming Xū.

Also, don't forget that Fire is the Child of Water because Fire is controlled by Water. In this instance the Child (Fire) will continually harass the Mother (Water) and this will lead to Xū in the Mother (Water).

The Wŭ cycle is often used in clinical practice to describe an imbalance between two or more organs/elements.[11] Again, this is a somewhat generalized statement because there are alternative views on this. See Chapter 10 for a more thorough analysis of the Wŭ cycle and acupuncture point combinations.

2. Wŭ Xíng Shū/Transporting points

The Five Shū/Transporting points were first mentioned in the 1st essay of *The Spiritual Pivot* (Líng Shū/靈樞).[12] They are a collection of five points on each of the twelve main channels which are all located between the elbows and fingers or the knees and toes. In clinical practice they are considered to be a very important special point category. They are called:

- Jǐng Well

- Yíng Spring

- Shù (Transport)[13] Stream

- Jīng (Flow)[14] River

- Hé (Unite)[15] Sea.

As you can see by their names, they have been referred to via the analogy of a flowing river – from the beginning at the top of a mountain in a well, onwards to a small spring, then a slightly larger stream as its flows down the mountain, picking up speed, on to a larger river with more power, before concluding at the river mouth meeting the sea. This analogy isn't just pretty Chinese poetry – there is substance to the flow, which will be discussed in more detail shortly.

Each of the Five Shū/Transporting points works on slightly different clinical applications as a result of being a different part of the river system: from the dynamic and fast-acting Jǐng Well points to the slower and deeper-flowing Hé (Unite) Sea points.

The 1st essay of *The Spiritual Pivot* also included the Yuán Source points (for both the Yīn and Yáng organs) as being a small part of the Shū/Transporting system of points. The Yuán Source points are the same as the Shù (Transport) Stream points on the Yīn channels, but the Yáng Yuán Source points are not. Table 8.1 lists the Yuán Source points.

Table 8.1 Yuán Source points[16]

Zàng Fǔ organs	Yuán Source points
Lung	LU 9
Heart	HT 7
Pericardium	PC 7
Spleen	SP 3
Kidney	KI 3
Liver	LR 3
Large Intestine	LI 4
Small Intestine	SI 4
Sān Jiāo	TE 4
Stomach	ST 42
Urinary Bladder	BL 64
Gall Bladder	GB 40

Before we discuss each of the Five Shū/Transporting points individually, I need to mention another contradiction in Chinese medicine. In Five Shū/Transporting theory, the flow of Qì is from the fingers to the elbows and the toes to the knees, whereas in channel theory not every channel flows that way. As we know, the Three Arm Yīn channels send Qì from the trunk to the fingers, and the Three Leg Yáng channels send Qì from the head to the toes. Personally, I'm not fussed about this and agree with what Deadman *et al.* (2007, pp.30–31) say:

> Whilst these two different perceptions of channel flow are another example of the readiness of Chinese medicine to embrace contradictory theories, we can say that

the direction of flow in the five shu-point theory is not as important as the quality of energy described at each of the points.

The Five Shū/Transporting points are listed in Table 8.2.

Table 8.2 Five Shū/Transporting points[17]

Zàng Fǔ channels	Jǐng Well point	Yíng Spring point	Shù (Transport) Stream point	Jīng (Flow) River point	Hé (Unite) Sea point
Lung	LU 11	LU 10	LU 9	LU 8	LU 5
Heart	HT 9	HT 8	HT 7	HT 4	HT 3
Pericardium	PC 9	PC 8	PC 7	PC 5	PC 3
Spleen	SP 1	SP 2	SP 3	SP 5	SP 9
Kidney	KI 1	KI 2	KI 3	KI 7	KI 10
Liver	LR 1	LR 2	LR 3	LR 4	LR 8
Large Intestine	LI 1	LI 2	LI 3	LI 5	LI 11
Small Intestine	SI 1	SI 2	SI 3	SI 5	SI 8
Sān Jiāo	TE 1	TE 2	TE 3	TE 6	TE 10
Stomach	ST 45	ST 44	ST 43	ST 41	ST 36
Urinary Bladder	BL 67	BL 66	BL 65	BL 60	BL 40
Gall Bladder	GB 44	GB 43	GB 41	GB 38	GB 34

Some of the classical theories on the use of the five shu-points are contradictory, some are scarcely borne out by clinical practice, and in some cases important clinical uses of these points are not referred to in the classical theories. (Deadman *et al.* 2007, p.32)

Bearing that previous statement in mind, the following are the different clinical applications for each of the Five Shū/Transporting points. Each of them treats quite a variety of disorders, some that are directly referred to in the classics, in particular *The Spiritual Pivot* and *The Classic of Difficulties* (*Canon of the Yellow Emperor's Eighty-One Difficult Issues*/Huáng Dì Bā Shí Yī Nán Jīng/黄帝八十一難經), and some that are more modern findings.

Jǐng Well points

The 1st essay in *The Spiritual Pivot* says, 'The point at which the qi emanates is known as the jing-well.'[18]

Jǐng translates as a 'water well'.[19]

All of the Jǐng Well points are located at the ends of fingers or toes, apart from KI 1, which is located under the foot. They are also the first or last points on their respective channels (see Table 8.2).

In no particular order, the Jǐng Well points can:[20]

- clear heat including acute fevers or internal organ heat

- restore consciousness

- work on the highest portion of the channel

- treat fullness below the Heart

- regulate the Shén – including irritability, mental restlessness/confusion, anxiety, insomnia/nightmares, manic depression, mania/hysteria

- treat diseases of the Yīn organs

- treat convulsions

- move stagnant Qì in the channels and organs

- tonify Yáng Xū in the organs

- clear External Pathogenic Factors

- expel Wind.

Of all the varied conditions/disorders that the Jǐng Well points treat, I would like to give one acupuncture point combination.

For frustration due to Liver Qì Stagnation, use the Jǐng Well point LR 1 along with LR 14.[21]

To make it a more thorough and balanced treatment, I would also include LR 3 as it's the Yuán Source point and can always be used in Five Shū/Transporting treatments. I would also consider GB 34, PC 6, LI 4 and GV 20 to round out the treatment.[22]

That gives a treatment with points on the legs/feet, arms/hands, trunk (front) and head for a total of 13 points if needled bilaterally.

Yíng Spring points

The 1st essay in *The Spiritual Pivot* says, 'The point at which the qi glides is known as the ying-spring.'[23]

Yíng translates as 'spring or pool'.[24]

All of the Yíng Spring points are located on the hands or feet. They are also the second or second-to-last points on their respective channels (see Table 8.2).

In no particular order, the Yíng Spring points can:[25]

- clear heat

- treat diseases of the Yáng channels

- treat diseases of the Yīn organs

- treat changes in complexion

- treat convulsions

- restore consciousness

- clear Internal or External Pathogenic Factors.

Of all the varied conditions/disorders that the Yíng Spring points treat, I would like to give one acupuncture point combination.

For clearing heat due to Stomach Fire Blazing, use the Yíng Spring point ST 44 along with ST 21, ST 36, CV 12, LI 4 and LI 11.[26]

I would also include ST 42 as it is the Yuán Source point and can always be used in Five Shū/Transporting treatments.

That gives a treatment with points on the legs/feet, arms/hands and trunk (front) with a total of 13 points if needled bilaterally.

Shù (Transport) Stream points

The 1st essay in *The Spiritual Pivot* says, 'The point at which the qi pours through is known as the shu-stream.'[27]

Shù translates as 'to transport'.[28]

All of the Shù (Transport) Stream points are located on the hands or feet. They are also the third or third-to-last points on their respective channels with the exception of the Gall Bladder channel, where it is the fourth point (GB 41) from the end of the channel (see Table 8.2).

Interestingly, all of the Yīn channel Shù (Transport) Stream points are also their Yuán Source points, making them very powerful points indeed.[29]

In no particular order, the Shù (Transport) Stream points can treat:[30]

- diseases of the Yīn organs

- diseases of the Yáng channels

- Bì syndrome (painful obstruction syndrome), particularly Damp Bì (but can treat all types) – including heaviness of the body and painful joints

- intermittent diseases – for example, malaria

- chronic diseases

- Damp or Phlegm.

Of all the varied conditions/disorders that the Shù (Transport) Stream points treat, I would like to give one acupuncture point combination.

For treating Damp Bì in the left knee due to Spleen and Kidney Yáng Xu, use the Shù (Transport) Stream points SP 3 and KI 3 respectively. These two points also happen to be the Yuán Source points for their respective organs, which can always be used in Five Shù/Transporting treatments.

I would also consider using some local left knee points such as SP 9, SP 10, ST 34, ST 36, MN-LE-16 (Xī Yǎn) and BL 40.[31]

To ensure that I also treat the Root/Běn of Spleen and Kidney Yáng Xū, I would include CV 4, CV 6, CV 9, CV 12, BL 20, BL 22, BL 23 and GV 4.[32]

This is quite possibly too many needles for one treatment, so I would split them across two treatments a few days apart – one face up and one face down, as shown in Tables 8.3 and 8.4.

Table 8.3 Shù (Transport) Stream treatment: Session 1 – face up

Location of point	Points	
Trunk (front)	CV 4 CV 6	CV 9 CV 12
Legs/feet	SP 3 SP 9 SP 10 KI 3	ST 34 ST 36 MN-LE-16 (Xī Yǎn)
Total points needled	20 needles used bilaterally	

Table 8.4 Shù (Transport) Stream treatment: Session 2 – face down

Location of point	Points	
Trunk (back)	BL 20 BL 22	BL 23 GV 4
Legs/feet	SP 3 SP 9 SP 10	KI 3 ST 36 BL 40
Total points needled	19 needles used bilaterally	

Jīng (Flow) River points

The 1st essay in *The Spiritual Pivot* says, 'The point at which the qi flows through is known as the jing-river.'[33]

Jīng translates as 'flow or pass'.[34]

All of the Jīng (Flow) River points are located on the wrists/forearms or ankles/lower legs. Unlike the previous three Shū/Transporting point groups, there is no consistent numbering system for the Jīng (Flow) River points (see Table 8.2).

In no particular order, the Jīng (Flow) River points can treat:[35]

- Lung disorders including cough, asthma or dyspnea

- chills and fevers/hot and cold sensations

- disorders of the voice

- diseases of the bones and tendons.

Of all the varied conditions/disorders that the Jīng (Flow) River points treat, I would like to give one acupuncture point combination.

For asthma and wheezing due to Lung Yīn Xū, use the Jīng (Flow) River point LU 8 along with LU 5, CV 17, BL 13, BL 43, KI 6 and HT 6.[36]

I would also include LU 9 as it is the Yuán Source point and can always be used in Five/Shū Transporting treatments.

That gives a treatment with points on the arms/hands, legs/feet, trunk (front) and trunk (back) with a total of 15 points if needled bilaterally.

Hé (Unite) Sea points

The 1st essay in *The Spiritual Pivot* says, 'The point at which the qi enters inwards is known as the he-sea.'[37]

Hé translates as 'to unite or join'.[38]

All of the Hé (Unite) Sea points are located on the elbows or knees. Similar to the Jīng (Flow) River, there is no consistent numbering system for the Hé (Unite) Sea points (see Table 8.2).

In no particular order, the Hé (Unite) Sea points can treat:[39]

- disorders of the Stomach, Small Intestine and Large Intestine

- counterflow Qì (Spleen Qì Sinking) leading to diarrhea

- disorders from poor eating and drinking

- diseases of the Yáng organs

- skin disorders

- cold expulsion

Of all the varied conditions/disorders that the Hé (Unite) Sea points treat, I would like to give one acupuncture point combination.

For itchiness and red-hot skin rashes due to Toxic Heat in the Xuè, use the Hé (Unite) Sea points LI 11, BL 40, PC 3, TE 10 and GB 34.[40]

I probably wouldn't worry about the Yuán Source points in this instance as there are already ten needles if done bilaterally. Instead, I would likely include M-LE-34 (Bǎi Chóng Wō), GB 31 and HT 7 for itchiness.[41]

That gives a treatment with points on the arms/hands and legs/feet with a total of 16 points if needled bilaterally.

3. Wǔ Xíng points

The Wǔ Xíng points are Wood, Fire, Earth, Metal and Water. Each of the twelve main channels has these points located on their channels between the elbows and fingers or the knees and toes.

The Yīn channels start at Wood and the Yáng at Metal, as confirmed by the 64th difficulty (Unschuld 1986, p.554) of *The Classic of Difficulties* (*Canon of the Yellow Emperor's Eighty-One Difficult Issues*/Huáng Dì Bā Shí Yī Nán Jīng/ 黃帝八十一難經), which states, 'The yin [Jǐng] wells are wood; the yang [Jǐng] wells are metal.'

As with the Five Shū/Transporting theory (discussed in Section 2 above), the flow of Qì is from the fingers to the elbows and the toes to the knees, whereas in channel theory not every channel flows that way. This obviously contradicts the normal channel flow for six of the twelve channels.

The six Yīn channels start their journey at the fingers/toes with the Wood point and move onwards to the Fire, Earth and Metal points before finishing with the Water point at the elbows/knees.

The six Yáng channels start their journey at the fingers/toes with the Metal point and move onwards to the Water, Wood and Fire points before finishing with the Earth point at the elbows/knees.

The Wǔ Xíng points are shown in Tables 8.5 and 8.6.

Table 8.5 Yīn Channel Five Element points[42]

Yīn channels	Wood point	Fire point	Earth point	Metal point	Water point
Lung	LU 11	LU 10	LU 9	LU 8	LU 5
Heart	HT 9	HT 8	HT 7	HT 4	HT 3
Pericardium	PC 9	PC 8	PC 7	PC 5	PC 3
Spleen	SP 1	SP 2	SP 3	SP 5	SP 9
Kidney	KI 1	KI 2	KI 3	KI 7	KI 10
Liver	LR 1	LR 2	LR 3	LR 4	LR 8

Table 8.6 Yáng Channel Five Element points[43]

Yáng channels	Metal point	Water point	Wood point	Fire point	Earth point
Large Intestine	LI 1	LI 2	LI 3	LI 5	LI 11
Small Intestine	SI 1	SI 2	SI 3	SI 5	SI 8
Sān Jiāo	TE 1	TE 2	TE 3	TE 6	TE 10
Stomach	ST 45	ST 44	ST 43	ST 41	ST 36
Urinary Bladder	BL 67	BL 66	BL 65	BL 60	BL 40
Gall Bladder	GB 44	GB 43	GB 41	GB 38	GB 34

The Wǔ Xíng points can be used for:

- treating the elements' related pathogen disorders
- treating multiple organ/channel disharmonies.

Treating the elements' related pathogen disorders

At the simplest level they work like this:[44]

- Wood points treat Wood element disorders including External or Internal Wind.

- Fire points treat Fire element disorders including External or Internal Heat/Fire.

- Earth points treat Earth element disorders including External or Internal Dampness.

- Metal points treat Metal element disorders; they don't treat Internal Dryness.

- Water points treat Water element disorders including External or Internal Cold.

Treat multiple organ/channel disharmonies

There are so many different possibilities depending on what diagnostic framework you use. I have listed seven Zàng Fǔ patterns of disharmony examples below.

Using the Metal point on the Kidney channel (KI 7) and the Water point on the Lung channel (LU 5) for asthma and wheezing (poor respiration) due to Lung Qì Xū and Kidney Yáng Xū

The Lungs belong to the Metal element, and the Kidneys belong to the Water element. Therefore, using this Shēng/Generating cycle combination ensures that the two organs directly responsible for strong breathing are strengthened by their connection (Diagram 8.5). This point combination can also be used to tonify Lung Qì and Kidney Yáng.

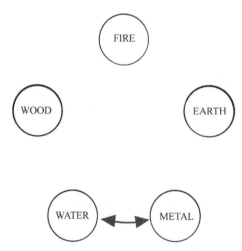

Diagram 8.5 Metal and Water Shēng/Generating cycle relationship

Using the Earth point on the Large Intestine channel (LI 11) and the Metal point on the Stomach channel (ST 45) for diverticulitis caused by Yáng Míng Fire Blazing

The Large Intestine belongs to the Metal element, and the Stomach belongs to the Earth element. Therefore, using this Shēng/Generating cycle combination ensures that the two organs directly affected by excess Fire are sedated with this connection (Diagram 8.6). This should also have a positive effect on the patient's diverticulitis.

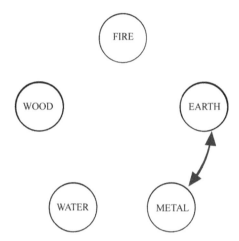

Diagram 8.6 Metal and Earth Shēng/Generating cycle relationship

Using the Fire point on the Kidney channel (KI 2) and the Water point on the Heart channel (HT 3) for menopause symptoms including night sweats and hot flushes/flashes due to Heart and Kidney Yīn Xū

The Kidneys belong to the Water element, and the Heart belongs to the Fire element. Therefore, using this Kè/Controlling cycle combination ensures that the two organs directly affected by Yīn Xū are tonified with this connection (Diagram 8.7). This should help reduce the menopause symptoms including hot flushes/flashes and night sweats.

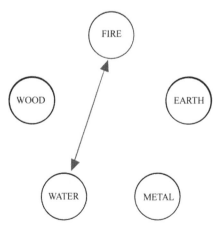

Diagram 8.7 Water and Fire Kè/Controlling cycle relationship

Using the Fire point on the Gall Bladder channel (GB 38) and the Wood point on the Heart channel (HT 9) for timidity, shyness, fear and anxiety due to Heart Xuè Xū and Gall Bladder Xū

The Gall Bladder belongs to the Wood element, and the Heart belongs to the Fire element. Therefore, using this Shēng/Generating cycle combination (Diagram 8.8) ensures that the two organs directly affected by their deficiencies/Xū are tonified. This should also help with the timidity, shyness, fear and anxiety.

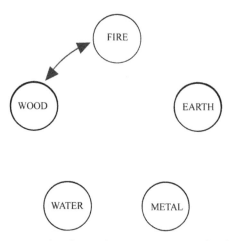

Diagram 8.8 Wood and Fire Shēng/Generating cycle relationship

Using the Metal point on the Spleen channel (SP 5) and the Earth point on the Lung channel (LU 9) for breathlessness, fatigue and tiredness due to Spleen and Lung Qì Xū

The Spleen belongs to the Earth element, and the Lungs belong to the Metal element. Therefore, using this Shēng/Generating cycle combination (Diagram 8.9) ensures that the two organs directly affected by Qì Xū are tonified with this connection, which should help correct the breathlessness, fatigue and tiredness.

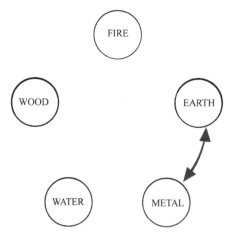

Diagram 8.9 Metal and Earth Shēng/Generating cycle relationship

Using the Fire point on the Urinary Bladder channel (BL 60) and the Water point on the Small Intestine channel (SI 2) for Full Heat in the Small Intestine leading to Damp Heat in the Urinary Bladder causing an acute urinary tract infection

The Urinary Bladder belongs to the Water element, and the Small Intestine belongs to the Fire element. Therefore, using this Kè/Controlling cycle combination (Diagram 8.10) ensures that the two organs directly affected by excess Fire and Damp are sedated with this connection. This should also have a positive effect on the patient's urinary tract infection.

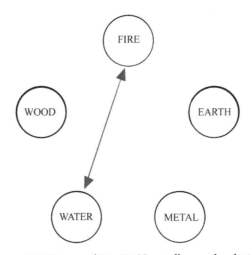

Diagram 8.10 Water and Fire Kè/Controlling cycle relationship

Using the Earth point on the Liver channel (LR 3), the Wood point on the Spleen channel (SP 1) and the Wood point on the Stomach channel (ST 43) for very poor digestion due to Rebellious Liver Qì overacting on the Stomach and Spleen

The Liver belongs to the Wood element, with the Spleen and Stomach belonging to the Earth element. Therefore, using this Kè/Controlling cycle combination (Diagram 8.11) ensures that the three organs directly affected by this imbalance should recover and help correct the poor digestion.

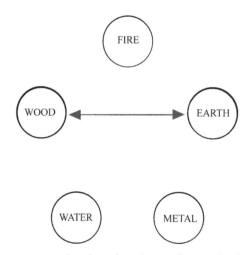

Diagram 8.11 Wood and Earth Kè/Controlling cycle relationship

4. Wǔ Xíng Horary points and the Chinese clock[45]

An Horary[46] point is the point on the channel that is the same as the channel itself – for example, the Wood point on the Wood channel. In this instance that would be the Wood point on the Liver channel (LR 1) and the Gall Bladder channel (GB 41).

This also applies for Fire points on Fire channels, Earth points on Earth channels, Metal points on Metal channels and Water points on Water channels.

Their function is to regulate or balance the associated organ and its individual organ functions. For example, the Horary point on the Lung channel is LU 8 and it can be used to:[47]

- govern Qì and respiration

- control the Jīng Luò and blood vessels

- control the dispersing and descending of Qì

- regulate the water passages

- control skin and hair

- regulate the nose

- regulate the Pò (Corporeal/Grounded/Earthly Soul)

- govern the voice

- regulate grief/sadness

- regulate External or Internal Pathogenic Dryness.

Horary points can be used at any time of the day in conjunction with other points for a more balanced treatment. Having said that, there is some credence to using the Horary points in their allocated Chinese clock two-hour period.[48]

The Chinese clock is a system of thinking in Chinese medicine where a two-hour segment (from every 24 hours) is allocated to each of the twelve Zàng Fǔ organs. In this two-hour period (the same time every day) the Vital Substances (Qì, Xuè, Jīn Yè and Jīng) are at their strongest vibration within each of the organs.[49]

For example, the Lungs have their daily boost of Vital Substances between 3 and 5am every day. That would mean treating your patient with LU 8 sometime between 3 and 5am. I'm not sure about you, but I'm not particularly keen to treat my patients at that time of the day.

The theory does suggest, however, that this would be like a triple shot to the organ you are wishing to treat. For example, using SP 3 between 9 and 11am would be the Earth point on the Earth channel in the Earth time.

See Diagram 8.12 for the times of each organ according to the Chinese clock.

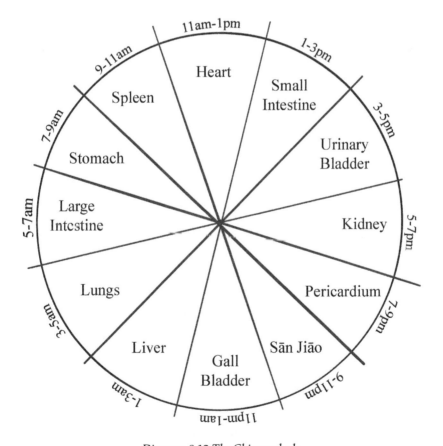

Diagram 8.12 The Chinese clock

See Table 8.7 for a list of the Horary points and the Chinese clock.

Table 8.7 Horary points and the Chinese clock[50]

Zàng Fǔ channels	Wǔ Xíng	Horary point	Chinese clock time
Lung	Metal point on Metal channel	LU 8	3–5am
Heart	Fire point on Fire channel	HT 8	11am–1pm
Pericardium	Fire point on Fire channel	PC 8	7–9pm
Spleen	Earth point on Earth channel	SP 3	9–11am
Kidney	Water point on Water channel	KI 10	5–7pm
Liver	Wood point on Wood channel	LR 1	1–3am
Large Intestine	Metal point on Metal channel	LI 1	5–7am
Small Intestine	Fire point on Fire channel	SI 5	1–3pm
Sān Jiāo	Fire point on Fire channel	TE 6	9–11pm
Stomach	Earth point on Earth channel	ST 36	7–9am
Urinary Bladder	Water point on Water channel	BL 66	3–5pm
Gall Bladder	Wood point on Wood channel	GB 41	11pm–1am

I have included two acupuncture point combinations for the Horary points below.

Heart organ

The Heart is part of the Fire element, so the Horary point would be the Fire point on the Heart (Fire) channel, which is HT 8.

It would make sense to include additional points to assist the Horary point. Some possible point options include:[51]

- HT 7 – Yuán Source point of the Heart

- CV 14 – Front Mù Collecting point of the Heart

- BL 15 – Back Shù Transporting point of the Heart

- SI 7 – Luò Connecting point of the Small Intestine (Yáng partner of the Heart)

- PC 7 – Yuán Source point of the Pericardium (Heart's bodyguard)

- CV 17 – Front Mù Collecting point of the Pericardium (Heart's bodyguard)

- BL 14 – Back Shù Transporting point of the Pericardium (Heart's bodyguard).

That gives a treatment with points on the arms/hands, trunk (front) and trunk (back) with a total of 14 points if needled bilaterally.

This treatment is designed to regulate or balance the Heart organ and its individual organ functions. In Chinese medicine the Heart:[52]

- governs Xuè

- controls the Xuè vessels

- manifests in the complexion

- houses the Shén

- opens into the tongue and controls speech

- controls sweat

- regulates joy

- regulates External/Internal Pathogenic Fire/Heat.

There is one last consideration when needling those points to regulate the Heart. If you felt so inclined, you could treat your patient between 11am and 1pm – the Heart time on the Chinese clock.

Gall Bladder organ

The Gall Bladder is part of the Wood element, so the Horary point would be the Wood point on the Gall Bladder (Wood) channel, which is GB 41.

It would make sense to include additional points to assist the Horary point. Some possible point options include:[53]

- GB 40 – Yuán Source point of the Gall Bladder

- GB 24 – Front Mù Collecting point of the Gall Bladder

- BL 19 – Back Shù Transporting point of the Gall Bladder

- LR 5 – Luò Connecting point of the Liver (Yīn partner of the Gall Bladder)

- LR 3 – Yuán Source point of the Liver (Yīn partner of the Gall Bladder)

- LR 14 – Front Mù Collecting point of the Liver (Yīn partner of the Gall Bladder)

- BL 18 – Back Shù Transporting point of the Liver (Yīn partner of the Gall Bladder).

That gives a treatment with points on the legs/feet, trunk (front) and trunk (back) with a total of 16 points if needled bilaterally.

This treatment is designed to regulate or balance the Gall Bladder organ and its individual organ functions. In Chinese medicine the Gall Bladder:[54]

- stores and excretes bile

- controls the tendons/sinews

- influences quality and length of sleep

- regulates anger

- regulates External/Internal Pathogenic Wind.

There is one last consideration when needling those points to regulate the Gall Bladder. If you felt so inclined, you could treat your patient between 11pm and 1am – the Gall Bladder time on the Chinese clock.

5. Wǔ Xíng Mother and Child points

The Wǔ Xíng Mother and Child points were first introduced in the 69th difficulty of *The Classic of Difficulties* (*Canon of the Yellow Emperor's Eighty-One Difficult Issues*/Huáng Dì Bā Shí Yī Nán Jīng/黃帝八十一難經).[55]

Using the Shēng/Generating cycle, each element has an element before it on the cycle and after it on the cycle. The one before is the Mother element, and the one after is the Child element. For example, the Earth element's Mother is the Fire element because it precedes it on the cycle, and the Earth element's Child is the Metal element because it follows it on the cycle. See Diagram 8.13.

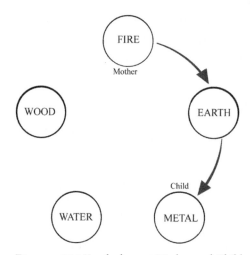

Diagram 8.13 Earth element Mother and Child

The Mother element can be used to tonify/nourish/support, and the Child element can be used to sedate/drain/deplete. The 69th difficulty (Unschuld 1986, p.583) of *The Classic of Difficulties* states: 'It is like this. In case of depletion, fill the respective [conduit's] mother. In case of repletion, drain the respective [conduit's] child.'

So how does that work in clinical practice? There are two approaches that have been given credence over the centuries:

- Use the affected channel's Mother or Child point.

- Use the Mother or Child element.

Use the affected channel's Mother or Child point

This is on the assumption that the affected organ/channel is the primary focus of your treatment. For example, your patient has Liver Xuè Xū and so you choose the

Mother point on the Liver channel because it will tonify Liver Xuè. That would be LR 8, which is the Water point on a Wood channel.

Alternatively, your patient has Liver Fire Blazing and so you choose the Child point on the Liver channel because it will sedate Liver Fire. That would be LR 2, which is the Fire point on a Wood channel.

Use the Mother or Child element

This assumes that you want to support the affected organ/channel by using a different organ/channel. For example, your patient has Lung Qì Xū and so you choose the Mother (Earth) point on the Mother (Earth) channel, which is the Spleen channel because it will tonify Lung Qì. That would be SP 3.

Another option is to use the Metal point on the Mother (Earth) channel, as this will strengthen the association between the two elements. On the Spleen channel it would be SP 5.

You could also use the Stomach channel as it's technically the Mother channel for the Metal element organs of Lung and Large Intestine. However, this rule usually runs with Yīn organs/channels treating Yīn organs/channels and Yáng organs/channels treating Yáng organs/channels.

So, to give you an example of a Yáng organ, your patient has Large Intestine Heat and so you choose the Child (Water) point on the Child (Water) channel, which is the Urinary Bladder channel because it will sedate Large Intestine Heat. That would be BL 66.

Another option is to use the Metal point on the Mother (Water) channel, as this will strengthen the association between the two elements. On the Urinary Bladder channel it would be BL 67.

If those examples were a little confusing, or even if they weren't, Table 8.8 has the full list of Mother and Child points for the Shēng/Generating cycle.

Table 8.8 Shēng/Generating cycle Mother and Child points[56]

Zàng Fǔ channels	Wǔ Xíng Mother point	Wǔ Xíng Child point
Lung	LU 9	LU 5
Heart	HT 9	HT 7
Pericardium	PC 9	PC 7
Spleen	SP 2	SP 5
Kidney	KI 7	KI 1
Liver	LR 8	LR 2
Large Intestine	LI 11	LI 2
Small Intestine	SI 3	SI 8
Sān Jiāo	TE 3	TE 10
Stomach	ST 41	ST 45
Urinary Bladder	BL 67	BL 65
Gall Bladder	GB 43	GB 38

Although the Shēng/Generating cycle is the most commonly used Wǔ Xíng cycle for Mother and Child theory, it can also be used on the Kè/Controlling cycle.

Shēng/Generating and Kè/Controlling cycles for treating acute and chronic disorders

Although the Shēng/Generating and Kè/Controlling cycles can be used in a multitude of different ways, one of the most common is to use the Shēng/Generating cycle for chronic disorders and the Kè/Controlling cycle for acute disorders.

For the Shēng/Generating cycle Mother and Child points, please refer to Table 8.8. For the Kè/Controlling cycle Mother and Child points, please see Table 8.9.

Table 8.9 Kè/Controlling cycle Mother and Child points

Zàng Fǔ channels	Wǔ Xíng Mother point	Wǔ Xíng Child point
Lung	LU 10	LU 11
Heart	HT 3	HT 4
Pericardium	PC 3	PC 5
Spleen	SP 1	SP 9
Kidney	KI 3	KI 2
Liver	LR 4	LR 3
Large Intestine	LI 5	LI 3
Small Intestine	SI 2	SI 1
Sān Jiāo	TE 2	TE 1
Stomach	ST 43	ST 44
Urinary Bladder	BL 40	BL 60
Gall Bladder	GB 44	GB 34

Point combination examples for Mother and Child treatments are covered in detail in Chapter 9.

Notes

1   Fung 1953, p.21. Dǒng Zhòng-shū (179–104 BCE) was a Confucian official who played a major role in ensuring that the newly implanted Han dynasty took Confucianism as its official ideology after the collapse of the Legalist-driven Qin dynasty.

2   Lau 2001, p.211 (Book Two, LII). The *Dào Dé Jīng*, the source of this quotation, was originally written anywhere from about 550 to 250 BCE. Lǎo Zǐ is generally considered to be the author of the *Dào Dé Jīng*, although this remains up for debate, as does when Lǎo Zǐ was actually alive. Reports suggest his birth was anywhere from

600 to 300 BCE. This quotation is taken from the Mǎ Wáng Duī version of the *Dào Dé Jīng*.

3   The translation of the Wǔ Xíng to Five Elements is not a particularly good one. Even the slightly less used Five Phases is not great. In fact, there isn't really one true translation that works best; as a result, Five Elements tends to continue to be the preferred choice for authors. As most people know the Wǔ Xíng as Five Elements, trying to change it now is possibly counterproductive. Further, it gives Western readers a term they have some base

level understanding of, because of the Four Elements concept from Greek antiquity.

4   Fung 1952, p.159. The Wŭ Xíng did exist prior to the development of this philosophical school, but from my research this was the first time that it was considered to be a legitimately developed theory.

5   Hinrichs and Barnes 2013, pp.65-96 (in particular pp.95-96).

6   Kaptchuk 2000, p.438.

7   Fung 1952, p.162.

8   Maciocia 2015, p.24.

9   Ibid., pp.24, 32.

10   Ibid., pp.24-25.

11   Ibid., pp.24-25, 32-33.

12   Wu 1993, pp.3-4: 1st chapter. *The Spiritual Pivot* (Líng Shū) was written somewhere between 200 and 0 BCE.

13   Marchment 2004, p.157. Shù doesn't translate as Stream. It translates as 'to transport'.

14   Marchment 2004, p.157. Jīng doesn't translate as River. It translates as 'flow' or 'pass'.

15   Ellis *et al.* 1989, p.369. Hé doesn't translate as Sea. It translates as 'to unite' or 'join'.

16   Flaws 2004, pp.120-121. *The Classic of Difficulties* (*Canon of the Yellow Emperor's Eighty-One Difficult Issues*/Huáng Dì Bā Shí Yī Nán Jīng) was originally written between 0 and 200 CE.

17   Ellis *et al.* 1991, p.65.

18   Deadman *et al.* 2007, p.29.

19   Ellis *et al.* 1989, p.375.

20   Deadman *et al.* 2007, pp.29-33; Flaws 2004, p.123; Maciocia 2015, pp.829-843; Ross 1995, pp.69-72; Wu 1993, p.157.

21   Ross 1995, p.72.

22   Hartmann 2009, p.9.

23   Deadman *et al.* 2007, p.29.

24   Marchment 2004, p.157.

25   Deadman *et al.* 2007, pp.29-34; Flaws 2004, p.123; Maciocia 2015, pp.829-843; Ross 1995, pp.69 72; Wu 1993, pp.24, 31, 157.

26   Ross 1995, p.72.

27   Deadman *et al.* 2007, p.29.

28   Marchment 2004, p.157.

29   Deadman *et al.* 2007, p.34.

30   Ibid., pp.29-32, 34-35; Flaws 2004, p.123; Maciocia 2015, pp.829-843; Ross 1995, pp.69-73; Wu 1993, pp.24, 31, 157.

31   Hartmann 2009, p.90.

32   Ibid., pp.5, 18.

33   Deadman *et al.* 2007, p.29.

34   Marchment 2004, p.157.

35   Deadman *et al.* 2007, pp.29-32, 35-36; Flaws 2004, p.123; Maciocia 2015, pp.829-843; Ross 1995, pp.69-71, 73; Wu 1993, p.157.

36   Ross 1995, p.72.

37   Deadman *et al.* 2007, p.29.

38   Ellis *et al.* 1989, p.369.

39   Deadman *et al.* 2007, pp.29-32, 36-37; Flaws 2004, p.123; Maciocia 2015, pp.829-843; Ross 1995, pp.69-71, 73; Wu 1993, pp.24, 31, 157.

40   Deadman *et al.* 2007, p.37; Ross 1995, p.73.

41   Hartmann 2009, p.9.

42   Flaws 2004, p.118: 64th difficulty. Deadman *et al.* 2007, p.29.

43   As previous note.

44   Maciocia 2015, p.840.

45   Franglen 2014, pp.86, 120-122; Hicks *et al.* 2010, pp.284-285; Ross 1995, pp.73-74, 77.

46   Horary means 'of an hour or hours'.

47   Kaptchuk 2000, pp.90-93; Maciocia 2015, pp.129-142.

48   Franglen 2014, pp.86, 120-122.

49   Hicks *et al.* 2010, pp.284-285.

50   Ibid.

51   Hartmann 2009, p.3.

52   Kaptchuk 2000, pp.88-90; Maciocia 2015, pp.107-116.

53   Hartmann 2009, p.2.

54   Kaptchuk 2000, p.95; Maciocia 2015, pp.209-213.

55   Unschuld 1986, p.583.

56   Maciocia 2015, pp.838-839.

Of the five elements, none is always predominant; of the four seasons, none lasts forever; of the days, some are long and some short, and the moon waxes and wanes.

Sūn Zǐ/孫子 (5th century BCE)[1]

It's when we start working together that the real healing takes place…it's when we start spilling our sweat, and not our blood.

David Hume (1711–1776 CE)[2]

9

Wǔ Xíng/Five Elements Point Category – Intermediate Concepts

Chapter 8 discussed concepts that were introductory and Chapter 10 will be discussing concepts that are advanced. This chapter will be discussing the concepts of the Wǔ Xíng Shēng/Generating and Kè/Controlling Cycles in the treatment of acute and chronic disorders.

1. Wǔ Xíng Shēng/Generating cycle for chronic disorders

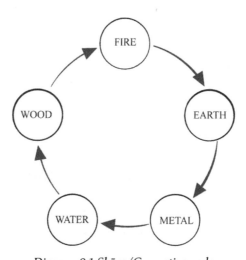

Diagram 9.1 Shēng/Generating cycle

When applying the Shēng/Generating cycle in clinical practice, it is often used for patients with chronic and gradually forming disorders.

The 67th chapter (Wang 1997, pp.322–323) of *The Yellow Emperor's Classic* (*Inner Canon of the Yellow Emperor*/Huáng Dì Nèi Jīng/黃帝內經) agrees when it talks about energy arriving at the Wǔ Xíng when it should not arrive.

If the energy arrives gradually, and more mildly, it will tend to only damage the Child along the Shēng/Generating cycle.

Conversely, a sudden and severe arrival can jump right past the Child on the Shēng/Generating cycle and instead attack the Grandchild along the Kè/Controlling cycle. In this sudden, severe and acute event, you treat the Kè/Controlling cycle.

This is a somewhat generalized statement because there are alternative views on this, but for the sake of the special point categories, this is the theory we will apply to the Shēng/Generating and Kè/Controlling cycles.

> [W]hen an element invades other element, it will be invaded by the evil energy, and the invasion is brought about by the running riot of itself. (Wang 1997, p.323)

Can you apply the Shēng/Generating cycle to all chronic conditions your patients present with? In theory, the answer is yes, because all organs/channels can be treated using the Shēng/Generating cycle. Therefore, it's up to you to decide which organ/s or channel/s are affected and then use the relevant Shēng/Generating cycle category listed in Table 9.1.

That means you can use the Shēng/Generating cycle for chronic musculoskeletal disorders by working out which channels are affected (and perhaps some organs too) and targeting those.

You could also use the Shēng/Generating cycle for chronic emotional imbalances affecting certain organs (and perhaps some channels too). As long as you can work out which organs and/or channels are affected, you can use the Shēng/Generating cycle for any of your patient's chronic complaints.

Once you have worked out which organ or channel is affected, you need to confirm which element it belongs to. Then you need to make note of which element is before and after your affected element. The element before is typically called the Mother, and the element after is typically called the Child.

For example, your patient has been suffering from chronic calf muscle tightness and cramping (both calves) for the past nine months, with the main area of concern located near BL 57. You determine that this is a Qì and Xuè stagnation primarily affecting the Urinary Bladder channel, which belongs to the Water element. You then make a note of the element before, which is Metal, and the element after, which is Wood. See Diagram 9.2.

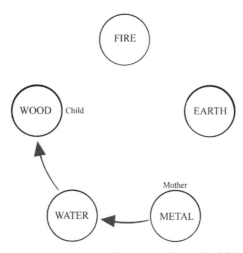

Diagram 9.2 Water element Mother and Child

My preference when using the Wŭ Xíng Mother and Child theory is to use both the Mother and Child points. This will be explained in more detail shortly.

Next you treat the Urinary Bladder channel because it's the main area of concern for the patient. Now this next bit can trip some practitioners up, so please pay attention. Because the Urinary Bladder channel is the main focus of the treatment, you would use the Metal point (BL 67) and Wood point (BL 65) on the Urinary Bladder channel. You don't use Metal or Wood channels. This will also be explained in a lot more detail shortly.

The 69th difficulty (Unschuld 1986, pp.583, 587) of *The Classic of Difficulties* (*Canon of the Yellow Emperor's Eighty-One Difficult Issues*/Huáng Dì Bā Shí Yī Nán Jīng/黃帝八十一難經) says it best: '[I]f a regular conduit has fallen ill by itself…one must select [for treatment] just this one conduit…one must prick the holes of the [sick] conduit itself.'[3]

Finally, you would needle some additional points in the local calf complaint as well as consider something higher up the body for a better body balance with your needles. Some possible points to consider are:

- Metal point – BL 67.

- Wood point – BL 65.

- Local calf points – BL 55, BL 56 and BL 57.

- Distal point on the trunk – BL 20 – is on the affected channel and is also the Back Shù Transporting point for the Spleen, which governs muscles.

- Distal point on the arm – SI 7 – the Small Intestine and Urinary Bladder are Tài Yáng (Six Division) partners. As such you can use the partnered channel as a mirror image with the calf corresponding to the forearm. SI 7 is the closest mirrored point to the main patient complaint.

- Needling these points bilaterally (because it's a bilateral complaint) would use a total of 14 needles.

The Shēng/Generating cycle point methods are listed in Table 9.1.

Table 9.1 Shēng/Generating cycle point methods

Wǔ Xíng/Five Element	Point method	Point element and name	Point element and name
Fire element: Heart Small Intestine Pericardium Sān Jiāo	Wood Earth	Wood points: HT 9 SI 3 PC 9 TE 3	Earth points: HT 7 SI 8 PC 7 TE 10
Earth element: Spleen Stomach	Fire Metal	Fire points: SP 2 ST 41	Metal points: SP 5 ST 45
Metal element: Lungs Large Intestine	Earth Water	Earth points: LU 9 LI 11	Water points: LU 5 LI 2
Water element: Kidneys Urinary Bladder	Metal Wood	Metal points: KI 7 BL 67	Wood points: KI 1 BL 65
Wood element: Liver Gall Bladder	Water Fire	Water points: LR 8 GB 43	Fire points: LR 2 GB 38

Next you need to decide how you will needle the points. There are generally four different strategies that could be employed:

- *You can needle both of the points with a balanced and nourishing method regardless of the diagnosis.*

  The idea here is that the body knows what needs to be done. You have started the process of healing by choosing the correct points and the patient's body will do the rest.

- *If there is stagnation, then you would flush/rush both points.*

  I like to use the terms 'flush' or 'rush' when referring to points that are excellent at rapidly moving/stimulating Qì. The points will rush (push or surge) the Qì to flush (break through) the stagnation.

- *If there is Excess/Shí, then sedate both points.*

  Sedating the Mother will force it to stop feeding the affected element because it needs to keep what it has left for itself. Sedating the Child will force the affected element to feed the Child, thereby naturally reducing its own supply.

- *If there is Deficiency/Xū, then tonify both points.*

Tonifying the Mother will give it a surplus which it can then pass on to the affected element, thereby helping to boost its supply. Tonifying the Child will reduce the need for the affected element to feed the Child, thereby naturally increasing its own supply.

The 69th difficulty (Unschuld 1986, p.583) of *The Classic of Difficulties* says: 'In case of depletion [Xū], fill the respective [conduit's] mother. In case of repletion [Shí], drain the respective [conduit's] child.'

Let's now look at each of the Shēng/Generating cycle point methods more closely to help cement the knowledge, and to give a few extra point combinations. Bear in mind that these are just one example of many that could be included in each of the elements.

Fire element

Use the 'Wood Earth' point method for chronic angina due to Heart Yīn Xū. In this instance the key channel to access is the Heart channel, which is part of the Fire element. Therefore, you use the Wood and Earth points on the Heart channel.

Wood point – HT 9.

Earth point – HT 7.

In this example, you would consider tonifying both points as discussed above. You would also consider using other points to tonify Heart Yīn and treat angina, ensuring a good body balance with the needles. An example of a full body treatment is:[4]

- Wood point – HT 9.

- Earth point – HT 7.

- Trunk (front) – CV 4, CV 14 and CV 15.

- Trunk (back) – BL 15.

- Legs/feet – SP 6.

- Needling these points bilaterally would use a total of 11 needles.

Earth element

Use the 'Fire Metal' point method for chronic anterior left knee pain and swelling due to Qì and Xuè stagnation in the Spleen and Stomach channels. Therefore, you use the Fire and Metal points on the Spleen and Stomach channels, which are part of the Earth element.

Fire point on the Spleen channel – SP 2.

Metal point on the Spleen channel – SP 5.

Fire point on the Stomach channel – ST 41.

Metal point on the Stomach channel – ST 45.

In this example, you would consider flushing/rushing all four points as discussed above. You would also consider using other points local to the knee joint as well as away from the leg, thereby ensuring a good body balance with the needles. An example of a full body treatment is:

- Fire point – SP 2.

- Metal point – SP 5.

- Fire point – ST 41.

- Metal point – ST 45.

- Local knee points[5] – SP 9, SP 10, ST 34, ST 35 and ST 36. All points are on the affected Earth element channels of Spleen and Stomach.

- Distal points on the trunk – CV 5 and CV 9. Used to draw the stagnation and swelling out of the knee and leg by opening/regulating the water passages.[6]

- Distal points on the arms/hands – LU 5 and LI 11. These two points are located on the right elbow, which is a mirrored joint to the left knee. They are also Six Division pairings for the Spleen (Tài Yīn pairing of Spleen and Lungs) and Stomach (Yáng Míng pairing of Stomach and Large Intestine).

- Needling these points unilaterally would use a total of 13 needles.[7]

Metal element

Use the 'Earth Water' point method for a chronic frozen right shoulder due to Qì and Xuè Stagnation in the Large Intestine channel. Therefore, you use the Earth and Water points on the Large Intestine channel, which is part of the Metal element.

Earth point – LI 11.

Water point – LI 2.

In this example, you would consider flushing/rushing both points as discussed above. You would also consider using other points local to the shoulder joint as well as away from the arm, thereby ensuring a good body balance with the needles. An example of a full body treatment is:

- Earth point – LI 11.

- Water point – LI 2.

- Local shoulder points – LI 14, LI 15, TE 14, HT 1, M-UE-48 (Jiān Qián) and N-UE-14 (Nào Shàng).[8]

- Distal points on the legs/feet – ST 31, ST 38, GB 39 and GB 42. ST 31 is needled on the left thigh/hip, which is the mirrored joint to the right shoulder. It is also a Six Division pairing for the Large Intestine (Yáng Míng pairing of Large Intestine and Stomach).

    ST 38, GB 39 and GB 42 are great distal points for shoulder problems.[9] ST 38 is probably the best known of these. The idea is that you needle the opposite leg (in this case the left leg) and stimulate the needles while the patient, or a third person, moves the shoulder gently.

- Needling these points unilaterally would use a total of 12 needles.

Water element

Use the 'Metal Wood' point method for chronic memory loss due to Kidney Jīng Xū. In this instance the key channel to access is the Kidney channel, which is part of the Water element. Therefore, you use the Metal and Wood points on the Kidney channel.

Metal point – KI 7.

Wood point – KI 1.

In this example, you would consider tonifying both points as discussed above. You would also consider using other points to tonify Kidney Jīng and treat memory loss, ensuring a good body balance with the needles. An example of a full body treatment is:[10]

- Metal point – KI 7.

- Wood point – KI 1.

- Trunk (front) – CV 4 and KI 12. Both treat Kidney Jīng Xū.

- Trunk (back) – BL 23. Treats Kidney Jīng Xū and memory loss.

- Arms/hands – TE 4 for Kidney Jīng Xū; HT 7 for memory loss.

- Legs/feet – SP 6. Treats Kidney Jīng Xū and memory loss.

- Needling these points bilaterally would use a total of 15 needles.

Wood element

Use the 'Water Fire' point method for chronic vertex headaches and anger outbursts due to Liver Fire Blazing. In this instance the key channel to access is the Liver channel, which is part of the Wood element. Therefore, you use the Water and Fire points on the Liver channel.

Water point – LR 8.

Fire point – LR 2.

In this example, you would consider sedating both points as discussed above. You would also consider using other points to sedate Liver Fire and treat vertex headaches with anger outbursts, ensuring a good body balance with the needles. An example of a full body treatment is:[11]

- Water point – LR 8.

- Fire point – LR 2.

- Head/face – GV 20, GB 20 and M-HN-3 (Yìn Táng). Apart from M-HN-3 (Yìn Táng), which can only treat anger, the other two points can treat all three issues.

- Trunk (front) – LR 14. Can treat Liver Fire Blazing and anger outbursts.

- Trunk (back) – BL 18. Can treat Liver Fire Blazing and anger outbursts.

- Arms/hands – LI 4 and LI 11. Can treat all three issues.

- Legs/feet – GB 37. Can treat all three issues.

- Needling these points bilaterally would use a total of 18 needles.

2. Wŭ Xíng Kè/Controlling cycle for acute disorders

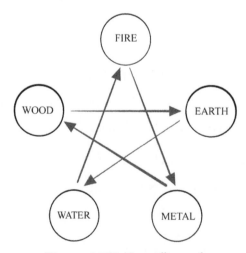

Diagram 9.3 Kè/Controlling cycle

The Kè/Controlling cycle is often used in clinical practice for patients with acute disorders. This is a somewhat generalized statement because there are alternative views on this, but for the sake of the special point categories, this is the theory we will apply to the Kè/Controlling cycle. See Section 1 above for a more in-depth explanation.

Can you apply the Kè/Controlling cycle to all acute conditions your patients present with? In theory, the answer is yes, because organs/channels can be treated using the Kè/Controlling cycle. Therefore, it's up to you to decide which organ/s or channel/s are affected and then use the relevant Kè/Controlling cycle category listed in Table 9.2.

That means you can use the Kè/Controlling cycle for acute musculoskeletal disorders by working out which channels are affected (and perhaps some organs too) and targeting those.

You can use the Kè/Controlling cycle for acute emotional imbalances affecting certain organs (and perhaps some channels too). As long as you can work out which organs and/or channels are affected, then you can use the Kè/Controlling cycle for any of your patient's acute complaints.

Once you have worked out which organ or channel is affected, you need to confirm which element it belongs to. Then you need to make note of which element is before and after your affected element. The element before is typically called the Mother, and the element after is typically called the Child.

For example, your patient has been suffering from acute acid reflux for the past five days. You determine that this is Stomach Fire Blazing, which belongs to the Earth element. You then make a note of the element before, which is Wood, and the element after, which is Water.

Next you treat the Stomach Fire Blazing because it's the main diagnosis for the patient. Now this next bit can trip some practitioners up, so please pay attention. Because Stomach Fire Blazing is the main focus of the treatment, you would use the Wood point (ST 43) and Water point (ST 44) on the Stomach channel. You don't use Wood or Water channels.

Finally, you would needle some additional local points in the chest area as well as consider something elsewhere in the body for a better balance with your needles. Some possible points are:

- Wood point – ST 43.

- Water point – ST 44.

- Local chest points – CV 17, CV 19 and CV 21.

- Distal point on trunk – CV 12 – is on the channel that already has points on the chest and is also the Front Mù Collecting point for the Stomach.

- Distal points on arm – LI 11 and TE 5 – clear heat anywhere in the body.

- Needling these points bilaterally would use a total of 12 needles.

The Kè/Controlling cycle point methods are listed in Table 9.2.

Table 9.2 Kè/Controlling cycle point method

Wŭ Xíng/Five Element	Point method	Point element and name	Point element and name
Fire element: Heart Small Intestine Pericardium Sān Jiāo	Water Metal	Water points: HT 3 SI 2 PC 3 TE 2	Metal points: HT 4 SI 1 PC 5 TE 1
Earth element: Spleen Stomach	Wood Water	Wood points: SP 1 ST 43	Water points: SP 9 ST 44
Metal element: Lungs Large Intestine	Fire Wood	Fire points: LU 10 LI 5	Wood points: LU 11 LI 3
Water element: Kidneys Urinary Bladder	Earth Fire	Earth points: KI 3 BL 40	Fire points: KI 2 BL 60
Wood element: Liver Gall Bladder	Metal Earth	Metal points: LR 4 GB 44	Earth points: LR 3 GB 34

Next you need to decide on how you will needle the points. There are generally four different strategies that could be employed (discussed in more detail in Section 1 above):

- You can needle both of the points with a balanced and nourishing method regardless of the diagnosis.

- If there is stagnation, you would flush/rush both points.

- If there is Excess/Shí, then sedate both points.

- If there is Deficiency/Xū, then tonify both points.

Let's look at each of the Kè/Controlling cycle point methods more closely to help cement the knowledge, and to give a few extra point combinations. Bear in mind that these are just one example of many that could be included in each of the elements.

Fire element

Use the 'Water Metal' point method for acute palpitations due to Heart Qì Xū. In this instance the key channel to access is the Heart channel, which is part of the Fire element. Therefore, you use the Water and Metal points on the Heart channel.

Water point – HT 3.

Metal point – HT 4.

In this example, you would consider tonifying both points as discussed above. You would also consider using other points to tonify Heart Qì and treat palpitations, ensuring a good body balance with the needles. An example of a full body treatment is:[12]

- Water point – HT 3.

- Metal point – HT 4.

- Trunk (front) – CV 6 can tonify Qì; CV 14 and CV 17 treat Heart Qì Xū and palpitations.

- Trunk (back) – BL 15. Treats Heart Qì Xū and palpitations.

- Arms/hands – PC 6. Treats Heart Qì Xū and palpitations.

- Legs/feet – SP 6 and ST 36 can tonify Qì and treat palpitations.

- Needling these points bilaterally would use a total of 15 needles.

Earth element

Use the 'Wood Water' point method for acute diarrhea due to Spleen Qì Xū. In this instance the key channel to access is the Spleen channel, which is part of the Earth element. Therefore, you use the Wood and Water points on the Spleen channel.

Wood point – SP 1.

Water point – SP 9.

In this example, you would consider tonifying both points as discussed above. You would also consider using other points to tonify Spleen Qì and treat diarrhea, ensuring a good body balance with the needles. An example of a full body treatment is:[13]

- Wood point – SP 1.

- Water point – SP 9.

- Trunk (front) – CV 12 and LR 13 treat Spleen Qì Xū and diarrhea.

- Trunk (back) – BL 20. Treats Spleen Qì Xū and diarrhea.

- Legs/feet – SP 6 and ST 36 can treat Spleen Qì Xū and diarrhea.

- Needling these points bilaterally would use a total of 13 needles.

Metal element

Use the 'Fire Wood' point method for acute tennis elbow (left) due to Qì and Xuè stagnation in the Lung and Large Intestine channels. Therefore, you use the Fire and Wood points on the Lung and Large Intestine channels, which are part of the Metal element.

Fire point on the Lung channel – LU 10.

Wood point on the Lung channel – LU 11.

Fire point on the Large Intestine channel – LI 5.

Wood point on the Large Intestine channel – LI 3.

In this example, you would consider flushing/rushing all four points as discussed above. You would also consider using other points local to the elbow joint as well as away from the arm, thereby ensuring a good body balance with the needles. An example of a full body treatment is:

- Fire point – LU 10.

- Wood point – LU 11.

- Fire point – LI 5.

- Wood point – LI 3.

- Local elbow points[14] – LU 5, LI 10, LI 11 and LI 12. All points are on the affected Metal element channels of Lung and Large Intestine.

- Distal points on the legs/feet – SP 9 and ST 35. These two points are located on the right knee, which is a mirrored joint to the left elbow. They are also Six Division pairings for the Lungs (Tài Yīn pairing of Lungs and Spleen) and Large Intestine (Yáng Míng pairing of Large Intestine and Stomach).

- Needling these points unilaterally would use a total of ten needles.[15]

Water element

Use the 'Earth Fire' point method for acute Achilles tendon strain (right) with swelling due to Qì and Xuè stagnation in the Kidney and Urinary Bladder channels. Therefore, you use the Earth and Fire points on the Kidney and Urinary Bladder channels, which are part of the Water element.

Earth point on the Kidney channel – KI 3.

Fire point on the Kidney channel – KI 2.

Earth point on the Urinary Bladder channel – BL 40.

Fire point on the Urinary Bladder channel – BL 60.

In this example, you would consider flushing/rushing all four points as discussed above. You would also consider using other points local to the ankle joint as well as away from the leg, thereby ensuring a good body balance with the needles. An example of a full body treatment is:

- Earth point – KI 3.

- Fire point – KI 2.

- Earth point – BL 40.

- Fire point – BL 60.

- Other local ankle points – KI 4 and BL 61. Both points are on the affected Water element channels of Kidney and Urinary Bladder.

- Distal points on the trunk – CV 5 and CV 9. Are used to draw the stagnation and swelling out of the ankle and leg by opening/regulating the water passages.[16]

- Distal points on the arms/hands – HT 7 and SI 5. These two points are located on the left wrist, which is a mirrored joint to the right ankle. They are also Six Division pairings for the Kidneys (Shào Yīn pairing of Kidneys and Heart) and Urinary Bladder (Tài Yáng pairing of Urinary Bladder and Small Intestine).

- Needling these points unilaterally would use a total of ten needles.[17]

Wood element

Use the 'Metal Earth' point method for acute stress due to Liver Qì Stagnation. In this instance the key channel to access is the Liver channel, which is part of the Wood element. Therefore, you use the Metal and Earth points on the Liver channel.

Metal point – LR 4.

Earth point – LR 3.

In this example, you would consider flushing/rushing both points as discussed above. You would also consider using other points to move Liver Qì and treat stress, ensuring a good body balance with the needles. An example of a full body treatment is:[18]

- Metal point – LR 4.

- Earth point – LR 3.

- Head/face – GV 20 and M-HN-3 (Yìn Táng) treat stress.

- Trunk (front) – LR 14. Treats Liver Qì Stagnation and stress.

- Trunk (back) – BL 18. Treats Liver Qì Stagnation and stress.

- Other leg/feet points – GB 34. Treats Liver Qì Stagnation and stress.

- Distal points on the arms/hands – PC 6 and LI 4. Both points treat Liver Qì Stagnation and stress. Also, when you combine LI 4 with LR 3, you 'open the Four Gates', which is an excellent point combination to treat stress and to move Qì.

- Needling these points bilaterally would use a total of 16 needles.

Notes

1   Sūn 2011, p.153. *The Art of War*, the source of this quotation, was originally written anywhere from about 450 to 350 BCE. Sūn Zǐ is generally considered to be the author of *The Art of War*, although this remains up for debate, as does when Sūn Zǐ was actually alive. Reports suggest his date of birth was anywhere from 500 to 400 BCE.

2   David Hume (1711–1776 CE) is one of my favorite philosophers of all time. The places he went to with his thinking continue to astound and inspire me. The quotation was retrieved from www.brainyquote.com/quotes/david_hume_389827.

3   This quotation is in two parts. The first part ('if a regular conduit has fallen ill by itself… one must select [for treatment] just this one conduit') is a direct translation of the 69th difficulty from Unschuld. The second part ('one must prick the holes of the [sick] conduit itself') is a commentary on the 69th difficulty.

4   Hartmann 2009, pp.4, 28. These are treatments for Heart Yīn Xū and angina. Not every point listed on those pages has been used in this formula. These are also not the only points that can be used.

5   Jarmey and Tindall 2005, p.78.

6   Deadman *et al.* 2007, pp.503, 509.

7   Personally, I would consider using some of the points bilaterally to create a more balanced treatment. This would likely include local knee points such as ST 34 and SP 9. That would be a combined total of 15 needles used.

8   Legge 2011, p.187; O'Connor and Bensky 1981, pp.227–229.

9   Hartmann 2009, p.49.

10   Ibid., pp.5, 100. These are treatments for Kidney Jīng Xū and memory loss. Not every point listed on those pages has been used in this formula. These are also not the only points that can be used.

11   Hartmann 2009, pp.9, 27, 74. These are treatments for Liver Fire Blazing, vertex headaches and anger outbursts. Not every point listed on those pages has been used in this formula. These are also not the only points that can be used.

12   Deadman *et al.* 2007, p.651; McDonald and Penner 1994, p.76. These are treatments for Heart Qì Xū and palpitations. Not every point listed on those pages has been used in this formula. These are also not the only points that can be used.

13   Deadman *et al.* 2007, p.645; McDonald and Penner 1994, p.40. These are treatments for Spleen Qì Xū and diarrhea. Not every point listed on those pages has been used in this formula. These are also not the only points that can be used.

14   Legge 2011, p.209.

15   Personally, I would consider using some of the points bilaterally to create a more balanced treatment. This would likely include local elbow points such as LU 5, LI 10 and LI 11. That would be a combined total of 13 needles used.

16   Deadman *et al.* 2007, pp.503, 509.

17   Personally, I would consider using some of the points bilaterally to create a more balanced treatment. This would likely include local ankle

points such as KI 3, KI 4 and BL 60. That would be a combined total of 13 needles used.

18   Hartmann 2009, pp.9, 149. These are treatments for Liver Qì Stagnation and stress. Not every point listed on those pages has been used in this formula. These are also not the only points that can be used.

[The wise] will start each day with the thought…

Fortune gives us nothing which we can really own.

Nothing, whether public or private, is stable; the destinies of men, no less than those of cities, are in a whirl…

We live in the middle of things which have all been destined to die. Mortal have you been born, to mortals have you given birth.

Reckon on everything, expect everything.

Seneca (4 BCE–65 CE)[1]

10

Wŭ Xíng/Five Elements Point Category – Advanced Concepts

This chapter will be discussing some of the more complicated or advanced concepts of the Wŭ Xíng. The acupuncture point combinations discussed will be for patients with internal environments that are inconsistent and unreliable.

'Reckon on everything, expect everything' should be the motto for this chapter!

Sections 1 and 2 look at the two Wŭ Xíng cycles of Chéng/Overacting and Wŭ/Insulting, which are already complicated in and of themselves. Section 3 discusses patients who have signs and symptoms pointing to an imbalance across more than one element.

This chapter is a fascinating journey into some very different ways of treating your patient's complaints.

1. Wŭ Xíng Chéng/Overacting cycle for complicated disorders

As discussed earlier, the Chéng/Overacting cycle tracks along the same pathway as the Kè/Controlling cycle. But rather than control/regulate the next element, the Chéng over-controls or overacts on the next element. This will cause the next element to become deficient/Xū, because it isn't being regulated by its Mother.

The Chéng/Overacting cycle is often used in clinical practice to describe an imbalance between two or more organs/elements.[2] This is a somewhat generalized statement because there are alternative views on this, but for the sake of the special point categories, this is the theory we will apply to the Chéng/Overacting cycle.

Can you apply the Chéng/Overacting cycle to any imbalance between two or more organs/elements that your patients present with? In theory, the answer is no, because not all multiple organs/channels complaints can be treated using the Chéng/Overacting cycle.

The key to using the Chéng/Overacting cycle is to decide which organs or channels are affected and then see whether there is a relevant Chéng/Overacting cycle category listed in Table 10.1. If there is, then you could theoretically use it; if not, then avoid using the Chéng/Overacting cycle.

There are five possible Chéng/Overacting cycle imbalances:[3]

- Fire overacting on Metal

- Metal overacting on Wood

- Wood overacting on Earth

- Earth overacting on Water

- Water overacting on Fire.

I have included a point combination example for each. Two are for Zàng Fǔ patterns and three are for Shén-based disorders. That way there is a point combination for all five Chéng/Overacting cycle imbalances.

The Chéng/Overacting cycle point methods are listed in Table 10.1.

Table 10.1 Chéng/Overacting cycle point method

Wǔ Xíng/Five Element	Point method	Point element and name	Point element and name
Fire element: Heart Small Intestine Pericardium Sān Jiāo	Water Metal	Water points: HT 3 SI 2 PC 3 TE 2	Metal points: HT 4 SI 1 PC 5 TE 1
Earth element: Spleen Stomach	Wood Water	Wood points: SP 1 ST 43	Water points: SP 9 ST 44
Metal element: Lungs Large Intestine	Fire Wood	Fire points: LU 10 LI 5	Wood points: LU 11 LI 3
Water element: Kidneys Urinary Bladder	Earth Fire	Earth points: KI 3 BL 40	Fire points: KI 2 BL 60
Wood element: Liver Gall Bladder	Metal Earth	Metal points: LR 4 GB 44	Earth points: LR 3 GB 34

Using the Chéng/Overacting cycle in clinical practice is a little different to the Shēng/Generating and Kè/Controlling cycles. Consequently, each point combination will list how each point can be needled.

There are also five considerations when deciding on the point combination. These are:

1. Use the Kè/Controlling cycle (to help balance the Chéng/Overacting cycle) as a clear link between the diseased organs. This will give the body clear instruction on what the points are being used for.

2. Use the Horary points for the diseased organs.

3. How many needles does that add up to once you have selected the Kè/Controlling cycle and Horary points? Is the number of needles in your accepted range?

4. Check to see where all the needles are located. Is there a good balance with the point combination?

5. Decide how you will needle each point. Do you want to nourish, flush, tonify or sedate?

I appreciate that this is a lot to consider when selecting points for an acupuncture point combination, but the more you do it, the faster you will get. I would also recommend having the subsequent tables (10.2–10.6) handy in clinic as a ready-reference guide.

Fire overacting on Metal

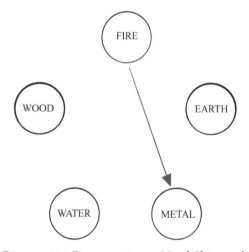

Diagram 10.1 Fire overacting on Metal Chéng cycle

You diagnose your patient with the Shén disorder of manic depression (Diān Kuáng) due to Heart Fire Blazing (mania) leading to Lung Qì Xū (depression). This is Fire overacting on Metal.

Use the Kè/Controlling cycle

This will be the Water and Metal points on the Heart channel (Water on Fire, Metal on Fire) as well as the Fire and Wood points on the Lung channel (Fire on Metal, Wood on Metal):

- Water on Fire – HT 3

- Metal on Fire – HT 4

- Fire on Metal – LU 10

- Wood on Metal – LU 11.

Use the Horary points

That would be the Fire point on the Heart channel (Fire on Fire) and the Metal point on the Lung channel (Metal on Metal):

- Fire on Fire – HT 8

- Metal on Metal – LU 8.

How many needles, and is that in your accepted range?

If needled bilaterally, this would be 12 needles.

Is there a good balance with the needle locations in the combination?

In this case, all of the points are on the arms/hands. However, the theory is sound, so it's up to you. If, like me, you would prefer to take a more body-balanced approach, then I suggest substituting the Horary points for the Front Mù Collecting points. That would then give you eight needles in the arms/hands and three needles on the front of the trunk.

How will you needle each point? Do you want to nourish, flush, tonify or sedate?

The points (including the Front Mù Collecting point options) are listed in Table 10.2 with an example of how you might choose to needle them. If you have a different approach to needling the points, feel free to stick with that approach.

Table 10.2 Fire overacting on Metal Chéng cycle

Point name	Special element/point	Needling method
HT 3	Water on Fire	Sedate the Mother
HT 4	Metal on Fire	These are associated elements, so they need to be needled in a balanced manner
HT 8	Fire on Fire	Sedate
LU 8	Metal on Metal	Tonify
LU 10	Fire on Metal	These are associated elements, so they need to be needled in a balanced manner
LU 11	Wood on Metal	Tonify the Child
CV 14	Front Mù Collecting point of the Heart	Sedate
LU 1	Front Mù Collecting point of the Lungs	Tonify

Metal overacting on Wood

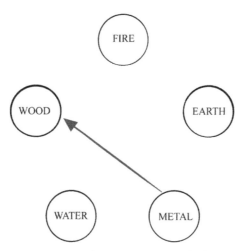

Diagram 10.2 Metal overacting on Wood Chéng cycle

You diagnose your patient with the Shén disorders of worry, stress and frustration due to Lung Qì Xū (worry) leading to Liver Qì Stagnation (stress and frustration). This is Metal overacting on Wood.

Use the Kè/Controlling cycle

This will be the Fire and Wood points on the Lung channel (Fire on Metal, Wood on Metal) and the Metal and Earth points on the Liver channel (Metal on Wood, Earth on Wood):

- Fire on Metal – LU 10

- Wood on Metal – LU 11

- Metal on Wood – LR 4

- Earth on Wood – LR 3.

Use the Horary points

That would be the Metal point on the Lung channel (Metal on Metal) as well as the Wood point on the Liver channel (Wood on Wood):

- Metal on Metal – LU 8

- Wood on Wood – LR 1.

How many needles, and is that in your accepted range?

If needled bilaterally, this would be 12 needles.

Is there a good balance with the needle locations in the combination?

In this case, all of the points are distributed across the arms/hands or legs/feet, which is a suitable body balance. However, you may like to add in some additional points on the trunk. Some good ones to consider would be the Front Mù Collecting points or the Back Shù Transporting points.

How will you needle each point? Do you want to nourish, flush, tonify or sedate?

The points are listed in Table 10.3 with an example of how you might choose to needle them. If you have a different approach to needling the points, then feel free to stick with that approach.

Table 10.3 Metal overacting on Wood Chéng cycle

Point name	Special element/point	Needling method
LU 8	Metal on Metal	Tonify
LU 10	Fire on Metal	Tonify the Mother
LU 11	Wood on Metal	These are associated elements, so they need to be needled in a balanced manner
LR 1	Wood on Wood	Flush
LR 3	Earth on Wood	Flush
LR 4	Metal on Wood	These are associated elements, so they need to be needled in a balanced manner

Wood overacting on Earth

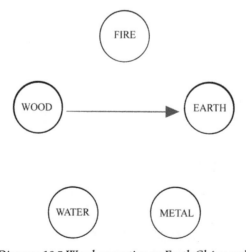

Diagram 10.3 Wood overacting on Earth Chéng cycle

You diagnose your patient with the Zàng Fǔ pattern of Liver overacting on/invading the Stomach and Spleen. This is Wood overacting on Earth. Further, it is either Liver Qì Stagnation or Liver Fire Blazing that is leading to the overacting/invading. This needs to be determined before an accurate needling method can be employed. If you are unsure, then utilize a balanced needling method.

Use the Kè/Controlling cycle

This will be the Metal and Earth points on the Liver channel (Metal on Wood, Earth on Wood), the Wood and Water points on the Stomach channel (Wood on Earth, Water on Earth) and the Wood and Water points on the Spleen channel (Wood on Earth, Water on Earth):

- Metal on Wood – LR 4
- Earth on Wood – LR 3
- Wood on Earth for the Stomach channel – ST 43
- Water on Earth for the Stomach channel – ST 44
- Wood on Earth for the Spleen channel – SP 1
- Water on Earth for the Spleen channel – SP 9.

Use the Horary points

That would be the Wood point on the Liver channel (Wood on Wood), the Earth point on the Stomach channel (Earth on Earth) and the Earth point on the Spleen channel (Earth on Earth):

- Wood on Wood – LR 1
- Earth on Earth for the Stomach channel – ST 36
- Earth on Earth for the Spleen channel – SP 3.

How many needles, and is that in your accepted range?

If needled bilaterally, this would be 18 needles.

Is there a good balance with the needle locations in the combination?

In this case, all of the points are on the legs/feet. However, the theory is sound, so it's up to you. If, like me, you would prefer to take a more body-balanced approach, then I suggest substituting the Horary points for the Front Mù Collecting points. That would then give you 12 needles in the legs/feet and five needles on the front of the trunk.

How will you needle each point? Do you want to nourish, flush, tonify or sedate?

The points (including the Front Mù Collecting point options) are listed in Table 10.4 with an example of how you might choose to needle them. If you have a different approach to needling the points, then feel free to stick with that approach.

Table 10.4 Wood overacting on Earth Chéng cycle

Point name	Special element/point	Needling method
LR 1	Wood on Wood	Balanced/nourish/flush – depends on the initial diagnosis
LR 3	Earth on Wood	These are associated elements, so they need to be needled in a balanced manner
LR 4	Metal on Wood	Balanced/nourish/flush – depends on initial diagnosis
SP 1	Wood on Earth	These are associated elements, so they need to be needled in a balanced manner
SP 3	Earth on Earth	Tonify – likely to be Spleen Qì Xū
SP 9	Water on Earth	Tonify the Child – likely to be Spleen Qì Xū
ST 36	Earth on Earth	Tonify – likely to be Stomach Qì Xū
ST 43	Wood on Earth	These are associated elements, so they need to be needled in a balanced manner
ST 44	Water on Earth	Tonify the Child – likely to be Stomach Qì Xū
LR 14	Front Mù Collecting point of the Liver	Balanced/nourish/flush – depends on the initial diagnosis
LR 13	Front Mù Collecting point of the Spleen	Tonify – likely to be Spleen Qì Xū
CV 12	Front Mù Collecting point of the Stomach	Tonify – likely to be Stomach Qì Xū

Earth overacting on Water

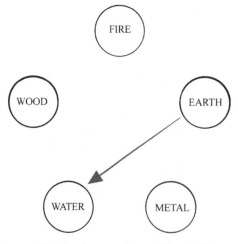

Diagram 10.4 Earth overacting on Water Chéng cycle

You diagnose your patient with the Zàng Fŭ pattern of Stomach Fire Blazing overacting on the Kidneys. This is Earth overacting on Water.

Use the Kè/Controlling cycle

This will be the Wood and Water points on the Stomach channel (Wood on Earth, Water on Earth) and the Earth and Fire points on the Kidney channel (Earth on Water, Fire on Water):

- Wood on Earth – ST 43

- Water on Earth – ST 44

- Earth on Water – KI 3

- Fire on Water – KI 2.

Use the Horary points

That would be the Earth point on the Stomach channel (Earth on Earth) and the Water point on the Kidney channel (Water on Water):

- Earth on Earth – ST 36

- Water on Water – KI 10.

How many needles, and is that in your accepted range?

If needled bilaterally, this would be 12 needles.

Is there a good balance with the needle locations in the combination?

In this case, all of the points are on the legs/feet. However, the theory is sound, so it's up to you. If, like me, you would prefer to take a more body-balanced approach, then I suggest substituting the Horary points for the Front Mù Collecting points. That would then give you eight needles in the legs/feet and three needles on the front of the trunk.

How will you needle each point? Do you want to nourish, flush, tonify or sedate?

The points (including the Front Mù Collecting point options) are listed in Table 10.5 with an example of how you might choose to needle them. If you have a different approach to needling the points, then feel free to stick with that approach.

Table 10.5 Earth overacting on Water Chéng cycle

Point name	Special element/point	Needling method
ST 36	Earth on Earth	Sedate
ST 43	Wood on Earth	Sedate the Mother

cont.

Point name	Special element/point	Needling method
ST 44	Water on Earth	These are associated elements, so they need to be needled in a balanced manner
KI 2	Fire on Water	Tonify the Child
KI 3	Earth on Water	These are associated elements, so they need to be needled in a balanced manner
KI 10	Water on Water	Tonify
CV 12	Front Mù Collecting point of the Stomach	Sedate
GB 25	Front Mù Collecting point of the Kidneys	Tonify

Water overacting on Fire

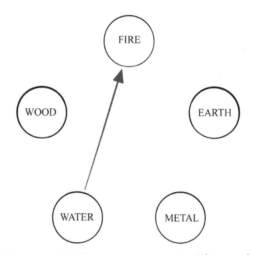

Diagram 10.5 Water overacting on Fire Chéng cycle

You diagnose your patient with the Shén disorders of fear/phobias and anxiety due to Kidney Yáng Xū (fear/phobias) leading to Heart Yáng Xū (anxiety). This is Water overacting on Fire.

Use the Kè/Controlling cycle
This will be the Earth and Fire points on the Kidney channel (Earth on Water, Fire on Water) and the Water and Metal points on the Heart channel (Water on Fire, Metal on Fire):

- Earth on Water – KI 3

- Fire on Water – KI 2

- Water on Fire – HT 3

- Metal on Fire – HT 4.

Use the Horary points

That would be the Water point on the Kidney channel (Water on Water) and the Fire point on the Heart channel (Fire on Fire):

- Water on Water – KI 10

- Fire on Fire – HT 8.

How many needles, and is that in your accepted range?

If needled bilaterally, this would be 12 needles.

Is there a good balance with the needle locations in the combination?

In this case, all of the points are distributed across the arms/hands or legs/feet, which is a suitable body balance. However, you may like to add in some additional points on the trunk. Some good ones to consider would be the Front Mù Collecting points or the Back Shù Transporting points.

How will you needle each point? Do you want to nourish, flush, tonify or sedate?

The points are listed in Table 10.6 with an example of how you might choose to needle them. If you have a different approach to needling the points, then feel free to stick with that approach.

Table 10.6 Water overacting on Fire Chéng cycle

Point name	Special element/point	Needling method
KI 2	Fire on Water	These are associated elements, so they need to be needled in a balanced manner
KI 3	Earth on Water	Tonify the Mother
KI 10	Water on Water	Tonify
HT 3	Water on Fire	These are associated elements, so they need to be needled in a balanced manner
HT 4	Metal on Fire	Tonify the Child
HT 8	Fire on Fire	Tonify

2. Wŭ Xíng Wŭ/Insulting cycle for complicated disorders

As discussed earlier, the Wŭ/Insulting cycle tracks along the same pathway as the Kè/Controlling cycle but in the opposite direction. Therefore, rather than the Kè cycle controlling/regulating the next element, the Wŭ insults the previous element. This will cause the previous element to become deficient/Xū, because it is being insulted by its Child.

The Wǔ/Insulting cycle is often used in clinical practice to describe an imbalance between two or more organs/elements.[4] Again, this is a somewhat generalized statement because there are alternative views on this, but for the sake of the special point categories, this is the theory we will apply to the Wǔ/Insulting cycle.

Can you apply the Wǔ/Insulting cycle to any imbalance between two or more organs/elements that your patients present with? In theory, the answer is no, because not all multiple organs/channels complaints can be treated using the Wǔ/Insulting cycle.

The key to using the Wǔ/Insulting cycle is to decide which organs or channels are affected and then see whether there is a relevant Wǔ/Insulting cycle category listed in Table 10.7. If there is, then you could theoretically use it; if not, then avoid using the Wǔ/Insulting cycle.

There are five possible Wǔ/Insulting cycle imbalances:[5]

• Fire insulting Water

• Water insulting Earth

• Earth insulting Wood

• Wood insulting Metal

• Metal insulting Fire.

I have included a point combination example for each. Two are for Zàng Fǔ patterns and three are for Shén-based disorders. That way there is a point combination for all five Wǔ/Insulting cycle imbalances.

The Wǔ/Insulting cycle point methods are listed in Table 10.7.

Table 10.7 Wǔ/Insulting cycle point method

Wǔ Xíng/Five Element	Point method	Point element and name	Point element and name
Fire element: Heart Small Intestine Pericardium Sān Jiāo	Water Metal	Water points: HT 3 SI 2 PC 3 TE 2	Metal points: HT 4 SI 1 PC 5 TE 1
Earth element: Spleen Stomach	Wood Water	Wood points: SP 1 ST 43	Water points: SP 9 ST 44
Metal element: Lungs Large Intestine	Fire Wood	Fire points: LU 10 LI 5	Wood points: LU 11 LI 3
Water element: Kidneys Urinary Bladder	Earth Fire	Earth points: KI 3 BL 40	Fire points: KI 2 BL 60
Wood element: Liver Gall Bladder	Metal Earth	Metal points: LR 4 GB 44	Earth points: LR 3 GB 34

Using the Wǔ/Insulting cycle in clinical practice is a little different to the Shēng/Generating and Kè/Controlling cycles. Consequently, each point combination will list how each point can be needled.

There are also five considerations when deciding on the point combination. These are:

1. Use the Kè/Controlling cycle (to help balance the Wǔ/Insulting cycle) as a clear link between the diseased organs. This will give the body clear instruction on what the points are being used for.

2. Use the Horary points for the diseased organs.

3. How many needles does that add up to once you have selected the Kè/Controlling cycle and Horary points? Is the number of needles in your accepted range?

4. Check to see where all the needles are located. Is there a good balance with the point combination?

5. Decide how you will needle each point. Do you want to nourish, flush, tonify or sedate?

I appreciate that this is a lot to consider when selecting points for an acupuncture point combination, but the more you do it, the faster you will get. I would also recommend having the subsequent tables (10.8–10.12) handy in clinic as a ready-reference guide.

Fire insulting Water

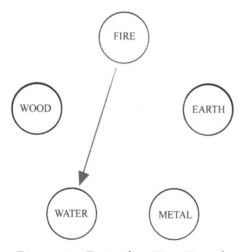

Diagram 10.6 Fire insulting Water Wǔ cycle

You diagnose your patient with the Zàng Fǔ pattern of Heart Fire Blazing insulting the Water element leading to Kidney Yáng Xū. This is Fire insulting Water.

Use the Kè/Controlling cycle

This will be the Water and Metal points on the Heart channel (Water on Fire, Metal on Fire) and the Earth and Fire points on the Kidney channel (Earth on Water, Fire on Water):

- Water on Fire – HT 3
- Metal on Fire – HT 4
- Earth on Water – KI 3
- Fire on Water – KI 2.

Use the Horary points

That would be the Fire point on the Heart channel (Fire on Fire) as well as the Water point on the Kidney channel (Water on Water):

- Fire on Fire – HT 8
- Water on Water – KI 10.

How many needles, and is that in your accepted range?

If needled bilaterally, this would be 12 needles.

Is there a good balance with the needle locations in the combination?

In this case, all of the points are distributed across the arms/hands or legs/feet, which is a suitable body balance. However, you may like to add in some additional points on the trunk. Some good ones to consider would be the Front Mù Collecting points or the Back Shù Transporting points.

How will you needle each point? Do you want to nourish, flush, tonify or sedate?

The points are listed in Table 10.8 with an example of how you might choose to needle them. If you have a different approach to needling the points, then feel free to stick with that approach.

Table 10.8 Fire insulting Water Wǔ cycle

Point name	Special element/point	Needling method
HT 3	Water on Fire	These are associated elements, so they need to be needled in a balanced manner
HT 4	Metal on Fire	Sedate the Child
HT 8	Fire on Fire	Sedate
KI 2	Fire on Water	These are associated elements, so they need to be needled in a balanced manner
KI 3	Earth on Water	Tonify the Mother
KI 10	Water on Water	Tonify

Water insulting Earth

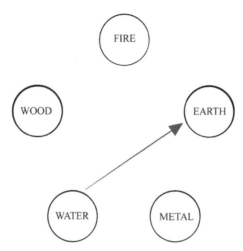

Diagram 10.7 Water insulting Earth Wŭ cycle

You diagnose your patient with the Shén disorders of fear/phobias and worry due to Kidney Yáng Xū (fear/phobias) insulting the Earth element and causing Spleen Yáng Xū (worry). This is Water insulting Earth.

Use the Kè/Controlling cycle

This will be the Earth and Fire points on the Kidney channel (Earth on Water, Fire on Water) and the Wood and Water points on the Spleen channel (Wood on Earth, Water on Earth):

- Earth on Water – KI 3
- Fire on Water – KI 2
- Wood on Earth – SP 1
- Water on Earth – SP 9.

Use the Horary points

That would be the Water point on the Kidney channel (Water on Water) and the Earth point on the Spleen channel (Earth on Earth):

- Water on Water – KI 10
- Earth on Earth – SP 3.

How many needles, and is that in your accepted range?

If needled bilaterally, this would be 12 needles.

Is there a good balance with the needle locations in the combination?

In this case, all of the points are on the legs/feet. However, the theory is sound, so it's up to you. If, like me, you would prefer to take a more body-balanced approach, then I suggest substituting the Horary points for the Front Mù Collecting points. That would then give you eight needles in the legs/feet and four needles on the front of the trunk.

How will you needle each point? Do you want to nourish, flush, tonify or sedate?

The points (including the Front Mù Collecting point options) are listed in Table 10.9 with an example of how you might choose to needle them. If you have a different approach to needling the points, then feel free to stick with that approach.

Table 10.9 Water insulting Earth Wǔ cycle

Point name	Special element/point	Needling method
KI 2	Fire on Water	Tonify the Child
KI 3	Earth on Water	These are associated elements, so they need to be needled in a balanced manner
KI 10	Water on Water	Tonify
SP 1	Wood on Earth	Tonify the Mother
SP 3	Earth on Earth	Tonify
SP 9	Water on Earth	These are associated elements, so they need to be needled in a balanced manner
GB 25	Front Mù Collecting point of the Kidneys	Tonify
LR 13	Front Mù Collecting point of the Spleen	Tonify

Earth insulting Wood

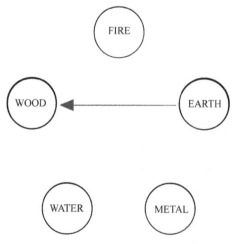

Diagram 10.8 Earth insulting Wood Wǔ cycle

You diagnose your patient with the Shén disorders of pensiveness and feeling overwhelmed/stressed due to Spleen Qì Xū (pensiveness) insulting the Wood element and causing Liver Xuè Xū (feeling overwhelmed/stressed). This is Earth insulting Wood.

Use the Kè/Controlling cycle

This will be the Wood and Water points on the Spleen channel (Wood on Earth, Water on Earth) and the Metal and Earth points on the Liver channel (Metal on Wood, Earth on Wood):

- Wood on Earth – SP 1
- Water on Earth – SP 9
- Metal on Wood – LR 4
- Earth on Wood – LR 3.

Use the Horary points

That would be the Earth point on the Spleen channel (Earth on Earth) and the Wood point on the Liver channel (Wood on Wood):

- Earth on Earth – SP 3
- Wood on Wood – LR 1.

How many needles, and is that in your accepted range?

If needled bilaterally, this would be 12 needles.

Is there a good balance with the needle locations in the combination?

In this case, all of the points are on the legs/feet. However, the theory is sound, so it's up to you. If, like me, you would prefer to take a more body-balanced approach, then I suggest substituting the Horary points for the Front Mù Collecting points. That would then give you eight needles in the legs/feet and four needles on the front of the trunk.

How will you needle each point? Do you want to nourish, flush, tonify or sedate?

The points (including the Front Mù Collecting point options) are listed in Table 10.10 with an example of how you might choose to needle them. If you have a different approach to needling the points, then feel free to stick with that approach.

Table 10.10 Earth insulting Wood Wŭ cycle

Point name	Special element/point	Needling method
SP 1	Wood on Earth	These are associated elements, so they need to be needled in a balanced manner
SP 3	Earth on Earth	Tonify
SP 9	Water on Earth	Tonify the Child
LR 1	Wood on Wood	Tonify
LR 3	Earth on Wood	These are associated elements, so they need to be needled in a balanced manner
LR 4	Metal on Wood	Tonify the Mother
LR 13	Front Mù Collecting point of the Spleen	Tonify
LR 14	Front Mù Collecting point of the Liver	Tonify

Wood insulting Metal

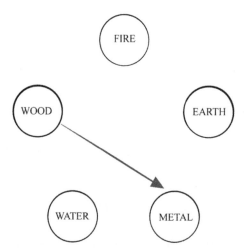

Diagram 10.9 Wood insulting Metal Wŭ cycle

You diagnose your patient with the Zàng Fŭ pattern of Liver Fire Blazing insulting the Metal element, leading to Lung Qì Xū. This is Wood insulting Metal.

Use the Kè/Controlling cycle

This will be the Metal and Earth points on the Liver channel (Metal on Wood, Earth on Wood) and the Fire and Wood points on the Lung channel (Fire on Metal, Wood on Metal):

- Metal on Wood – LR 4

- Earth on Wood – LR 3

- Fire on Metal – LU 10

- Wood on Metal – LU 11.

Use the Horary points

That would be the Wood point on the Liver channel (Wood on Wood) and the Metal point on the Lung channel (Metal on Metal):

- Wood on Wood – LR 1

- Metal on Metal – LU 8.

How many needles, and is that in your accepted range?

If needled bilaterally, this would be 12 needles.

Is there a good balance with the needle locations in the combination?

In this case, all of the points are distributed across the arms/hands or legs/feet, which is a suitable body balance. However, you may like to add in some additional points on the trunk. Some good ones to consider would be the Front Mù Collecting points or the Back Shù Transporting points.

How will you needle each point? Do you want to nourish, flush, tonify or sedate?

The points are listed in Table 10.11 with an example of how you might choose to needle them. If you have a different approach to needling the points, then feel free to stick with that approach.

Table 10.11 Wood insulting Metal Wŭ cycle

Point name	Special element/point	Needling method
LR 1	Wood on Wood	Sedate
LR 3	Earth on Wood	Sedate the Child
LR 4	Metal on Wood	These are associated elements, so they need to be needled in a balanced manner
LU 8	Metal on Metal	Tonify
LU 10	Fire on Metal	Tonify the Mother
LU 11	Wood on Metal	These are associated elements, so they need to be needled in a balanced manner

Metal insulting Fire

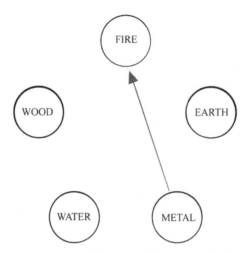

Diagram 10.10 Metal insulting Fire Wŭ cycle

You diagnose your patient with the Shén disorders of grief and sadness due to Lung Qì Xū (grief) insulting the Fire element and causing Heart Qì Xū (sadness). This is Metal insulting Fire.

Use the Kè/Controlling cycle

This will be the Fire and Wood points on the Lung channel (Fire on Metal, Wood on Metal) and the Water and Metal points on the Heart channel (Water on Fire, Metal on Fire):

- Fire on Metal – LU 10

- Wood on Metal – LU 11

- Water on Fire – HT 3

- Metal on Fire – HT 4.

Use the Horary points

That would be the Metal point on the Lung channel (Metal on Metal) and the Fire point on the Heart channel (Fire on Fire):

- Metal on Metal – LU 8

- Fire on Fire – HT 8.

How many needles, and is that in your accepted range?

If needled bilaterally, this would be 12 needles.

Is there a good balance with the needle locations in the combination?

In this case, all of the points are on the arms/hands. However, the theory is sound, so it's up to you. If, like me, you would prefer to take a more body-balanced approach, then I suggest substituting the Horary points for the Front Mù Collecting points. That would then give you eight needles in the legs/feet and three needles on the front of the trunk.

How will you needle each point? Do you want to nourish, flush, tonify or sedate?

The points (including the Front Mù Collecting point options) are listed in Table 10.12 with an example of how you might choose to needle them. If you have a different approach to needling the points, then feel free to stick with that approach.

Table 10.12 Metal insulting Fire Wŭ cycle

Point name	Special element/point	Needling method
LU 8	Metal on Metal	Tonify
LU 10	Fire on Metal	These are associated elements, so they need to be needled in a balanced manner
LU 11	Wood on Metal	Tonify the Child
HT 3	Water on Fire	Tonify the Mother
HT 4	Metal on Fire	These are associated elements, so they need to be needled in a balanced manner
HT 8	Fire on Fire	Tonify
LU 1	Front Mù Collecting point of the Lungs	Tonify
CV 14	Front Mù Collecting point of the Heart	Tonify

3. Wŭ Xíng mix and match

Sometimes the patient complains of a mix of signs and symptoms that don't fit nicely into just one organ or element. Occasionally, this will result in disorders occurring in two elements (across multiple organs) at the same time.

For example, Liver Fire Blazing can lead to Heart Qì Xū. Here, the Wood element (Mother) has depleted the Fire element (Child) along the Shēng/Generating cycle. In this example, you actually treat the Mother organ/channel because it is actively injuring its Child. This is different to the point combination examples given previously for the Shēng, Kè, Chéng and Wŭ cycles. As you may recall, those point combinations were used exclusively for the element/channel affected – that is, you used the Mother or Child point on the injured organ/channel.

The 69th difficulty (Unschuld 1986, p.584) of *The Classic of Difficulties* (*Canon of the Yellow Emperor's Eighty-One Difficult Issues*/Huáng Dì Bā Shí Yī Nán Jīng/黄帝八十一難經) confirms this when it says:

> If in spring one feels a [movement in the] vessels that is [associated with] the kidneys, this represents a depletion [Xū] evil. In such a situation the kidneys are depleted and cannot transmit any influences to the liver. Hence one fills the kidneys... The liver is the child of the kidneys. Hence [the text] states: 'Fill the mother.' If in spring one feels a [movement in the] vessels that is [associated with] the heart, this represents a repletion [Shí] evil. In such a situation the heart is replete with abundant influences. These [influences] move contrary to their proper direction and come to seize the liver. Hence one drains the heart... The liver represents the mother of the heart. Hence [the text] states: 'Drain the child.'[6]

Let's explore the example above in a little more detail. This will be done via two different patients with the same main complaints of palpitations and tiredness:

- *Patient 1: Zàng Fǔ pattern diagnosis of Heart Qì Xū, which is the cause of their palpitations and tiredness.*

  The treatment for this patient could be via the use of the Shēng/Generating cycle. That would use the 'Wood Earth' point method on the affected organ/channel. The Wood point is HT 9 and the Earth point is HT 7. Additional points would need to be selected to align with this patient's main complaints and Zàng Fǔ pattern.

- *Patient 2: Zàng Fǔ pattern diagnosis of Liver Fire Blazing which is leading to Heart Qì Xū, and this is what is causing the palpitations and tiredness.*

  The treatment for this patient would potentially need to be different to the one chosen for patient 1.[7] This is because a different organ (and element) are the main cause of your patient's complaints. So even though the Heart Qì Xū is causing your patient's main complaints (manifestation/Biāo), you might still focus on the Liver Fire Blazing because it started everything (the root cause/Běn). In this instance, you don't treat the Heart but the Liver. This style of point combination is discussed further below.

We also need to consider that sometimes (quite often actually) three elements can be diseased simultaneously. A good example of that is Spleen and Lung Qì Xū with Liver Yáng Rising. Here we have the Earth element (Spleen), Metal element (Lungs) and Wood element (Liver) affected along both the Shēng/Generating and Kè/Controlling cycles. This results in a mix and match of Mother and Child organs which poses a range of questions for the practitioner, including:

- Which organ do you treat first?

- Can you treat more than one organ in the same treatment?

- Was there an organ that was the instigator, or root cause, of the other organs becoming diseased?

- Which organ is most acute and potentially easiest to treat? This organ is often the one that produces the main complaints for which the patient seeks treatment. If that is the case, then this organ is considered to be the manifestation.[8]

- How often do I need to treat them?

- Do I have to treat the patient's chief complaint? What if I think something else is more important?

These questions are outside the scope of this book, but there does need to be a brief discussion on it nonetheless. This is because it dictates what point combination you might employ; and that is an important part of this book. I will incorporate this discussion into five treatment examples for the Wŭ Xíng mix and match. This will include two examples I have already touched on plus three more:

- Liver Fire Blazing leading to Heart Qì Xū (Wood and Fire)

- Spleen and Kidney Yáng Xū (Earth and Water)

- Kidney Yīn Xū leading to Heart Yīn Xū (Water and Fire)

- Stomach and Large Intestine (Yáng Míng) Fire Blazing (Earth and Metal)

- Spleen and Lung Qì Xū with Liver Yáng Rising (Earth, Metal and Wood).

There are also three considerations when deciding on the point combination. These are:

1. Use the opposing element point on each channel. For example, in the case of Kidney Yáng Xū (Water) leading to Lung Qì Xū (Metal), you do the Water point on the Lung channel (Water on Metal) and the Metal point on the Kidney channel (Metal on Water).

2. Use the Horary points for the diseased organs.

3. Do you treat the root or manifestation, or both at the same time? Ultimately, your point combination will be different depending on whether you plan to treat the root or the manifestation, or try to treat both at the same time.

Liver Fire Blazing leading to Heart Qì Xū

Shēng/Generating cycle – Wood depleting Fire (see Diagram 10.11).

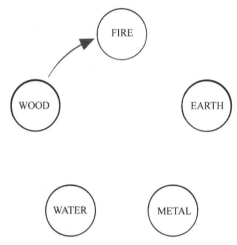

Diagram 10.11 Wood depleting Fire Shēng cycle

In this instance it has been established that Liver Fire Blazing was the root cause of Heart Qì Xū, which is the manifestation. Wood (Mother) is therefore depleting the Fire (Child) along the Shēng/Generating cycle.

In all likelihood your patient has presented to you with signs and symptoms of palpitations, tiredness, anger/irritability, stress/mental restlessness, red/dry eyes and headaches, to name but a few.[9]

Use the opposing element point on each channel

That would be the Fire point on the Liver channel (Fire on Wood) and the Wood point on the Heart channel (Wood on Fire) done via the Shēng/Generating cycle:

- Fire on Wood – LR 2

- Wood on Fire – HT 9.

Use the Horary points

That would be the Wood point on the Liver channel (Wood on Wood) and the Fire point on the Heart channel (Fire on Fire):

- Wood on Wood – LR 1

- Fire on Fire – HT 8.

Treat the root or manifestation, or both at the same time?

If you target the root of Liver Fire Blazing first, then you could include the points in Table 10.13 to sedate Liver Fire (I have included the Fire Wood, Wood Fire and Horary points).

Table 10.13 Liver Fire Blazing treatment[10]

Location of point	Points	
Head/face/neck	GB 20	
Trunk (back)	BL 18	
Arms/hands	LI 11 HT 8	HT 9
Legs/feet	LR 1 LR 2	GB 37
Total points needled	16 needles used bilaterally	

If you target the manifestation of Heart Qì Xū first, then you could include the points in Table 10.14 to tonify Heart Qì (I have included the Fire Wood, Wood Fire and Horary points).

Table 10.14 Heart Qì Xū treatment[11]

Location of point	Points	
Trunk (front)	CV 6 CV 14	CV 17
Trunk (back)	BL 15	
Arms/hands	HT 7 HT 8	HT 9
Legs/feet	LR 1 LR 2	ST 36
Total points needled	17 needles used bilaterally	

You might even try to target the root and manifestation of Liver Fire Blazing and Heart Qì Xū in the same treatment. If that is the case, you might do a treatment similar to that shown in Table 10.15.

Table 10.15 Liver Fire Blazing and Heart Qì Xū treatment

Location of point	Points	
Head/face/neck	GB 20	
Trunk (front)	CV 6 CV 14	CV 17
Trunk (back)	BL 15	BL 18
Arms/hands	LI 11 HT 7	HT 8 HT 9
Legs/feet	LR 1 LR 2	ST 36 GB 37
Total points needled	25 needles used bilaterally	

At 25 needles, that might be too many to use in one treatment. If that is the case, then you might look to split the points across two separate treatments.[12] Or a unilateral treatment would bring it down to 14 needles.

Spleen and Kidney Yáng Xū

Kè/Controlling cycle and Wǔ/Insulting cycle – Earth and Water (see Diagram 10.12).

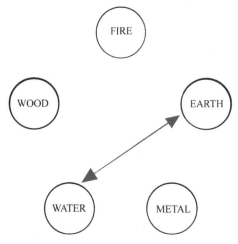

Diagram 10.12 Earth and Water imbalance on the Kè and Wǔ cycles

In this instance your focus is to treat the Earth (Spleen Yáng Xū) and Water (Kidney Yáng Xū) elements. Unlike the previous example, where it was established which organ was the root cause, this diagnosis doesn't indicate that. Therefore, your emphasis depends on which organ is the root and which is the manifestation.

From my clinical experience, the likelihood is that the Spleen becomes depleted first and the Kidneys follow. In this instance, the Earth (Mother) is depleting the Water (Child) along the Kè/Controlling cycle.

It is, however, not unusual for the Kidneys to become deficient/Xū first, especially in genetic diseases or in the elderly.[13] In this scenario, the Water is still the Child but is insulting the Earth (Mother) along the Wǔ cycle.

In a clinical setting, your patient has likely presented with signs and symptoms of coldness, low back pain, edema and loose stools, to name but a few.[14]

Use the opposing element point on each channel

That would be the Water point on the Spleen channel (Water on Earth) and the Earth point on the Kidney channel (Earth on Water) done along the Kè/Controlling cycle:

- Water on Earth – SP 9

- Earth on Water – KI 3.

Use the Horary points

That would be the Earth point on the Spleen channel (Earth on Earth) and the Water point on the Kidney channel (Water on Water):

- Earth on Earth – SP 3

- Water on Water – KI 10.

Treat the root or manifestation, or both at the same time?

If you target Spleen Yáng Xū first, then you could include the points in Table 10.16 to tonify Spleen Yáng (I have included the Water Earth, Earth Water and Horary points).

Table 10.16 Spleen Yáng Xū treatment[15]

Location of point	Points	
Trunk (front)	CV 9	ST 28
Trunk (back)	BL 20	BL 22
Arms/hands	TE 6	
Legs/feet	SP 3 SP 9	KI 3 KI 10
Total points needled	17 needles used bilaterally	

If you target Kidney Yáng Xū first, then you could include the points in Table 10.17 to tonify Kidney Yáng (I have included the Water Earth, Earth Water and Horary points).

Table 10.17 Kidney Yáng Xū treatment[16]

Location of point	Points	
Trunk (front)	CV 4	CV 6
Trunk (back)	BL 23	GV 4
Arms/hands	TE 4	
Legs/feet	SP 3 SP 9	KI 3 KI 10
Total points needled	15 needles used bilaterally	

You might even try to target the Spleen and Kidney Yáng Xū in the same treatment. If that is the case, you might do a treatment similar to that shown in Table 10.18.

Table 10.18 Spleen and Kidney Yáng Xū treatment

Location of point	Points	
Trunk (front)	CV 4	CV 9
	CV 6	ST 28
Trunk (back)	BL 20	BL 23
	BL 22	GV 4
Arms/hands	TE 4	TE 6
Legs/feet	SP 3	KI 3
	SP 9	KI 10
Total points needled	24 needles used bilaterally	

At 24 needles, that might be too many to use in one treatment. If you don't have a problem with that, then go for it; otherwise, consider a unilateral treatment, as that would reduce it to 14 needles.

Kidney Yīn Xū leading to Heart Yīn Xū

Kè/Controlling cycle and Chéng/Overacting cycle – Water controlling Fire (see Diagram 10.13).

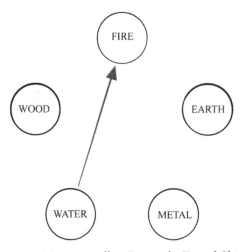

Diagram 10.13 Water controlling Fire on the Kè and Chéng cycles

In this instance it has been established that Kidney Yīn Xū was the root cause of Heart Yīn Xū, which is the manifestation. Water (Mother) is therefore depleting the Fire (Child) along the Kè/Controlling cycle, which actually makes it a Chéng/Overacting cycle issue.

In all likelihood your patient has presented to you with signs and symptoms of insomnia with nightmares, palpitations, poor memory, dizziness, tinnitus, night sweats and low back pain, to name but a few.[17]

Use the opposing element point on each channel

That would be the Fire point on the Kidney channel (Fire on Water) and the Water point on the Heart channel (Water on Fire) done via the Kè/Controlling cycle:

- Fire on Water – KI 2

- Water on Fire – HT 3.

Use the Horary points

That would be the Water point on the Kidney channel (Water on Water) and the Fire point on the Heart channel (Fire on Fire):

- Water on Water – KI 10

- Fire on Fire – HT 8.

Treat the root or manifestation, or both at the same time?

If you target the root of Kidney Yīn Xū first, then you could include the points in Table 10.19 to tonify Kidney Yīn (I have included the Fire Water, Water Fire and Horary points).

Table 10.19 Kidney Yīn Xū treatment[18]

Location of point	Points	
Trunk (front)	CV 4	CV 6
Trunk (back)	BL 23	
Arms/hands	HT 3 HT 6	HT 8
Legs/feet	KI 2 KI 10	SP 6
Total points needled	16 needles used bilaterally	

If you target the manifestation of Heart Yīn Xū first, then you could include the points in Table 10.20 to tonify Heart Yīn (I have included the Fire Water, Water Fire and Horary points).

Table 10.20 Heart Yīn Xū treatment[19]

Location of point	Points	
Trunk (front)	CV 14	CV 15
Trunk (back)	BL 15	
Arms/hands	HT 3 HT 6	HT 8
Legs/feet	KI 2 KI 10	SP 6
Total points needled	16 needles used bilaterally	

You might even try to target the root and manifestation of Kidney and Heart Yīn Xū in the same treatment. If that is the case, you might do a treatment similar to that shown in Table 10.21.

Table 10.21 Kidney and Heart Yīn Xū treatment

Location of point	Points	
Trunk (front)	CV 4 CV 6	CV 14 CV 15
Trunk (back)	BL 15	BL 23
Arms/hands	HT 3 HT 6	HT 8
Legs/feet	KI 2 KI 10	SP 6
Total points needled	20 needles used bilaterally	

At 20 needles, that might be too many to use in one treatment. If you don't have a problem with that, then go for it; otherwise, consider a unilateral treatment, as that would reduce it to 12 needles.

Stomach and Large Intestine (Yáng Míng) Fire Blazing

Shēng/Generating cycle – Earth and Metal (see Diagram 10.14).

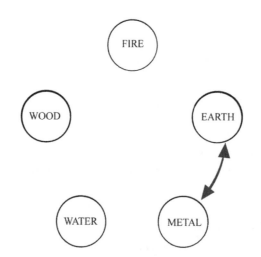

Diagram 10.14 Earth and Metal imbalance Shēng cycle

In this instance your focus is to treat the Earth (Stomach Fire Blazing) and Metal (Large Intestine Fire Blazing) elements. Unlike the previous example, where it was established which organ was the root cause, this diagnosis doesn't indicate that. Therefore, your emphasis depends on which organ is the root and which is the manifestation.

From my clinical experience, the likelihood is that the Stomach becomes Excess/Shí first and the Large Intestine follows. In this instance, the Earth (Mother) is sending Shí heat to the Metal (Child) along the Shēng/Generating cycle.

In a clinical setting, your patient has likely presented to you with signs and symptoms of red face, fevers, heartburn, bleeding gums, bad breath, constipation or much worse.[20]

Use the opposing element point on each channel

That would be the Metal point on the Stomach channel (Metal on Earth) and the Earth point on the Large Intestine channel (Earth on Metal) done along the Shēng/Generating cycle:

- Metal on Earth – ST 45

- Earth on Metal – LI 11.

Use the Horary points

That would be the Earth point on the Stomach channel (Earth on Earth) and the Metal point on the Large Intestine channel (Metal on Metal):

- Earth on Earth – ST 36

- Metal on Metal – LI 1.

Treat the root or manifestation, or both at the same time?

If you target Stomach Fire Blazing first, then you could include the points in Table 10.22 to sedate Stomach Fire (I have included the Metal Earth, Earth Metal and Horary points).

Table 10.22 Stomach Fire Blazing treatment[21]

Location of point	Points	
Head/face/neck	ST 6	
Trunk (front)	CV 12	ST 21
Trunk (back)	BL 21	
Arms/hands	LI 1 LI 11	PC 8
Legs/feet	ST 36	ST 45
Total points needled	17 needles used bilaterally	

If you target Large Intestine Fire Blazing, then you could include the points in Table 10.23 to sedate Large Intestine Fire (I have included the Metal Earth, Earth Metal and Horary points).

Table 10.23 Large Intestine Fire Blazing treatment[22]

Location of point	Points	
Trunk (front)	ST 25	
Trunk (back)	BL 25	
Arms/hands	LI 1 LI 11	TE 6
Legs/feet	ST 36	ST 45
Total points needled	14 needles used bilaterally	

You might even try to target the Stomach and Large Intestine Fire Blazing in the same treatment. If that is the case, you might do a treatment similar to that shown in Table 10.24.

Table 10.24 Stomach and Large Intestine Fire Blazing treatment

Location of point	Points	
Head/face/neck	ST 6	
Trunk (front)	CV 12 ST 21	ST 25
Trunk (back)	BL 21	BL 25
Arms/hands	LI 1 LI 11	PC 8 TE 6
Legs/feet	ST 36	ST 45
Total points needled	23 needles used bilaterally	

At 23 needles, that might be too many to use in one treatment. If you don't have a problem with that, then go for it; otherwise, consider a unilateral treatment as that would reduce it to 12 needles.

Spleen and Lung Qì Xū with Liver Yáng Rising

Shēng/Generating and Kè/Controlling cycle – Earth, Metal and Wood (see Diagram 10.15).

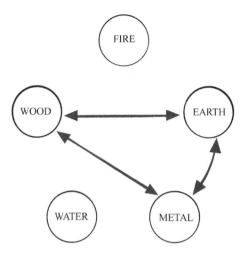

Diagram 10.15 Earth, Metal and Wood imbalances on the Shēng and Kè cycles

Unlike the previous examples in this mix-and-match method, which only had two organs injured, this imbalance has three organs that have been affected.

Unlike previous examples, where it was established which organ was the root cause, this diagnosis doesn't indicate that. Therefore, your emphasis depends on which organ is the root, which is the manifestation and which is sitting in the middle.

In this scenario, one organ started all of the problems, and this organ is considered the root cause. Over time it injures a second organ, which is the one sitting in the middle, before both damaged organs trigger injury to a third. This is considered the most recent and is therefore called the manifestation.

In Spleen and Lung Qì Xū with Liver Yáng Rising there are six possible scenarios:

- Spleen Qì Xū (root) leading to Lung Qì Xū and then Liver Yáng Rising (manifestation)

- Spleen Qì Xū (root) leading to Liver Yáng Rising and then Lung Qì Xū (manifestation)

- Lung Qì Xū (root) leading to Spleen Qì Xū and then Liver Yáng Rising (manifestation)

- Lung Qì Xū (root) leading to Liver Yáng Rising and then Spleen Qì Xū (manifestation)

- Liver Yáng Rising (root) leading to Spleen Qì Xū and then Lung Qì Xū (manifestation)

- Liver Yáng Rising (root) leading to Lung Qì Xū and then Spleen Qì Xū (manifestation).

Use the opposing element point on each channel

That would be the Metal and Wood points on the Spleen channel (Metal on Earth and Wood on Earth), the Earth and Wood points on the Lung channel (Earth on Metal and Wood on Metal) and the Earth and Metal points on the Liver channel (Earth on Wood and Metal on Wood) along the Shēng/Generating and Kè/Controlling cycles:

- Metal on Earth – SP 5

- Wood on Earth – SP 1

- Earth on Metal – LU 9

- Wood on Metal – LU 11

- Earth on Wood – LR 3

- Metal on Wood – LR 4.

Use the Horary points

That would be the Earth point on the Spleen channel (Earth on Earth), the Metal point on the Lung channel (Metal on Metal) and the Wood point on the Liver channel (Wood on Wood):

- Earth on Earth – SP 3

- Metal on Metal – LU 8

- Wood on Wood – LR 1.

Treat the root or manifestation, or both at the same time?

This will depend on whether you plan to treat Spleen Qì Xū, Lung Qì Xū or Liver Yáng Rising, or try to treat all three at the same time. We will discuss this further now.

Point combination treatments are shown in Tables 10.25–10.28.

SPLEEN QÌ XŪ (ROOT) LEADING TO LUNG QÌ XŪ AND THEN LIVER YÁNG RISING (MANIFESTATION)

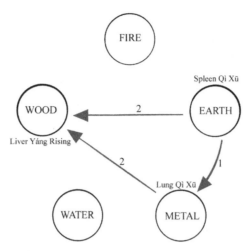

Diagram 10.16 Spleen Qì Xū leading to Lung Qì Xū and then Liver Yáng Rising

In this patient diagnosis, Spleen Qì became Xū and is the root cause of all other organ problems. Over time it injures Lung Qì along the Shēng/Generating cycle before both injure the Liver, leading to Liver Yáng Rising, which is the manifestation. This final double organ act works on:

- the Chéng cycle with the Lungs overacting on the Liver; Metal overacting on Wood

- the Wŭ cycle with the Spleen insulting the Liver; Earth insulting Wood.

SPLEEN QÌ XŪ (ROOT) LEADING TO LIVER YÁNG RISING AND THEN LUNG QÌ XŪ (MANIFESTATION)

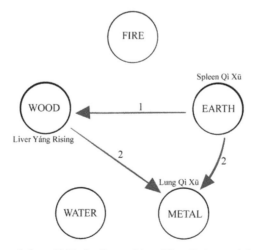

Diagram 10.17 Spleen Qì Xū leading to Liver Yáng Rising and then Lung Qì Xū

In this patient diagnosis, Spleen Qì became Xū and is the root cause of all other organ problems. Over time it injures Liver Yáng along the Kè/Controlling cycle (but is actually a Wǔ/Insulting cycle issue). The final act is when both injure the Lungs, leading to Lung Qì Xū, which is the manifestation. This final double organ act works on:

- the Wǔ cycle with the Liver insulting the Lungs; Wood insulting Metal

- the Shēng cycle with the Spleen depleting the Lungs; Earth depleting Metal.

LUNG QÌ XŪ (ROOT) LEADING TO SPLEEN QÌ XŪ AND THEN LIVER YÁNG RISING (MANIFESTATION)

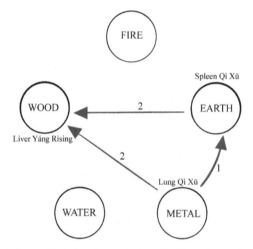

Diagram 10.18 Lung Qì Xū leading to Spleen Qì Xū and then Liver Yáng Rising

In this patient diagnosis, Lung Qì became Xū and is the root cause of all other organ problems. Over time it injures Spleen Qì along the Shēng/Generating cycle before both injure the Liver, leading to Liver Yáng Rising, which is the manifestation. This final double organ act works on:

- the Chéng cycle with the Lungs overacting on the Liver; Metal overacting on Wood

- the Wǔ cycle with the Spleen insulting the Liver; Earth insulting Wood.

LUNG QÌ XŪ (ROOT) LEADING TO LIVER YÁNG RISING AND THEN SPLEEN QÌ XŪ (MANIFESTATION)

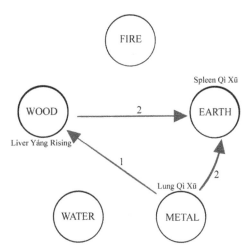

Diagram 10.19 Lung Qì Xū leading to Liver Yáng Rising and then Spleen Qì Xū

In this patient diagnosis, Lung Qì became Xū and is the root cause of all other organ problems. Over time it injures Liver Yáng along the Kè/Controlling cycle (but is actually a Chéng/Overacting cycle issue). The final act is when both injure the Spleen, leading to Spleen Qì Xū, which is the manifestation. This final double organ act works on:

- the Chéng cycle with the Liver overacting on the Spleen; Wood overacting on Earth

- the Shēng cycle with the Lungs depleting the Spleen; Metal depleting Earth.

LIVER YÁNG RISING (ROOT) LEADING TO SPLEEN QÌ XŪ AND THEN LUNG QÌ XŪ (MANIFESTATION)

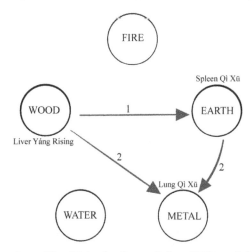

Diagram 10.20 Liver Yáng Rising leading to Spleen Qì Xū and then Lung Qì Xū

In this patient diagnosis, the Liver becomes Xū before (gradually) becoming Shí as well (Liver Yáng Rising – Shí on Xū). It is the root cause of all other organ problems. Over time it injures Spleen Qì along the Kè/Controlling cycle (but is actually a Chéng/Overacting cycle issue), before both injure the Lungs, leading to Lung Qì Xū, which is the manifestation. This final double organ act works on:

- the Wǔ cycle with the Liver insulting the Lungs; Wood insulting Metal

- the Shēng cycle with the Spleen depleting the Lungs; Earth depleting Metal.

LIVER YÁNG RISING (ROOT) LEADING TO LUNG QÌ XŪ AND THEN SPLEEN QÌ XŪ (MANIFESTATION)

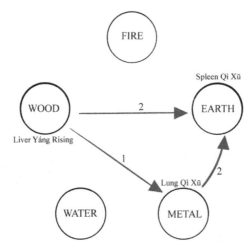

Diagram 10.21 Liver Yáng Rising leading to Lung Qì Xū and then Spleen Qì Xū

In this patient diagnosis, the Liver becomes Xū before (gradually) becoming Shí as well (Liver Yáng Rising – Shí on Xū). It is the root cause of all other organ problems. Over time it injures Lung Qì along the Kè/Controlling cycle (but is actually a Wǔ/Insulting cycle issue), before both injure the Spleen, leading to Spleen Qì Xū, which is the manifestation. This final double organ act works on:

- the Chéng cycle with the Liver overacting on the Spleen; Wood overacting on Earth

- the Shēng cycle with the Lungs depleting the Spleen; Metal depleting Earth.

A good base-level treatment that works on all three organs equally, as well as providing a distinct link between the three main elements of Earth, Metal and Wood, is shown in Table 10.25. The treatment includes the Metal Earth, Wood Earth, Earth Metal, Wood Metal, Earth Wood, Metal Wood and Horary points.

Table 10.25 Spleen and Lung Qì Xū with Liver Yáng Rising treatment

Location of point	Points	
Arms/hands	LU 8 LU 9	LU 11

Legs/feet	SP 1	LR 1
	SP 3	LR 3
	SP 5	LR 4
Total points needled	18 needles used bilaterally	

If you decide to tonify Spleen Qì Xū first, then you could include the points in Table 10.26. You could also consider using some points from Table 10.25.

Table 10.26 Spleen Qì Xū treatment[23]

Location of point	Points	
Trunk (front)	LR 13	CV 12
	CV 9	
Trunk (back)	BL 20	
Arms/hands	LU 7	
Legs/feet	SP 3	ST 36
	SP 6	
Total points needled	14 needles used bilaterally	

If you decide to tonify Lung Qì Xū first, then you could include the points in Table 10.27. You could also consider using some points from Table 10.25.

Table 10.27 Lung Qì Xū treatment[24]

Location of point	Points	
Trunk (front)	CV 6	CV 17
Trunk (back)	BL 13	BL 43
Arms/hands	LU 7	LU 9
Legs/feet	ST 36	SP 6
Total points needled	14 needles used bilaterally	

If you decide to treat Liver Yáng Rising first, then you could include the points in Table 10.28. You could also consider using some points from Table 10.25.

Table 10.28 Liver Yáng Rising treatment[25]

Location of point	Points	
Head/face/neck	GV 20	GB 20
Trunk (front)	CV 4	
Trunk (back)	BL 18	
Legs/feet	LR 2	GB 43
	LR 3	KI 3
Total points needled	14 needles used bilaterally	

Regardless of your choice, you need to commit to a theme with the treatment. What are you treating first? Are you treating the root? Or treating the manifestation first? Are you treating the middle organ first? Or are you trying to do it all at the same time?

Every choice provided is a proven and legitimate approach, so choose one and commit.

Over the past three chapters (8–10) we have analyzed Wǔ Xíng acupuncture point combinations in depth. Yet we have still barely touched the surface of an extremely complex, intricate, yet fascinating school of thought. For more information, please refer to my references from these three chapters. Then consider reading those books, as well as referring to their reference lists.

Notes

1   De Botton 2000, p.91. This is only part of Seneca's *Praemeditatio*; the entire meditation is, in my opinion, one of the greatest philosophical pieces of all time. Seneca (4 BCE–65 CE) is, currently, my favorite Western philosopher ever. His ideas, thoughts and actions were unforgettable. The battles he had with the Goddess Fortune were, though quite unorthodox, simply breathtaking. I actually don't agree with a fair chunk of what he wrote, but that doesn't make him any less amazing in my eyes. For example, he preferred to focus on the worst possible outcome in any given situation, whereas I prefer to focus on the best possible outcome. Regardless, he is the King of Western philosophy!

2   Maciocia 2015, pp.24, 32.

3   Ibid., p.24.

4   Ibid., pp.24–25, 32–33.

5   Ibid., pp.24–25.

6   'The text' that is being referred to is *The Yellow Emperor's Classic* (*Inner Canon of the Yellow Emperor*/Huáng Dì Nèi Jīng).

7   It is possible for you to use the same treatment for both patients because you are still treating a component of their diagnosis – and it's still a very important component. Typically, however, if you can be as specific as possible with your acupuncture point combination, this will give you a greater chance of patient recovery.

8   This statement, although technically correct, does have a small issue attached to it. Typically, when you refer to the root and manifestation, you are talking about an underlying organ that is diseased (root) which has a range of signs and symptoms associated with it. Over time, if left untreated, this organ negatively impacts on other organs. The most recent organ will then have a range of different signs and symptoms which the patient is needing priority treatment for; it is these signs and symptoms that are considered the manifestation, and not necessarily the organ that is associated with

those main patient complaints. But when you think about it, that most recent organ that's diseased is actually the one producing the signs and symptoms, so technically it can still be referred to as the manifestation, with the original cause of everything considered to be the root.

9   McDonald and Penner 1994, pp.75, 129; Maciocia 2015, pp.491, 542.

10 McDonald and Penner 1994, p.131; Maciocia 2015, p.544.

11 McDonald and Penner 1994, p.76.

12 Doing two separate treatments with that one group of 25 needles seems a little pointless if you ask me. This is because you could do the same by treating the Liver Fire Blazing in one treatment and treating the Heart Qì Xū in the next treatment. To me, this would actually be more target-specific. The points have a greater affinity in those separate groupings too, making it a lot clearer to the patient's body what you are trying to do. So I would alternate between Liver Fire Blazing and Heart Qì Xū, or simply target one pattern for a period of time, rather than try to needle those 25 points across two separate treatments.

13 McDonald and Penner 1994, p.189.

14 Ross 1985, p.200.

15 Hartmann 2009, p.18.

16 Ibid., p.5.

17 McDonald and Penner 1994, p.198.

18 Hartmann 2009, p.5.

19 Ibid., p.4.

20 Yáng Míng Fire Blazing can present with severe bowel disorders such as irritable bowel syndrome, ulcerative colitis and even Crohn's disease.

21 McDonald and Penner 1994, p.64; Ross 1985, p.99.

22 McDonald and Penner 1994, p.21.

23 Hartmann 2009, p.18.

24 Ibid., p.11; McDonald and Penner 1994, p.16.

25 Hartmann 2009, p.9; Ross 1985, p.111.

Part 4

Chinese Medicine Esoteric Categories and Acupuncture Point Combinations

[The Goddess Fortune asks Boethius], Why do you burden me each day, mortal man, with your querulous accusations? What harm have I done you? ... When nature brought you forth from your mother's womb I received you naked and devoid of everything and fed you from my own resources. I was inclined to favour you, and I brought you up – and this is what makes you lose patience with me – with a measure of indulgence, surrounding you with all the splendour and affluence at my command. Now I have decided to withdraw my hand. You have been receiving a favour as one who has had the use of another's possessions, and you have no right to complain as if what you have lost was fully your own. You have no cause to begin groaning at me: I have done you no violence... Shall man's insatiable greed bind me to a constancy which is alien to my ways? Inconstancy is my very essence; it is the game I never cease to play as I turn my wheel in its ever-changing circle, filled with joy as I bring the top to the bottom and the bottom to the top. Yes, rise up on my wheel if you like, but don't count it an injury when by the same token you begin to fall, as the rules of the game will require.

Boethius (480–524 CE)[1]

Welcome to Part 4 of *The Principles and Practical Application of Acupuncture Point Combinations*. Over the next four chapters I will be exploring some of the more esoteric ideas/topics in Chinese medicine. These topics are full of fascinating discussion, which I hope you enjoy reading as much as I enjoyed writing it.

It is worth noting that these four topics of the Qī Qíng/Seven Emotions, Qí Jīng Bā Mài/Eight Extraordinary Vessels, Wǔ Shén/Five Spirits and Wǔ Xíng/Five Element Archetypes do tend to get people talking. I know some of you will probably have strong views about them, which may oppose others' views. Regardless, these topics rarely disappoint!

Finally, like the Goddess Fortune implies (in the quotation above), life runs in cycles, and that is perfect symmetry for the four topics in Part 4. If you go into these chapters with that in mind, I think you will find that the chapters will read better and make more sense.

Why? Because they are polarizing and therefore tend to create strong discussion. I can't claim to know everyone's thoughts on why they have such strong views; although from personal experience, one of the biggest differentiating factors seems to be the medicine's history. Some people just don't consider these topics to be relevant because they haven't enough written history and clinical experience behind them.

I can comfortably say that this doesn't stand up on in-depth analysis for the Qī Qíng/Seven Emotions and the Wǔ Shén/Five Spirits, but it does, somewhat, for the Qí Jīng Bā Mài/Eight Extraordinary Vessels and Wǔ Xíng/Five Element Archetypes.

But when I find myself in these polarizing conversations, I often suggest to the other person that not every disease that was in ancient China can be applied to modern diseases. Therefore, we need newer interpretations on the wide range of different Chinese medicine concepts. So, whilst the Wǔ Xíng/Five Element Archetypes might be a more recent development in Chinese medicine and philosophy, it doesn't mean that we should automatically discount it for that reason alone.

It's not like we have treated all of the ancient Chinese diseases, therefore we need to consider how ancient Chinese medicine can be incorporated into our modern diseases. This may require us to look at the concepts and bring them into our modern world.

So, what can you expect from these four chapters?

Chapter 11 is on the Qī Qíng/Seven Emotions, and even though the title suggests seven emotions will be discussed, there are in fact twelve. I did this because I felt that the Seven Emotions creates restriction in clinical practice because not everyone fits into those headings.

Chapter 12 analyzes the Qí Jīng Bā Mài/Eight Extraordinary Vessels. It is worth noting that it's impossible to thoroughly discuss the Qí Jīng Bā Mài in one chapter so I have been target-specific with my acupuncture point combinations. I have also stripped away all the padding and given a very concise and easy-to-follow discussion on the Eight Extraordinary Vessels.

Chapter 13 discusses the Wŭ Shén/Five Spirits, which I consider vitally important. I have this view because researching the literature has shown me a real lack in this area.

Chapter 14 takes you on a journey through the Wŭ Xíng/Five Element Archetypes. This is perhaps the most controversial chapter in Part 4. All I ask is that you read it with an open mind before making a judgement. You might find that the material gives you food for thought.

Note

1   Boethius 1999, pp.24–25. Anicius Boethius (480–524 CE) wrote *The Consolation of Philosophy* in 524 CE while in prison awaiting execution for conspiracy against his king. The quotation in question is part of that incredible text. It is worth noting that I did edit it somewhat because it was rather lengthy. In my opinion it's truly one of the more remarkable pieces of philosophy I have ever come across.

How much more damage anger and grief do than the things that cause them.

Marcus Aurelius (121–180 CE)[1]

How can someone's human nature be corrupted? By the emotions... When the emotions are out of control human nature lives in obscurity. It is not that human nature should be blamed. Rather it is the coming and going, by turn, of the seven emotions which prevents human nature from being fully developed... When emotions are not aroused, human nature will be fully developed. Yet human nature and emotions cannot be separated from each other.

Lǐ Áo/李翱 (772–841 CE)[2]

11

Qī Qíng/Seven Emotions

So far throughout this book you have been given a lot of acupuncture point combinations for a wide range of different signs and symptoms, as well as Zàng Fǔ patterns. Some of these point combinations have included the emotions.

This chapter is dedicated to point combinations for the Qī Qíng or Seven Emotions, which will make it easier for you to find treatment options for the emotions quickly. In this chapter you will be given a list of the different emotions that will be discussed. These will include the original seven (Qī Qíng), as well as a range of additional emotions and emotional states.

Apart from discussing point combinations, this chapter will also be dedicated to a range of different topics related to the emotions.

1. Brief history of emotions

Emotions have been around since the very beginnings of time. Whatever your belief system is, emotions are a part of that belief system. Different religious texts, philosophical musings and ancient fables, myths and legends have been hypothesizing about emotions for thousands of years.

The Chinese, Greeks and Romans even had demons, gods and goddesses that were responsible for the monitoring of our fortune, which, by default, could manifest in severe emotional upheaval – one of the most famous of which was Pandora's Box.

According to this wonderful myth, at the beginning of humanity everyone was happy. There was no sadness, no anger, no anxiety or fears, just joyful prancing and dancing and singing – all day, every day! One day Hermes, the trickster god, was traveling past Pandora's home carrying a very heavy box. He was sweating and panting and looking quite distressed. Pandora offered Hermes water and food to help him recover and to aid him on his long journey. She also offered to look after the box for him because it was heavy and cumbersome and he still had far to go. Hermes agreed on one condition: that Pandora was not to open the box under any circumstance. She happily agreed and Hermes went on his way.

Almost as soon as Hermes left, Pandora started hearing noises coming from the box. She asked her husband about it and he told her to stop concerning herself about it and to come outside to sing, dance and be merry. But Pandora stayed near the box, listening curiously to the quiet noises. She concluded that they were voices and that creatures were trapped inside the box. Crucially, Pandora stopped being merry and joyful. She wouldn't go outside, she wouldn't eat and she wouldn't sleep. She became completely fixated on the box.

After a few days the local community staged an intervention in an attempt to free Pandora from this obvious addiction. The intervention didn't work, and Pandora decided that the voices in the box were asking to be rescued. Not only that, but they claimed they had been unfairly imprisoned and desired to be freed from their jail.

In the end, Pandora couldn't handle it anymore and she opened the box. Ultimately, she had been correct because there were imprisoned creatures, but she was wrong to think that these sprites were nice and deserving of their freedom. You see, these creatures had names – and their names were pain, fear, anger, desire, anxiety, envy, sadness… All these winged beasts were charged with destroying people's merriness and joy.

The people closest to Pandora were struck first and they either started arguing with each other or began weeping. Upon seeing this, Pandora slammed the box shut, but she heard another voice in the box asking to be freed with the others. And that's when Pandora made her only good decision in days: she reopened the box, and out came the sprite called hope.

Regardless of which ancient or modern religious or philosophical musings you adhere to, what I find most interesting about all of them is that we are still cogitating about emotions. So, either humanity hasn't worked out how to transcend emotions or we aren't supposed to, and, in fact, we *need* to be aroused by emotions.

2. Chinese medicine view of emotions

Chinese medicine has been telling us for thousands of years that emotions are an important part of our existence and that we should never transcend any emotion.

Emotions are a valid and important part of our day-to-day lives. When it is appropriate to be angry – when you bang your shin on a low coffee table – then you should be angry. When it is appropriate to be pensive – when you are studying for your next big exam – then you should be pensive.

The Chinese people have been treating emotions for at least the past 2000 years, ever since *The Yellow Emperor's Classic* (*Inner Canon of the Yellow Emperor*/Huáng Dì Nèi Jīng/黃帝內經) was written around 200–0 BCE. Prior to that the Chinese believed that following a variety of different philosophical precepts could assist one with regulating emotions and improving one's lot in life.

Chinese medicine also believes that you can have either a disease that, over time, causes/triggers an emotion or an emotion that, over time, can cause/trigger a disease. This is important to understand because it tells you that emotions and disease are interchangeable.

The other thing worth noting is that Chinese medicine believes that each emotion has the potential to damage specific organs, depending on the emotion. This helps to break down how different emotions are triggered, depending on which organ is diseased, and vice versa.

For example, I have had the occasional client who is an alcoholic, with the alcohol injuring their Liver. When the Liver gets diseased, the typical emotional response is anger. Therefore, the more the person drinks, the angrier they could get.

Emotions are only a problem when they become consistent enough for the person (or people around them) to recognize the emotion as being what defines them. This becomes very apparent when a different emotional response was warranted and yet the person still emotes the same way every time. For example, the patient is angry all the time, even when they should be exhibiting other emotions such as sadness, fear or shock. The point is that the patient emotes in the same manner almost all the time, to the detriment of all other emotions.

In excellent news, all emotions can be treated with Chinese medicine, some more effectively than others.

3. The Heart Shén and emotions
In a basic sense the Shén is our:

- memory – short-term and long-term

- consciousness – semi-conscious, unconscious

- sleep – insomnia, narcolepsy, dreaming/nightmares

- emotions – all of them, not just joy

- Hún – Ethereal/Heavenly/Dream-Big Soul

- Pò – Corporeal/Grounded/Earthly/Do-Big-Be-Big Soul

- Yì – Thought/Post-Heaven Intellect

- Zhì – Willpower/Pre-Heaven Intellect.

Therefore, by default, any emotional imbalance in the body can have the Heart (and Heart Shén) as its primary source. Having said that, each organ does have a more dynamic relationship with an emotion. These are discussed in Table 11.1 as well as within each of the emotion sections.

4. The emotions and their associated Yīn and Yáng organs and Wǔ Xíng/Five Elements
Each of the emotions has the potential to injure or be injured by certain organs and elements. Table 11.1 lists the main organs and elements, but bear in mind that there

are almost always secondary organs and elements that can be affected too. For these secondary organs/elements, please refer directly to each emotion further below.

Table 11.1 Qí Qíng/Seven Emotions[3]

Emotion/emotional state	Yīn organs	Yáng organs	Wǔ Xíng/Five Elements
Anger and frustration	Liver	Gall Bladder	Wood
Joy/mania	Heart		Fire
Pensiveness	Spleen	Stomach	Earth
Worry	Spleen Lungs		Earth Metal
Sadness and grief	Lungs Heart		Metal Fire
Fear	Kidneys	Urinary Bladder Gall Bladder	Water Wood
Shock	Kidneys Heart		Water Fire
Depression	Liver Heart Lungs	Gall Bladder	Wood Fire Metal
Manic depression/Diān Kuáng	Heart plus others		Fire plus others
Anxiety	Heart Kidneys		Fire Water
Stress	Liver Heart	Gall Bladder	Wood Fire

5. Zàng Fǔ patterns and emotions

Pretty much every single Zàng Fǔ pattern has the potential for an emotion to be attached to it. Obviously, some are a lot more likely than others. For example, any Heart pattern is likely because the Heart houses the Shén.[4] Another common pattern is Liver Qì Stagnation.[5] Some of the less likely patterns include Damp Heat in the Urinary Bladder or Small Intestine Xū and Cold.

For specific Zàng Fǔ patterns, please refer to the individual emotions below. For each of these emotions the following headings will be included:

- Discussion

- Wǔ Xíng/Five Elements; Yīn and Yáng organs

- Zàng Fǔ patterns

- Specific Zàng Fǔ pattern discussion – including additional comments, treatment principles and treatment

- General acupuncture point combination – including comments for why the points were chosen.

Anger and frustration
Discussion[6]

Anger is considered a Yáng on Yīn or Young Yáng emotion and is the second most Yáng emotion that can be displayed, behind only joy. As a result, it can't sustain itself for long and will burn up quickly. However, over time anger can self-seed and this usually results in the patient exhibiting Heat signs in the body. This self-seeding (anger feeds on anger) results in more consistent and longer outbursts of anger, even when a different emotion would be expected.

Occasionally, patients present with repressed anger and will probably claim they have no anger at all. This repression is unhealthy in Chinese medicine because it means the patient isn't expressing anger and instead is locking it away internally. This is concerning because the anger can start to build up like molten lava inside a dormant volcano. If the anger isn't allowed to release itself, it can explode violently, often at the most unexpected time.

Anger and frustration go hand in hand in Chinese medicine.[7]

Wǔ Xíng/Five Elements; Yīn and Yáng organs for anger and frustration

- Wǔ Xíng/Five Elements = Wood.

- Main organs = Liver and Gall Bladder.

- Secondary organs = Heart and Stomach.

Zàng Fǔ patterns for anger and frustration

Anger and/or frustration tend to create Yáng Shí or Stagnation patterns.

The following are some of the more likely Zàng Fǔ patterns for anger and/or frustration:[8]

- Liver Fire Blazing

- Liver Yáng Rising

- Liver Qì Stagnation

- Damp Heat in the Liver and Gall Bladder

- Liver Invading the Stomach

- Heart Fire Blazing.

Of the patterns above, I will provide additional notes for four of them.

Specific Zàng Fǔ pattern discussion for anger and frustration[9]
LIVER FIRE BLAZING

Type of anger: Acute and verbally aggressive anger outbursts that are usually unexpected by the recipient. The patient will describe the anger as being a gradual build-up that then explodes, or will come from nowhere and surprise everyone, including themselves. They are likely to recognize anger as being a key disorder that they wish to have treated.

Treatment principle: Sedate Liver Fire; calm the anger.

Treatment:

- Head/face/neck – GB 20.

- Trunk (front) – CV 14.

- Arms/hands – LI 11, TE 5.

- Legs/feet – LR 2, LR 5.

- Total needles used bilaterally = 11.

DAMP HEAT IN THE LIVER AND GALL BLADDER

Type of anger: Acute angry outbursts that can sustain themselves longer than with the other patterns discussed here. This is because they have the Damp which clogs their senses, thereby clouding sensible judgement. Even so, anger is a Yáng emotion and therefore will burn up quicker than all other emotions (with the exception of manic joy). Word of warning: be *very* careful with these patients because the anger could be part of a psychosis.

Treatment principle: Clear Damp Heat in the Liver and Gall Bladder; calm the anger.

Treatment:

- Trunk (front) – CV 14, LR 14, GB 24.

- Arms/hands – PC 5.

- Legs/feet – LR 2, LR 5, GB 34.

- Total needles used bilaterally = 13.

LIVER QÌ STAGNATION

Type of anger: Cyclical emotional imbalance that will include anger outbursts accompanied by stress, frustration, unhappiness and feeling overwhelmed. The key with this anger is that it's just one emotion among many others, and the patient is likely to request treatment for stress (not anger) as the primary disorder.

Treatment principle: Move Qì; regulate the Liver; regulate the anger.

Treatment:

- Trunk (front) – CV 14, LR 14.
- Arms/hands – PC 6.
- Legs/feet – LR 2, LR 3, GB 34.
- Total needles used bilaterally = 11.

HEART FIRE BLAZING

Type of anger: Acute and verbally/physically aggressive anger outbursts that are usually unexpected by the recipient and, in all likelihood, undeserved. The patient will describe the anger as being a gradual build-up that then explodes, or that it comes from nowhere and surprises everyone, including themselves.

Treatment principle: Sedate Heart Fire; calm the anger.

Treatment:

- Trunk (front) – CV 14.
- Arms/hands – HT 3, HT 8, PC 8, LI 11.
- Legs/feet – LR 2.
- Total needles used bilaterally = 11.

Anger and frustration point combination – general

See Table 11.2.

Table 11.2 Anger and frustration point combination – general[10]

Location of point	Point	Reasoning
Head/face/neck	GV 20	Highest point on the body – helps to regulate energy in and out of the head.
	M-HN-3 (Yìn Táng)	Supports GV 20 in its functions.
Trunk (front)	CV 14	Front Mù Collecting point of the Heart; nourishing the Heart can balance the Shén.
	CV 17	Front Mù Collecting point of the Pericardium; supports the Heart Shén.
Trunk (back)	GV 8	Level with the Back Shù Transporting point of the Liver (BL 18); soothes the Liver.
Arms/hands	HT 5	Nourishes the Heart Shén.
	HT 7	Yuán Source point of the Heart; nourishing the Heart can balance the Shén.

cont.

Location of point	Point	Reasoning
Legs/feet	LR 2	Yíng Spring point of the Liver. In my opinion, the best point for anger.
	LR 3	Yuán Source point of the Liver.
	KI 1	Lowest point on the body – helps to regulate energy in and out of the head; supports GV 20 in its functions.
Total points needled		15 needles used bilaterally

Joy/mania
Discussion[11]

Joy is considered a Yáng on Yáng or Mature Yáng emotion and is the most Yáng emotion that can be displayed. It therefore sustains itself for even less time than anger (already discussed). Joy is also a very addictive emotion that tends to want to display itself at every possible opportunity.

Joy isn't typically a cause of disease. However, joy is problematic when a person strives to stay joyful all the time because it becomes unachievable. Joy that is diseased is usually termed as someone who is over-excited, addicted, agitated, restless, mentally stimulated, hypervigilant or manic. They will also obsessively crave/desire things.

Alternatively, the patient falls below the joy mark once too often and sinks into depression.

Wǔ Xíng/Five Elements; Yīn and Yáng organs for joy/mania

- Wǔ Xíng/Five Elements = Fire.

- Main organs = Heart and Heart Shén.

Zàng Fǔ patterns for joy/mania

Joy/mania tends to create Shí patterns.

The following are some of the more likely Zàng Fǔ patterns for joy/mania:[12]

- Heart Fire Blazing

- Phlegm Fire Harassing the Heart

- Phlegm Misting the Heart Shén

- Heart Qì Xū

- Heart Xuè Xū.

Of the patterns above, I will provide additional notes for four of them.

Specific Zàng Fǔ pattern discussion for joy/mania[13]
HEART FIRE BLAZING

Type of joy: Loud, funny, great salesman, draws a crowd, incredibly entertaining, can be flighty, but most importantly harmless. Will struggle to unwind, as chasing the next 'joyful' moment.

Treatment principle: Sedate Heart Fire; calm the manic joy.

Treatment:

- Head/face/neck – GV 20.

- Trunk (front) – CV 14.

- Trunk (back) – BL 15.

- Arms/hands – HT 3, HT 8, PC 8, LI 11.

- Legs/feet – KI 1.

- Total needles used bilaterally = 14.

PHLEGM FIRE HARASSING THE HEART

Type of joy: Agitated, incoherent speech, tendency to hit or scold people, uncontrolled laughter or crying, wanting to maim, injure or kill. Very dangerous people!

Treatment principle: Sedate Heart Fire; disperse Phlegm from the Heart; disperse Phlegm Fire from the Shén; calm the manic joy.

Treatment:

- Head/face/neck – GV 24.

- Trunk (front) – CV 14.

- Trunk (back) – BL 15.

- Arms/hands – HT 3, HT 7, PC 5.

- Legs/feet – ST 40.

- Total needles used bilaterally = 12.

HEART QÌ XŪ

Type of joy: Will strive for joy but regularly falls below the mark. Knowing what it feels like to be happy, they recognize the depression and therefore want treatment.

Treatment principle: Tonify Heart Qì; reintroduce joy.

Treatment:

- Trunk (front) – CV 6, CV 14, CV 17.

- Trunk (back) – BL 15.

- Arms/hands – HT 5, HT 7.

- Legs/feet – SP 6.

- Total needles used bilaterally = 11.

Heart Xuè Xū

Type of joy: Similar to Heart Qì Xū, but more chronic, and therefore harder to treat. They will also have longer episodes of depression.

Treatment principle: Tonify Heart Xuè; reintroduce joy.

Treatment:

- Trunk (front) – CV 4.

- Trunk (back) – BL 15, BL 17.

- Arms/hands – HT 6, HT 7.

- Legs/feet – SP 4.

- Total needles used bilaterally = 11.

Joy/mania point combination – general
See Table 11.3.

Table 11.3 Joy/mania point combination – general[14]

Location of point	Point	Reasoning
Head/face/neck	M-HN-3 (Yìn Táng) GV 16 GV 26 BL 10	Calms the Shén; regulates joy. Calms the Shén; regulates joy. Settles an acute manic episode. Calms the Shén; regulates joy.
Trunk (back)	GV 14	Settles an acute manic episode.
Arms/hands	LI 11 PC 6 PC 7 HT 7	Settles an acute manic episode. Calms the Shén; regulates joy. Yuán Source point of the Pericardium; supports the Heart and Heart Shén. Yuán Source point of the Heart; calms the Shén; regulates joy.
Legs/feet	ST 40	Settles an acute manic episode.
Total points needled		16 needles used bilaterally

Pensiveness
Discussion[15]

Pensiveness is the most neutral emotion and is, in some respects, not really an emotion at all. It is defined as being plunged in thought, and thought is Yì, which is one of the Wǔ Shén/Five Spirits. Yì is housed in the Earth element,[16] which is why the Stomach and Spleen can be negatively affected by over-thinking, especially in terms of over-studying/concentrating or of over-analyzing/reflecting on past or future events. If this occurs, the natural instinct is for the Spleen to become Xū/Deficient and for the Stomach to become Shí/Excess.

The Heart and Kidney can also be adversely affected by pensiveness. These two organs are responsible for short-term and long-term memory.[17] Over-thinking from an early age can injure the Heart and Kidney, exhausting them and leading to Xū patterns.

Wǔ Xíng/Five Elements; Yīn and Yáng organs for pensiveness

- Wǔ Xíng/Five Elements = Earth.

- Main organs = Spleen and Stomach.

- Secondary organs = Heart, Lungs and Kidneys.

Zàng Fǔ patterns for pensiveness

Pensiveness tends to create Shí, Xū or Stagnant patterns.
The following are some of the more likely Zàng Fǔ patterns for pensiveness:[18]

- Spleen Qì Xū

- Heart Qì Xū

- Lung Qì Xū

- Stomach Fire Blazing

- Stomach Qì Rebelling Upwards

- Kidney Xū (any type).

Of the patterns above, I will provide additional notes for four of them.

Specific Zàng Fǔ pattern discussion for pensiveness[19]
Spleen Qì Xū

Type of pensiveness: Over-studying, over-analyzing, over-thinking and concentrating for too long without a long-enough break. This might be related to a task for work, college exams or even reflecting on past or future events and not living in the present moment.

Treatment principle: Tonify Spleen Qì; balance the Yì/Thought.

Treatment:

- Trunk (front) – LR 13.

- Trunk (back) – BL 20, BL 49.

- Arms/hands – LU 9.

- Legs/feet – ST 36, SP 3.

- Total needles used bilaterally = 12.

HEART QÌ XŪ

Type of pensiveness: Related to poor short-term and/or long-term memory. Can be a precursor to dementia or even Alzheimer's disease, especially if both the Heart and Kidneys are diseased.[20]

Treatment principle: Tonify Heart Qì; balance the Yì/Thought.

Treatment:

- Trunk (front) – CV 6, CV 14, CV 17.

- Trunk (back) – BL 15, BL 49.

- Arms/hands – HT 5.

- Legs/feet – ST 36, SP 6.

- Total needles used bilaterally = 13.

STOMACH QÌ REBELLING UPWARDS

Type of pensiveness: Episodic and related to eating. This is going to be problematic if the patient eats while thinking, analyzing or stressing over a particular thing. Alternatively, it will be triggered by severe emotional thinking while eating, leading to heartburn/reflux.[21]

Treatment principle: Descend Rebellious Stomach Qì; balance the Yì/Thought.

Treatment:

- Trunk (front) – ST 21, CV 12, CV 17.

- Trunk (back) – BL 21, BL 49.

- Legs/feet – ST 34, ST 44.

- Total needles used bilaterally = 12.

KIDNEY XŪ (ANY TYPE)

Type of pensiveness: Related to poor short-term and/or long-term memory. Can be a precursor to dementia or even Alzheimer's disease, especially if both the Heart and Kidneys are diseased.[22]

Treatment principle: Tonify the Kidneys; balance the Yì/Thought.

Treatment:

- Trunk (front) – GB 25.

- Trunk (back) – BL 23, BL 49.

- Arms/hands – TE 4.

- Legs/feet – KI 3, KI 6, SP 6.

- Total needles used bilaterally = 14.

Pensiveness point combination – general

See Table 11.4.

Table 11.4 Pensiveness point combination – general[23]

Location of point	Point	Reasoning
Head/face/neck	GV 20 ST 8 M-HN-3 (Yìn Táng) BL 10	Regulates the Yì and Shén. Clears the head to help with mental clarity. Regulates the Yì and Shén. Clears the head to help with mental clarity.
Trunk (back)	BL 49	Yì Shè = House of the Yì.[24]
Arms/hands	PC 6 HT 7	Regulates the Heart Shén and, by default, the Yì. Regulates the Heart Shén and, by default, the Yì.
Legs/feet	SP 3 SP 6	Yuán Source point of the Spleen; regulates the Yì. Regulates the Yì and Shén.
Total points needled		16 needles used bilaterally

Worry
Discussion[25]

Worry is considered a Yīn on Yáng or Young Yīn emotion. Although it is predominantly a neutral emotion, it is still Yīn; therefore, it will be able to sustain itself for a long time, arriving gradually and burning up just as slowly.

When worry strikes, it knots Qì, which leads to Stagnation. This Stagnation affects the smooth flow of Qì, Xuè, Jīn Yè and even Jīng, which quickly leads to Xū/Deficient patterns in the organs that make Qì and Xuè, namely the Spleen, Lungs and Heart.

The Gall Bladder can also be affected because, when a patient is excessively worried, they never achieve anything, and the Gall Bladder is an organ that loves getting things done via strong decision making. The Gall Bladder is also the Yáng partner of the Liver, which is the first organ affected when Qì stagnates, resulting in both organs becoming stuck and further limiting the ability to get stuff done.[26]

Wǔ Xíng/Five Elements; Yīn and Yáng organs for worry

- Wǔ Xíng/Five Elements = Earth and Metal.

- Main organs = Spleen and Lungs.

- Secondary organs = Heart, Liver and Gall Bladder.

Zàng Fǔ patterns for worry

Worry tends to create Xū or Stagnant patterns.

The following are some of the more likely Zàng Fǔ patterns for worry:[27]

- Spleen Qì Xū

- Lung Qì Xū

- Heart Qì Xū

- Heart Xuè Xū

- Liver Qì Stagnation

- Liver Yáng Rising

- Gall Bladder Xū.

Of the patterns above, I will provide additional notes for four of them.

Specific Zàng Fǔ pattern discussion for worry[28]

Lung Qì Xū

Type of worry: The patient may specifically state that worry is the primary emotion in their life. An episode of worry may also be accompanied by breathing difficulties such as shortness of breath, wheezing or even an asthmatic attack. They may also have a cough, fatigue very easily and have a very quiet demeanor/voice.[29]

Treatment principle: Tonify Lung Qì; balance the Qì flow; reduce worry.

Treatment:

- Trunk (front) – LU 1, CV 17.

- Trunk (back) – BL 13.

- Arms/hands – LU 7, LU 9.

- Legs/feet – ST 36, SP 6.

- Total needles used bilaterally = 13.

SPLEEN QÌ XŪ

Type of worry: Episodic and usually related to eating while worried. This can lead to feeling full after not eating very much, ascites or even an acute episode of diarrhea within a few hours of eating. The worry 'knot' can also create upward rebelling Qì leading to heartburn/reflux.[30]

Treatment principle: Tonify Spleen Qì; balance the Qì flow; reduce worry.

Treatment:

- Trunk (front) – LR 13.

- Trunk (back) – BL 20.

- Arms/hands – LU 9.

- Legs/feet – ST 36, SP 3, SP 6.

- Total needles used bilaterally = 12.

GALL BLADDER XŪ

Type of worry: Consider this pattern if the patient describes being excessively worried about never achieving anything, because the Gall Bladder is an organ that loves getting things done. Also consider this pattern if the patient explains that during an attack of worry they get a 'stuck feeling in their throat'.

Treatment principle: Tonify the Gall Bladder; balance the Qì flow; reduce worry.

Treatment:

- Trunk (front) – GB 24.

- Trunk (back) – BL 19, BL 48.

- Arms/hands – LU 7, HT 7.

- Legs/feet – GB 40.

- Total needles used bilaterally = 12.

HEART XUÈ XŪ

Type of worry: This is the likely pattern for a patient who is worried but doesn't fit into any of the other categories. This is particularly the case if they complain about multiple emotions because the Heart Shén isn't being nourished; or because multiple emotions are damaging the Heart Shén.[31] Also consider this pattern if they suggest that their worry is worse after an episode of insomnia. As *The Systematic Classic of Acupuncture and Moxibustion* (Zhēn Jiǔ Jiá Yǐ Jīng/ 針灸甲乙經) states in book 1, chapter 1 (Mi 2004, p.6): 'If the heart is affected by apprehension, thought, and worry, this injures the spirit [Shén].'

Treatment principle: Tonify Heart Xuè; balance the Qì flow; reduce worry.

Treatment:

- Trunk (front) – CV 4, CV 14, CV 17.

- Trunk (back) – BL 17.

- Arms/hands – HT 6, HT 7.

- Legs/feet – SP 4.

- Total needles used bilaterally = 11.

Worry point combination – general
See Table 11.5.

Table 11.5 Worry point combination – general[32]

Location of point	Point	Reasoning
Head/face/neck	GV 20 M-HN-3 (Yìn Táng) BL 10	Calms the Shén; reduces worry. Calms the Shén; reduces worry. Calms the Shén; reduces worry.
Trunk (front)	CV 14 CV 17	Front Mù Collecting point of the Heart; nourishing the Heart can balance the Shén. Front Mù Collecting point of the Pericardium; supports the Heart Shén.
Arms/hands	PC 6 LU 7 HT 4 HT 7	Calms the Shén; reduces worry. Calms the Shén; reduces worry. Calms the Shén; reduces worry. Yuán Source point of the Heart; nourishing the Heart can balance the Shén.
Legs/feet	SP 6	Calms the Shén; reduces worry.
Total points needled		16 needles used bilaterally

Sadness and grief
Discussion[33]
Sadness and/or grief are considered Yīn on Yáng or Young Yīn emotions. Although they are predominantly neutral emotions, they are still Yīn; therefore, they will be able to sustain themselves for a long time, arriving gradually and burning up just as slowly.

As a result, the patient will present with Xū patterns predominantly. These will likely occur in:

- the Lungs – presenting as severe sadness/grief/depression/worry

- the Liver – with the patient cycling between anger, depression and frustration (the diagnosis might also be Liver Qì Stagnation)

- the Heart – with the patient exhibiting a depressed state that is usually accompanied (and aggravated) by anxiety, insomnia and palpitations.

Wŭ Xíng/Five Elements; Yīn and Yáng organs for sadness and grief

- Wŭ Xíng/Five Elements = Fire and Metal.

- Main organs = Heart and Lungs.

- Secondary organs = Liver.

Zàng Fŭ patterns for sadness and grief

Sadness and/or grief tend to create Xū patterns.

The following are some of the more likely Zàng Fŭ patterns for sadness and/or grief:[34]

- Heart Qì Xū

- Heart Xuè Xū

- Lung Qì Xū

- Liver Xuè Xū

- Liver Qì Stagnation.

Of the patterns above, I will provide additional notes for four of them.

Specific Zàng Fŭ pattern discussion for sadness and grief[35]
Lung Qì Xū

Type of sadness/grief: Severe sadness, which is clearly described as depression by the patient. They know what it is because they are 'in it' all the time. This depression is sometimes described as (or accompanied by) grief, sadness or worry.

Treatment principle: Tonify Lung Qì; reintroduce joy; reduce sadness and grief.

Treatment:

- Trunk (front) – LU 1, CV 17.

- Trunk (back) – BL 13, BL 42.

- Arms/hands – LU 3, LU 9.

- Legs/feet – SP 3.

- Total needles used bilaterally = 13.

HEART QÌ XŪ

Type of sadness/grief: The patient may use the word 'depression' to describe the 'funk' they are in, or even suggest a 'lack of joy' in their life. This sadness is usually accompanied (and aggravated) by anxiety, insomnia and palpitations.

Treatment principle: Tonify Heart Qì; reintroduce joy; reduce sadness and grief.

Treatment:

- Trunk (front) – CV 6, CV 14, CV 17.

- Trunk (back) – BL 15.

- Arms/hands – HT 5, HT 7.

- Legs/feet – ST 36, SP 6.

- Total needles used bilaterally = 13.

LIVER XUÈ XŪ

Type of sadness/grief: The patient may describe a feeling of unhappiness, sadness or feeling 'off', or even a vague sense of unease, but are unlikely to use the word 'depression'. They are also likely to describe the trigger as stress and overwork occurring the day before the onset of sadness.

Treatment principle: Tonify Liver Xuè; reintroduce joy; reduce sadness and grief.

Treatment:

- Trunk (front) – CV 4, CV 14.

- Trunk (back) – BL 17, BL 18.

- Arms/hands – HT 6, HT 7.

- Legs/feet – LR 3, SP 4.

- Total needles used bilaterally = 14.

LIVER QÌ STAGNATION

Type of sadness/grief: Cyclical emotional imbalance that will include anger, stress, frustration, unhappiness, feeling overwhelmed and pretty much any other emotion possible.[36] The key with this sadness is that it's just one emotion among many others, and the patient is likely to request treatment for stress rather than sadness or grief.

Treatment principle: Move Qì; regulate the Liver; reintroduce joy; reduce sadness and grief.

Treatment:

- Trunk (front) – LR 14.

- Trunk (back) – BL 18, BL 42.

- Arms/hands – LU 3, PC 6.

- Legs/feet – GB 34, LR 3.

- Total needles used bilaterally = 14.

Sadness and grief point combination - general
See Table 11.6.

Table 11.6 Sadness and grief point combination – general[37]

Location of point	Point	Reasoning
Head/face/neck	GV 20 M-HN-3 (Yìn Táng)	Calms the Shén; reduces sadness or grief. Calms the Shén; reduces sadness or grief.
Trunk (front)	CV 14 CV 17	Front Mù Collecting point of the Heart; nourishing the Heart can balance the Shén. Front Mù Collecting point of the Pericardium; supports the Heart Shén.
Trunk (back)	BL 42 BL 47	Pò Hù = Corporeal Soul Door.[38] Hún Mén = Ethereal Soul Gate.[39] Both back points help to reduce sadness or grief.
Arms/hands	LU 3 PC 6 HT 3 HT 7	Calms the Pò to reduce sadness or grief. Regulates the Heart Shén and, by default, the Pò. Stimulates endorphins to help regulate the mood. Regulates the Heart Shén and, by default, the Pò.
Total points needled		16 needles used bilaterally

Fear
Discussion[40]
Fear is considered a Yīn on Yīn or Mature Yīn emotion and is the most Yīn emotion that can be displayed. It's a pure Yīn emotion and therefore it will be able to sustain itself for a long time. It will typically arrive gradually and burn up just as slowly.

Interestingly, though, the fear can manifest itself in two ways (via an acute or chronic build-up). An acute fear response is an event that is sudden and shocking, which scatters Qì. It's also a very Yáng response which quickly drains Qì, leaving the patient Xū. The chronic fear gradually develops over many years and may not be from a sudden, single event. This vague feeling of unease is also very draining on Qì, which leaves the patient with a Xū pattern.

As a result, the patient will present with Xū patterns predominantly. These will likely occur in:

- the Kidneys – leaving them Yīn and/or Yáng Xū

- the Heart – any type, because, as previously mentioned, the Heart can be negatively affected by any of the emotions

- the Gall Bladder – via the patient having a distinct lack of courage. This timidity and cowardice blocks the Gall Bladder's free spirit of drive, determination, decision making and courage, leaving it decidedly Xū.

Wǔ Xíng/Five Elements; Yīn and Yáng organs for fear

- Wǔ Xíng/Five Elements = Water and Wood.

- Main organs = Kidneys, Urinary Bladder and Gall Bladder.

- Secondary organs = Heart and Liver.

Zàng Fǔ patterns for fear

Fear tends to create Xū patterns.

The following are some of the more likely Zàng Fǔ patterns for fear:[41]

- Kidney Xū (any type)

- Heart and Kidney not Communicating

- Heart Xū (any type)

- Gall Bladder Xū

- Liver Xuè Xū.

Of the patterns above, I will provide additional notes for four of them.

Specific Zàng Fǔ pattern discussion for fear[42]
KIDNEY YĪN XŪ

Type of fear: Fear can injure the Kidneys regardless of whether it's from a sudden onset event or long-term build-up (which the patient will describe as a vague unease). If the patient is happy to describe the fear, then watch their body language, because a Kidney Xū fear response is usually an urgent need to urinate.

Treatment principle: Tonify Kidney Yīn; reduce the fear.

Treatment:

- Trunk (front) – GB 25, CV 4.
- Trunk (back) – BL 23, BL 52.
- Arms/hands – HT 6, TE 4.
- Legs/feet – SP 6, KI 6.
- Total needles used bilaterally = 15.

Kidney Yáng Xū

Type of fear: As for Kidney Yīn Xū; the main differences, though, are the obvious Yīn Xū versus Yáng Xū signs and symptoms.

Treatment principle: Tonify Kidney Yáng; reduce the fear.

Treatment:

- Trunk (front) – GB 25, CV 6.
- Trunk (back) – BL 23, BL 52, GV 4.
- Arms/hands – TE 4.
- Legs/feet – KI 3, KI 7.
- Total needles used bilaterally = 14.

Gall Bladder Xū

Type of fear: Fear can injure the Gall Bladder by targeting its courage. This can be via a sudden onset event or long-term. Regardless, this Xū results in timidity and cowardice and the patient is likely to complain of plum-stone throat and indigestion when they discuss the fear.

Treatment principle: Tonify the Gall Bladder; reduce the fear.

Treatment:

- Trunk (front) – GB 24.
- Trunk (back) – BL 18, BL 19, BL 48.
- Arms/hands – HT 7.
- Legs/feet – GB 40.
- Total needles used bilaterally = 12.

Heart Xū (any type)

Type of fear: This is the likely pattern for a patient who is fearful but doesn't fit into any of the other categories. This is particularly the case if the patient complains about multiple emotions. Also consider this pattern if they suggest that their fear is worse after an episode of insomnia.

Treatment principle: Tonify the Heart; reduce the fear.

Treatment:

- Trunk (front) – CV 14, CV 17.

- Trunk (back) – BL 15.

- Arms/hands – PC 6, HT 7.

- Legs/feet – ST 36, SP 6.

- Total needles used bilaterally = 12.

Fear point combination – general

See Table 11.7.

Table 11.7 Fear point combination – general[43]

Location of point	Point	Reasoning
Head/face/neck	GV 20 M-HN-3 (Yìn Táng)	Calms the Shén; reduces fear. Calms the Shén; reduces fear.
Trunk (back)	BL 15 BL 19 BL 23 BL 52	Back Shù Transporting point of the Heart; nourishing the Heart can balance the Shén. Back Shù Transporting point of the Gall Bladder; reduces GB fear. Back Shù Transporting point of the Kidneys; reduces fear. Zhì Shì = Will Residence.[44] Reduces fear.
Arms/hands	HT 7	Calms the Shén; reduces fear.
Legs/feet	GB 40 KI 3	Yuán Source point of the Gall Bladder; reduces GB fear. Yuán Source point of the Kidneys; reduces fear.
Total points needled		16 needles used bilaterally

Shock

Discussion[45]

Shock scatters Qì, which is a very Yáng response, but then it leaves the patient incredibly drained and Xū, which is the Yīn backfire. This negatively impacts on the Heart and Kidneys.

The Heart is the 'Emperor' organ,[46] and is, according to the Mandate of Heaven/ Tiān Mìng, the most altruistic, noble and human-hearted organ in the body.

As such, it is the organ most affected by what occurs in its empire (the body), and what happens to the Emperor transpires in his subjects.

According to Cotterell (1995, p.73), Mencius said:

> When a king rejoices in the joy of his people, they rejoice in his joy; when he grieves in the sorrow of his people, they also grieve at his sorrow. A common bond of joy will pervade the kingdom; a common bond of sorrow will do the same.

Shock is like a severe earthquake that has just rocked the empire and the Heart is distraught. He[47] goes out into his realm to survey the damage, passing on gifts of food, drink and equipment, which leaves him physically drained. Then he sees all the death and destruction, and this leaves him mentally drained. Should we be surprised, then, when shock leaves the Heart Xū?

The Kidneys are the most generous organ in the body, always happy to give out energy to help sustain the other organs in the body. They do this on the assumption that the organs will return the favor. When shock scatters Qì and leaves the body Xū, the Kidneys go into overdrive to support the other organs, which will leave them Xū if they are not supported themselves.

Overall, shock is considered an inconsistent emotion that causes Qì to scatter, leading to some organs being Xū and some being Stagnant.

Wǔ Xíng/Five Elements; Yīn and Yáng organs for shock

- Wǔ Xíng/Five Elements = Fire and Water.

- Main organs = Heart and Kidneys.

- Secondary organs = any other organ.

Zàng Fǔ patterns for shock

Shock tends to create Xu patterns.

The following are some of the more likely Zàng Fǔ patterns for shock:[48]

- Heart Qì Xū

- Heart Xuè Xū

- Kidney Qì Xū

- Yīn Xū (multiple organs including the Heart and Kidneys)

- Yáng Xū (multiple organs including the Heart and Kidneys)

- a combination of a variety of other organ patterns.

Of the patterns above, I will provide additional notes for four of them.

Specific Zàng Fǔ pattern discussion for shock[49]
HEART QÌ XŪ

Type of shock: The Heart becomes Xū because it's providing so much support to the rest of the body; like an altruistic Emperor, the Heart is looking after its subjects (Zàng Fǔ organs), resulting in fatigue and Xū.

Treatment principle: Tonify Heart Qì; balance the Qì flow; settle the shock.

Treatment:

- Trunk (front) – CV 6, CV 14, CV 17.
- Trunk (back) – BL 15.
- Arms/hands – HT 5, HT 7.
- Legs/feet – ST 36, SP 6.
- Total needles used bilaterally = 13.

HEART XUÈ XŪ

Type of shock: Similar to Heart Qì Xū but more chronic and therefore harder to treat.

Treatment principle: Tonify Heart Xuè; balance the Qì flow; settle the shock.

Treatment:

- Trunk (front) – CV 4, CV 14.
- Trunk (back) – BL 15, BL 17.
- Arms/hands – HT 6, HT 7.
- Legs/feet – SP 4, SP 6.
- Total needles used bilaterally = 14.

KIDNEY YĪN XŪ

Type of shock: The Kidneys become Xū because they provide so much support to the rest of the body. The Kidneys expect it back in return, but in this instance it clearly doesn't happen, leading to Kidney Xū.

Treatment principle: Tonify Kidney Yīn; balance the Qì flow; settle the shock.

Treatment:

- Trunk (front) – CV 4, GB 25.
- Trunk (back) – BL 23.
- Arms/hands – HT 6, TE 4.

- Legs/feet – SP 6, KI 6.

- Total needles used bilaterally = 13.

KIDNEY YÁNG XŪ

Type of shock: As for Kidney Yīn Xū; the main differences, though, are the obvious Yīn Xū versus Yáng Xū signs and symptoms.

Treatment principle: Tonify Kidney Yáng; balance the Qì flow; settle the shock.

Treatment:

- Trunk (front) – CV 6, GB 25.

- Trunk (back) – BL 23, GV 4.

- Arms/hands – TE 4.

- Legs/feet – KI 3, KI 6.

- Total needles used bilaterally = 12.

Shock point combination – general

The four Zàng Fǔ patterns discussed above are typically more chronic, so I have included a point combination in Table 11.8 for the treatment of acute shock.

Table 11.8 Shock point combination – general[50]

Location of point	Point	Reasoning
Head/face/neck	GV 20 GV 25 GV 26	All of these points treat acute shock. They target the following to achieve this: • Heart Shén
Trunk (front)	CV 4 CV 6	• the Heart organ • the Kidney organ
Arms/hands	PC 6 PC 9	• fast-acting points at the top and bottom of the body • a balance throughout the body with the remaining points.
Legs/feet	ST 36 KI 1	
Total points needled		13 needles used bilaterally

Depression
Discussion[51]
Depression is considered a Yīn on Yīn or Mature Yīn emotion and is one of the most Yīn emotions that can be displayed. It's a pure Yīn emotion and therefore it will be able to sustain itself for a long time. It will typically arrive gradually and burn up just as slowly.

From a Chinese medicine perspective, depression is not as simple to diagnose as other emotions. The three most likely organs are the Liver, Heart and Lungs. Having said that, the Spleen, Kidneys and Gall Bladder can get involved too.

Therefore, each of the organs will receive special attention below.

There are three other main problems with depression:

- *The patient doesn't recognize that they are depressed.*

  Depression is quite a sneaky emotion and can often be portrayed by the patient as any number of other emotional states, including, but not limited to, stress, anger, frustration, dis-ease, feeling overwhelmed, feeling a little 'off in the head', feeling 'off color', feeling 'not quite right'.

  Whatever label they give it, it's still a possibility that it is depression. Regardless, treat the patient using your preferred diagnostic tool, or isolate which of the Zàng Fǔ patterns below is the cause and treat accordingly.

- *The patient is severely depressed and is contemplating suicide outwardly.*

  Be very careful here. The patient should also be seeing a psychiatrist or psychologist. Look for a slow heal rather than a fast fix; they are likely to be very Xū/Deficient and so they don't have the energy to follow through with their talk on suicide. But if you give them a huge boost of energy, this might be the catalyst for them to follow through with their threat.

  Be very careful with these patients. If in doubt, refer them to someone else more experienced. There is no shame in that; in fact, it's a duty-of-care issue.

- *The patient is severely depressed and is contemplating suicide inwardly.*

  This is the biggest problem because you don't know they are contemplating taking their own life. They have put up a mask which fools even their closest family and friends. Chances are, they have planned how they are going to commit suicide but they just haven't got the energy to do it yet.

  The treatment approach is exactly the same as for the previous bullet point.

Wǔ Xíng/Five Elements; Yīn and Yáng organs for depression

- Wǔ Xíng/Five Elements = Wood, Fire and Metal.

- Main organs = Liver, Heart, Lungs and Gall Bladder.

- Secondary organs = Spleen and Kidneys.

Zàng Fǔ patterns for depression

Depression tends to create Xū patterns.

The following are some of the more likely Zàng Fǔ patterns for depression:[52]

- Liver Xuè Xū

- Liver Yáng Rising

- Liver Qì Stagnation

- Heart Qì Xū

- Heart Xuè Xū

- Lung Qì Xū

- Gall Bladder Xū

- Spleen Qì/Yáng Xū with Damp Accumulation

- Kidney Xū (any type).

I won't be discussing these specifically. Instead, I will be discussing organ depression for the six organs most likely to be affected by depression.

Specific Zàng Fŭ pattern discussion for depression[53]

The following six organ depressions aren't your traditional Zàng Fŭ patterns. Rather, I am discussing the type of depression in a specific organ sense.

LIVER TYPE

Type of depression:

- Cyclical depression with the predominant emotions of anger and frustration, and feeling overwhelmed and stressed.

- Patients are unlikely to say they are depressed and instead will use phrases such as 'feeling a little off today', 'I'm just not in the mood to do anything', 'I'm just not in the groove', 'I'm just not with it' or 'I don't feel quite right'.

- However, if they recognize this as depression, they will tell you. Can be severe.

- May use alcohol to stabilize their mood after a hard day's work. This could build up to significant amounts as the years progress.

Treatment principle: Move and tonify the Liver Qì and Xuè; although unlikely, if there are any Shí/Excess signs, sedate them first; lift the mood/spirits.

Treatment:

- Trunk (front) – LR 14.

- Trunk (back) – BL 18, BL 47.

- Arms/hands – PC 6, HT 7.

- Legs/feet – LR 3, SP 6, GB 34.

- Total needles used bilaterally = 16.

HEART TYPE

Type of depression:

- Any type of depression can result from Heart and/or Heart Shén imbalances.

- Typically, Heart depression will straddle anxiety and insomnia; any other emotion may also be present.

- Likely to use stimulants/uppers/gambling to keep them away from depression; of course, there is a catch, because too many stimulants will negatively impact on their sleep. Unlikely to use alcohol unless it's just a few drinks to give them a surge.

- May surprise everyone by committing suicide because they had been seen as the life of the party (happy-go-lucky individuals).

Treatment principle: Tonify the Heart; although unlikely, if there are any Shí/Excess signs, sedate them first; lift the mood/spirits.

Treatment:

- Trunk (front) – CV 14, CV 15, CV 17.

- Trunk (back) – BL 15, BL 44.

- Arms/hands – HT 3, HT 7, PC 6.

- Legs/feet – SP 6.

- Total needles used bilaterally = 15.

SPLEEN TYPE

Type of depression:

- When we are healthy, we live in the present moment. However, when the Spleen becomes Xū/Deficient, we tend to live in the past, and when it is Shí/Excess, we live in the future.

- Breaking away from the present can leave us not just reflective but also worried, pensive and broody in our daily lives. We have lost the whole point of the present being a 'present'!

- Our Spleen loves to feel valued and important, but to do that we need to be in the present moment. By spending too much time away from daily activities, we get a disconnect with those around us, and this is what creates the depression.

Treatment principle: Move and tonify the Spleen Qì and Xuè; although unlikely, if there are any Shí/Excess signs, sedate them first; lift the mood/spirits.

Treatment:

- Trunk (front) – LR 13, CV 12.
- Trunk (back) – BL 20, BL 49.
- Arms/hands – HT 7, LU 9.
- Legs/feet – ST 36, SP 6.
- Total needles used bilaterally = 15.

Lung type

Type of depression:

- This is a distinct depression. The patient knows about it, and the likelihood is that the people around them will also know about it.
- It is severe grief/sadness/depression; what I call 'pit' depression. They are in it, they know what it is, and they will likely tell you all about it.
- The problem is that some of these people won't tell you and hide their true feelings. If they do commit suicide, it comes as a shock to everyone.
- Worry may be present, as well as suicidal thoughts/planning.
- They are unlikely to be addicted to anything and will tend to retreat away from the world and sit in their 'pit'.

Treatment principle: Tonify the Lung Qì; although unlikely, if there are any Shí/Excess signs, sedate them first; lift the mood/spirits.

Treatment:

- Trunk (front) – LU 1, CV 17.
- Trunk (back) – BL 13, BL 42.
- Arms/hands – LU 3, LU 9.
- Legs/feet – SP 6.
- Total needles used bilaterally = 13.

Kidney type

Type of depression:

- This type of depression is almost an emotional after-thought. It comes as a direct result of the breakdown of the Kidneys' driving forces. These are our willpower, drive, determination, enthusiasm and initiative. When these forces aren't stimulated, we can 'give up' on life. This can lead to a severe Xū/Deficient depression.

- Alternatively, the patient starts out as depressed and this eventually leads to a Kidney Xū, which intensifies the depression because the patient now has issues with willpower, drive, determination, enthusiasm and initiative.

Treatment principle: Tonify the Kidneys; lift the mood/spirits.

Treatment:

- Trunk (front) – CV 4, CV 6.

- Trunk (back) – BL 23, BL 52.

- Arms/hands – TE 4, HT 7.

- Legs/feet – SP 6, KI 3, KI 6.

- Total needles used bilaterally = 16.

GALL BLADDER TYPE

Type of depression:

- This depression is accompanied by a range of the following: timidity, shyness, withdrawing from society, nervousness, being easily startled, lacking courage/initiative/drive/determination, poor decision making, insomnia with restlessness/vivid dreams/early waking, sighing, floaters in the eyes, dizziness and blurry vision.

- Typically, this person is aware they are depressed but are unlikely to tell anyone about it.

- They will also hide as many of the above signs and symptoms from people because they consider them to be personal faults.

- These personal faults have, however, developed over years and years, and they blame the world for their faults.

- Therefore, they are dangerous individuals who could rage/snap at any moment.

Treatment principle: Tonify the Gall Bladder; although unlikely, if there are any Shí/Excess signs, sedate them first; lift the mood/spirits.

Treatment:

- Trunk (front) – GB 24.

- Trunk (back) – BL 18, BL 19.

- Arms/hands – HT 7, LU 9.

- Legs/feet – GB 40, LR 3.

- Total needles used bilaterally = 14.

Depression point combination – general
See Table 11.9.

Table 11.9 Depression point combination – general[54]

Location of point	Point	Reasoning
Head/face/neck	GV 20 M-HN-3 (Yìn Táng)	Calms the Shén; lifts the mood/spirits. Calms the Shén; lifts the mood/spirits.
Trunk (front)	CV 14 CV 17	Front Mù Collecting point of the Heart; nourishing the Heart can balance the Shén. Front Mù Collecting point of the Pericardium; supports the Heart Shén.
Trunk (back)	BL 42 BL 47	Pò Hù = Corporeal Soul Door.[55] Hún Mén = Ethereal Soul Gate.[56] Both back points help to lift the mood/spirits.
Arms/hands	LU 3 PC 6 HT 3 HT 7	Calms the Pò; lifts the mood/spirits. Calms the Shén; lifts the mood/spirits. Stimulates endorphins to help lift the mood/spirits. Calms the Shén; lifts the mood/spirits.
Total points needled		16 needles used bilaterally

Manic depression/Diān Kuáng
Discussion[57]

Diān = depression.

Kuáng = manic.

Manic depression is defined as a group of mental disorders that feature loss of contact with reality. Psychotic disorders manifest some of the following:[58]

- delusions

- hallucinations

- severe thought disturbances

- abnormal alteration of mood

- grossly abnormal behavior.

Diān and Kuáng co-exist like Yīn and Yáng. This Chinese medicine diagnosis is a mutual relationship between the raging mania and the lethargic depression. If a person is diagnosed as just manic or just depressed, then they are not Diān Kuáng.

It is typical for a patient with this diagnosis to be sitting predominantly in either Diān or Kuáng, but there will still be a small part of the other manifesting in them at the same time. They will then roll over into the opposite for a time; this is repeated over and over again as they cycle from one to the other.

Wŭ Xíng/Five Elements; Yīn and Yáng organs for manic depression

- Wŭ Xíng/Five Elements = Fire plus others.

- Main organs = Heart plus others.

- Secondary organs = any other organ, in particular the Stomach and Gall Bladder.

Zàng Fŭ patterns for manic depression

Diān Kuáng tends to create Shí, Xū or Stagnant patterns.
    The following are some of the more likely Zàng Fŭ patterns for Diān Kuáng:[59]

- Stomach Phlegm Fire Blazing

- Phlegm Fire Harassing the Heart

- Heart Xuè Xū and Spleen Qì Xū

- Gall Bladder Xū.

I will provide additional notes for all of these patterns.

Specific Zàng Fŭ pattern discussion for manic depression[60]
STOMACH PHLEGM FIRE BLAZING

Type of Diān Kuáng:

- Mild form – loud, funny, 'life of the party', boisterous, discards clothing and runs around; most importantly, harmless.

- Severe form – aggressive, violent, scary, rough, abusive, uncontrollable rage, wanting to maim, injure or kill. This type of aggression is typically directed towards a particular person/people who 'did them wrong'. This is targeted hostility and it is unlikely strangers will be targeted, unless they are caught in the cross-fire.

Treatment principle: Clear Phlegm and Fire from the Stomach; clear Phlegm and Fire from the Shén.

Treatment:

- Head/face/neck – GV 20.

- Trunk (front) – CV 15.

- Arms/hands – LI 11, PC 5, HT 7.

- Legs/feet – ST 40, ST 44.

- Total needles used bilaterally = 12.

PHLEGM FIRE HARASSING THE HEART

Type of Diān Kuáng:

- Mild form – loud, funny, great salesman, 'draws a crowd', can be flighty; most importantly, harmless.

- Severe form – agitated, incoherent speech, uncontrolled laughter or crying, tendency to hit or scold people, wanting to maim, injure or kill. This type of aggression is directed towards 'everyone on the planet'; because everyone they have met has treated them poorly, they see no reason to think the people they haven't met are different. This is untargeted hostility towards anyone/everyone.

Treatment principle: Clear Phlegm and Fire from the Heart; clear Phlegm and Fire from the Shén.

Treatment:

- Head/face/neck – GV 20.

- Trunk (front) – CV 14, CV 15, CV 17.

- Trunk (back) – GV 12.

- Arms/hands – PC 7, HT 7.

- Legs/feet – ST 40.

- Total needles used bilaterally = 11.

GALL BLADDER XŪ

Type of Diān Kuáng:

- Mild form – nervous, timid, shy, withdrawn but polite, 'people pleaser' but resentful about that, so feels like a 'door-mat' for others; most importantly, harmless to themselves or others.

- Severe form – repressed anger leading to significant resentment towards 'everyone on the planet'. Believes that everyone is against them, which they consider to be unfair because they feel they are so giving. They are still harmless but could 'blow their top' at any time, making them incredibly dangerous individuals to others or themselves (suicide).

    As long as they don't 'blow their top' they will do no physical harm to themselves or others. They are damaging their Shén internally, though, with a brain that just won't switch off, and this brain will be harboring ill will towards others. If they explode, they are potentially the most dangerous people on the planet, and their hostility will be directed towards anyone and everyone, including themselves.

Treatment principle: Regulate the Gall Bladder and Liver organs; build Heart Xuè; build Spleen Qì; regulate the Shén.

Treatment:

- Head/face/neck – GV 20.

- Trunk (front) – GB 24, CV 14, CV 15, CV 17.

- Trunk (back) – BL 19.

- Arms/hands – HT 7.

- Legs/feet – GB 40, SP 6.

- Total needles used bilaterally = 14.

HEART XUÈ XŪ WITH SPLEEN QÌ XŪ

Type of Diān Kuáng:

- Mild form – anxious, easily startled, on edge, loss of contact with reality, emotionally unstable with inconsistent forays into anger, laughter or crying; most importantly, harmless.

- Severe form – all mild forms will be worsened and, along with a serious tiredness/insomnia cycle, they will be very unpredictable. They are still harmless but could 'blow their top' at any time, making them incredibly dangerous individuals.

  Similar to Gall Bladder Xū, but with less harboring of ill will towards anyone and everyone. Having said that, if they 'blow their top', they will likely react in exactly the same manner as both the Gall Bladder Xū and the Phlegm Fire Harassing the Heart patterns already discussed.

Treatment principle: Build Heart Xuè; build Spleen Qì; regulate the Shén.

Treatment:

- Head/face/neck – GV 20.

- Trunk (front) – CV 14, CV 15, LR 13.

- Trunk (back) – BL 15, BL 20.

- Arms/hands – HT 7.

- Legs/feet – ST 36, SP 6.

- Total needles used bilaterally = 15.

Manic depression/Diān Kuáng point combination - general

The four Zàng Fǔ patterns discussed above are typically more chronic, so I have included a point combination in Table 11.10 for the treatment of acute Diān flare-up and in Table 11.11 for the treatment of acute Kuáng flare-up.

Table 11.10 Manic depression/Diān point combination - general[61]

Location of point	Point	Reasoning
Head/face/neck	GV 20	All of these points treat acute Diān. They target the following to achieve this:
Trunk (front)	CV 17	
Trunk (back)	BL 15 BL 18 BL 20	• Heart Shén • the Heart organ • fast-acting points at the top and bottom of the body
Arms/hands	PC 6 HT 3 HT 7	• a balance throughout the body with the remaining points.
Legs/feet	ST 40	
Total points needled		16 needles used bilaterally

Table 11.11 Manic depression/Kuáng point combination - general[62]

Location of point	Point	Reasoning
Head/face/neck	GV 16 GV 26 BL 10 M-HN-3 (Yìn Táng)	All of these points treat acute Kuáng. They target the following to achieve this: • Heart Shén • the Heart organ
Trunk (back)	GV 14	• fast-acting points at the top and bottom of the body
Arms/hands	LI 11 PC 6 PC 7 HT 7	• a balance throughout the body with the remaining points.
Legs/feet	ST 40	
Total points needled		16 needles used bilaterally

Anxiety

Discussion[63]

Anxiety is described as a feeling of worry, nervousness or unease about something with an uncertain outcome.[64]

From a Chinese medicine perspective, it's almost always a Heart emotion. Therefore, it would be useful to confirm (or rule out) the Heart by asking a series of questions pointing to a Heart pattern.

It's also quite common for anxiety to be attached to other emotions, in particular fear and phobias.

Alternatively, there will be certain triggers that the patient has probably associated with an anxiety attack. These triggers are important to establish with the patient in order to get a better understanding of what the underlying Zàng Fǔ pattern is.

Wǔ Xíng/Five Elements; Yīn and Yáng organs for anxiety

- Wǔ Xíng/Five Elements = Fire and Water.

- Main organs = Heart and Kidneys.

Zàng Fǔ patterns for anxiety

Anxiety tends to create Shí, Xū or Stagnant patterns.

The following are some of the more likely Zàng Fǔ patterns for anxiety:[65]

- Heart Qì Xū

- Heart Xuè Xū

- Heart Fire Blazing

- Phlegm Fire Harassing the Heart

- Phlegm Misting the Heart Shén

- Gall Bladder Xū

- Heart and Gall Bladder Qì Xū

- Heart and Kidney Yīn Xū

- Heart Xuè Xū and Spleen Qì Xū.

Of the patterns above, I will provide additional notes for four of them.

Specific Zàng Fǔ pattern discussion for anxiety[66]
HEART XUÈ XŪ

Type of anxiety: The mildest form of anxiety out of the four discussed, although Heart Qì Xū (on its own) is technically less severe. Is often accompanied by insomnia, palpitations, poor memory and dizziness. If the patient has any form of phobia, then this pattern is more severe, and harder to treat, than if anxiety was on its own. If they do have a phobia/fear, then you need to clarify that there isn't a second pattern involved.

Treatment principle: Tonify the Heart Xuè; settle the anxiety.

Treatment:

- Trunk (front) – CV 14.

- Trunk (back) – BL 15, BL 17, BL 20.

- Arms/hands – HT 6, HT 7.

- Legs/feet – SP 4, SP 6.

- Total needles used bilaterally = 15.

HEART AND GALL BLADDER QÌ XŪ

Type of anxiety: If it was just Heart Qì Xū, the patient would almost certainly be coping, with a very minor anxiety – perhaps one so slight that they don't even have a name to describe the way they feel. With the addition of the Gall Bladder comes timidity, shyness, withdrawal from society, 'people pleasing', sighing and indecisiveness. Further, they will probably be fearful and be suffering from a phobia of some sort. This may include panic attacks.

Treatment principle: Tonify the Heart Qì; tonify the Gall Bladder; settle the anxiety.

Treatment:

- Trunk (front) – GB 24, CV 14.

- Trunk (back) – BL 15, BL 19.

- Arms/hands – HT 5, HT 7.

- Legs/feet – GB 40, SP 6.

- Total needles used bilaterally = 15.

HEART AND KIDNEY YĪN XŪ

Type of anxiety: Probably the most chronic anxiety possible, which will, almost certainly, be straddled with a severe phobia. You will rarely get the opportunity to treat this person because they will almost never leave their house and, unless they know you, will have significant trust issues. All your usual Heart and Kidney Yīn Xū signs will be present, so an accurate diagnosis won't be difficult, as long as they are honest when they talk to you. The other issue is their memory, which will be very poor, either as a result of the deficiency or because of long-term drug use.

Treatment principle: Tonify the Heart Yīn; tonify the Kidney Yīn; settle the anxiety.

Treatment:

- Trunk (front) – CV 4, CV 6, CV 14, CV 17.

- Trunk (back) – BL 15, BL 23.

- Arms/hands – HT 6, HT 7.

- Legs/feet – KI 3, KI 6.

- Total needles used bilaterally = 16.

Phlegm Fire Harassing the Heart

Type of anxiety: Will be an acute, yet chronic, anxiety, which will almost certainly straddle psychotic behavior. They will be jittery, nervous, restless, agitated and confused. Internally, they will suffer from palpitations, insomnia, nightmares, dizziness or vertigo, and poor memory/focus/concentration. They may also have sensory perception issues, such as seeing things that aren't there or hearing things that weren't said. Word of warning: be *very* careful with these patients. If in any doubt, refer them on; they should almost certainly be seeing a psychiatrist or psychologist.

Treatment principle: Sedate the Heart; disperse Phlegm Heat from the Heart; settle the anxiety.

Treatment:

- Trunk (front) – CV 9, CV 12, CV 14, CV 17.

- Trunk (back) – BL 15, BL 44.

- Arms/hands – PC 5, HT 7.

- Legs/feet – ST 40, SP 6.

- Total needles used bilaterally = 16.

Anxiety point combination – general
See Table 11.12.

Table 11.12 Anxiety point combination – general[67]

Location of point	Point	Reasoning
Head/face/neck	GV 20 M-HN-3 (Yìn Táng)	Calms the Shén; settles anxiety. Calms the Shén; settles anxiety.
Trunk (front)	CV 14 CV 15 CV 17	Front Mù Collecting point of the Heart; nourishing the Heart can balance the Shén. An excellent point to balance the Shén. Front Mù Collecting point of the Pericardium; supports the Heart Shén.
Trunk (back)	BL 15 BL 44	Back Shù Transporting point of the Heart; nourishing the Heart can balance the Shén. Shén Táng = Spirit Hall.[68]

Arms/hands	PC 6 HT 3 HT 7	Calms the Shén; settles anxiety. Calms the Shén; settles anxiety. Yuán Source point of the Heart; nourishing the Heart can balance the Shén.
Total points needled		15 needles used bilaterally

Stress

Discussion[69]

Stress is considered a state of mental or emotional strain or tension resulting from adverse or demanding circumstances.[70]

Stress is considered a Yáng on Yīn or Young Yáng emotion and is the second most Yáng emotion that can be displayed, behind only joy. It is equal with anger and frustration; in fact, some lecturers, authors and practitioners lump the three terms together under the 'anger' banner.

I don't put the three emotions/emotional terms together because stress is a little different in the way it reacts. Where anger and frustration charge like a 'bull out of a gate', stress is more sneaky, subtle and persistent. But, similar to anger and frustration, stress can self-seed, which results in more consistent, and longer-lasting, stress even when a different emotion would be expected.

From a Chinese medicine perspective, it's almost always a Liver emotion. Therefore, it would be useful to confirm (or rule out) the Liver by asking a series of questions pointing to a Liver pattern.

It's also quite common for stress to be attached to other emotions, in particular anger, depression and/or frustration.

Wǔ Xíng/Five Elements; Yīn and Yáng organs for stress

- Wǔ Xíng/Five Elements = Wood and Fire.

- Main organs = Liver, Gall Bladder and Heart.

Zàng Fǔ patterns for stress

Stress tends to create Shí, Xū or Stagnant patterns.

The following are some of the more likely Zàng Fǔ patterns for stress:[71]

- Liver Qì Stagnation

- Liver Yáng Rising

- Liver Fire Blazing

- Liver Xuè Xū

- Damp Heat in the Liver and Gall Bladder

- Gall Bladder Xū

- Heart Fire Blazing

- Heart Xuè Xū

- Stomach and Gall Bladder Phlegm Accumulation

- Kidney Xū (any type).

Of the patterns above, I will provide additional notes for four of them.

Specific Zàng Fǔ pattern discussion for stress[72]
LIVER QÌ STAGNATION

Type of stress: The most common form. It typically results in a person feeling mildly angry, frustrated, overwhelmed, mildly disjointed, wired and struggling to cope. It can hang around for a while but will tend to disappear quickly if the person does something active, because this forces the Qì to move.

Treatment principle: Move Liver Qì; ease the stress.

Treatment:

- Head/face/neck – GV 20, GB 20.

- Trunk (front) – LR 14.

- Trunk (back) – BL 18.

- Arms/hands – PC 6, LI 4.

- Legs/feet – GB 34, LR 3.

- Total needles used bilaterally = 15.

GALL BLADDER XŪ AND HEART XUÈ XŪ

Type of stress: More severe and chronic than for Liver Qì Stagnation. Apart from stress, the person will likely suffer from insomnia, mood swings, anxiety, restlessness, palpitations and social withdrawal; because they are Xū, it will also take them longer to get into a stressful state, but it will also take them a lot longer to move back out of it again.

Treatment principle: Tonify the Gall Bladder; tonify the Heart Xuè; ease the stress.

Treatment:

- Trunk (front) – CV 14, GB 24.

- Trunk (back) – BL 15, BL 19.

- Arms/hands – HT 6, HT 7.

- Legs/feet – GB 40, SP 4.

- Total needles used bilaterally = 15.

Stomach and Gall Bladder Phlegm Accumulation

Type of stress: This is a much more significant and explosive stress. This stress is noticed by family members, friends, work colleagues – everyone! The person can't keep this stress hidden. They are loud, abrupt, rude, inconsiderate, selfish, wired, vague and forgetful. A very strange combination indeed! The Phlegm gives them Fire, which generates the activity, momentum and noise, but it also gives them the Damp, which clogs up the Shén, making them vague and forgetful.

Treatment principle: Sedate the Stomach; disperse Phlegm from the Stomach; sedate the Gall Bladder; disperse Phlegm from the Gall Bladder; ease the stress.

Treatment:

- Head/face/neck – GV 20.

- Trunk (front) – GB 24, CV 12.

- Trunk (back) – BL 19, BL 21.

- Arms/hands – PC 5, PC 6.

- Legs/feet – GB 34, ST 40.

- Total needles used bilaterally = 16.

Kidney Xū (any type)

Type of stress: Typically the chronic form, which appears after years of stressful work and/or play. The Kidneys are our most generous organ and, as such, give out to those organs in need. They expect it back, but in this instance it doesn't occur. The big clue for this pattern is the word 'chronic'. That means the patient has been doing something their body/mind doesn't like for years and years. It's unlikely that the Kidneys will be the only organ injured, so make sure you take a thorough case history of your patient to ensure that there are, or aren't, other organs diseased.

Treatment principle: Tonify the Kidneys; ease the stress.

Treatment:

- Trunk (front) – CV 4, CV 6, GB 25.

- Trunk (back) – BL 23.

- Arms/hands – TE 4, HT 7.

- Legs/feet – KI 3, KI 6, SP 6.

- Total needles used bilaterally = 16.

Stress point combination - general
See Table 11.13.

Table 11.13 Stress point combination - general[73]

Location of point	Point	Reasoning
Head/face/neck	GV 20 M-HN-3 (Yìn Táng) GB 20	Calms the Shén; eases the stress. Calms the Shén; eases the stress. Calms the Shén; eases the stress.
Trunk (front)	CV 17	Front Mù Collecting point of the Pericardium; supports the Heart Shén.
Arms/hands	PC 6 HT 7 LI 4	Calms the Shén; eases the stress. Yuán Source point of the Heart; nourishing the Heart can balance the Shén. 'Opens the Four Gates' with LR 3.[74]
Legs/feet	GB 34 LR 3	Moves the Qì to ease the stress. 'Opens the Four Gates' with LI 4.
Total points needled		15 needles used bilaterally

Treating patients with emotional disturbances is one of the most rewarding aspects of Chinese medicine. Although there is no denying the satisfaction you get when you help someone with a sore low back or neck tension with headaches, helping a patient with severe emotional turmoil is just so gratifying.

Notes

1   Aurelius 2004, p.181. Marcus Aurelius wrote *Meditations* around 170 CE while he was the Emperor of Rome. A lot of what he wrote was not original. Having said that, he was one of the most powerful people on the planet at the time, so when he spoke, people listened. Therefore, he was able to bring previous philosophical ideas to the forefront of people's thinking.

2   Chang 1977, pp.105–106. Lǐ Áo (772–841 CE) was a Confucian scholar during the Tang dynasty (618–907 CE), which was dominated by Daoist and Buddhist thought. He was very big on dissecting every aspect of human nature, including the Seven Emotions. Interestingly, Lǐ Áo had a different set of Seven Emotions to the traditional Chinese medicine view, but he was a philosopher, not a medical practitioner. The Seven Emotions Lǐ Áo ascribed to were anger, joy, grief, fear, desire, disgust and love.

3   Hartmann 2009, pp.27, 29, 50, 62, 66, 136, 140, 149, 156, 172, 183–184; Hicks *et al.* 2010, pp.13–17; Maciocia 2009, pp.115–159; Mi 2004, pp.3–7; Wang and Robertson 2008, p.77.

4   Dechar 2006, pp.169–192.

5   Rossi 2007, p.171.

6   Maciocia 2004, pp.385–386; Maciocia 2009, pp.122–125.

7   Maciocia 2009, p.122.

8   Cheng 2010, pp.269, 450–452; Hartmann 2009, p.27; Maciocia 2004, pp.791, 800–802; Maciocia 2009, pp.122–125; Ross 1995, pp.438–439, 441, 453; Rossi 2007, pp.171–183.

9   As previous note.

10 Hartmann 2009, p.27.

11 Maciocia 2004, pp.388–389; Maciocia 2009, pp.126–127.

12 Cheng 2010, pp.269, 451; Hartmann 2009, p.98; Maciocia 2004, p.794; Maciocia 2009, pp.126–127; Ross 1995, pp.439–440, 453–454; Rossi 2007, pp.171–183, 185–189.

13 As previous note.

14 Hartmann 2009, p.184.

15 Maciocia 2004, pp.386–387; Maciocia 2009, pp.129–131.

16 Dechar 2006, p.220.

17 Maclean and Lyttleton 1998, p.850.

18 Hartmann 2009, p.113; Maciocia 2009, pp.129–131; Ross 1995, p.441; Rossi 2007, pp.171–183, 185–189.

19 As previous note.

20 Maclean and Lyttleton 1998, pp.849–864.

21 Maclean and Lyttleton 2002, pp.105–106.

22 Maclean and Lyttleton 1998, pp.849–864; Rossi 2007, p.219.

23 Hartmann 2009, p.156.
24 Ellis *et al*. 1989, pp.178-179.
25 Maciocia 2004, pp.386-387; Maciocia 2009, pp.127-129.
26 Wang and Robertson 2008, pp.232-234.
27 Cheng 2010, p.269; Hartmann 2009, p.172; Maciocia 2004, pp.791-792; Maciocia 2009, pp.127-129; Ross 1995, pp.438, 441, 453-456; Rossi 2007, pp.171-183, 185-189.
28 As previous note.
29 Cheng 2010, pp.313-314.
30 Maclean and Lyttleton 2002, pp.105-106.
31 Mi 2004, p.6. *The Systematic Classic of Acupuncture and Moxibustion* (Zhēn Jiǔ Jiá Yǐ Jīng) was written by Huang Fu Mi in 282 CE.
32 Hartmann 2009, p.172.
33 Maciocia 2004, pp.387-388; Maciocia 2009, pp.131-133.
34 Cheng 2010, pp.269, 451; Hartmann 2009, p.136; Maciocia 2004, p.792; Maciocia 2009, pp.131-133; Ross 1995, pp.438, 441, 453-454; Rossi 2007, pp.171-183, 185-189, 204-215, 219-221.
35 As previous note.
36 Rossi 2007, p.171.
37 Hartmann 2009, p.136.
38 Ellis *et al*. 1989, pp.173-174.
39 Deadman *et al*. 2007, p.306.
40 Maciocia 2004, pp.384-386; Maciocia 2009, pp.133-134.
41 Cheng 2010, p.269; Hartmann 2009, p.62; Maciocia 2004, pp.792-793; Maciocia 2009, pp.133-134; Ross 1995, pp.438-439, 441, 453-457; Rossi 2007, pp.171-183, 214-221.
42 As previous note.
43 Hartmann 2009, p.62.
44 Deadman *et al*. 2007, p.310.
45 Maciocia 2009, pp.134-135.
46 Ni 1995, p.34: 8th chapter. *The Yellow Emperor's Classic* (*Inner Canon of the Yellow Emperor*/ Huáng Dì Nèi Jīng) was written somewhere between 200 and 0 BCE.
47 This is not a sexist use of the word 'He'; all Emperors in ancient China were male.
48 Hartmann 2009, p.140; Maciocia 2009, pp.134-135; O'Connor and Bensky 1981, p.571; Rossi 2007, pp.171-183.
49 As previous note.
50 Hartmann 2009, p.140.
51 Maciocia 2004, pp.380-384; Maciocia 2009, pp.341-356; Maclean and Lyttleton 2010, pp.95-105.
52 Cheng 2010, pp.269, 450-452; Hartmann 2009, p.50; Maciocia 2004, pp.797-799; Maciocia 2009, pp.341-416; Maclean and Lyttleton 2010, pp.95-155; Ross 1995, pp.437-441, 453-456; Rossi 2007, pp.171-183; Schnyer and Allen 2001.
53 Ross 1995, p.438. This reference doesn't include the Gall Bladder.
54 Hartmann 2009, p.50.
55 Ellis *et al*. 1989, pp.173-174.
56 Deadman *et al*. 2007, p.306.
57 Maciocia 2009, pp.497-509; Rossi 2007, pp.125-134.
58 Martin 1994, p.547.
59 Cheng 2010, pp.445-446; Hartmann 2009, pp.183-185; Maciocia 2004, pp.798-799, 802; Maciocia 2009, pp.497-534; O'Connor and Bensky 1981, pp.629-630; Ross 1995, pp.437, 440-441; Rossi 2007, pp.125-140, 171-183, 185-189, 351-362.
60 As previous note.
61 Hartmann 2009, p.51.
62 Ibid., p.91.
63 Maciocia 2004, pp.384-386; Maciocia 2009, pp.417-427; Maclean and Lyttleton 1998, pp.865-869.
64 https://en.oxforddictionaries.com/definition/anxiety.
65 Hartmann 2009, p.29; Maciocia 2004, pp.792-793, 799-800; Maciocia 2009, pp.417-446; Maclean and Lyttleton 1998, pp.865-885; Ross 1995, pp.437-441, 453-457; Rossi 2007, pp.171-183, 204-221.
66 As previous note.
67 Hartmann 2009, p.29.
68 Lade 1989, p.163.
69 https://en.oxforddictionaries.com/definition/stress.
70 https://en.oxforddictionaries.com/definition/stress.
71 Hartmann 2009, p.149; Ross 1995, pp.453-454; Rossi 2007, pp.171-183, 313-329.
72 As previous note.
73 Hartmann 2009, p.149.
74 The Four Gates is discussed further in Chapter 6.

Serenus [friend of Seneca's]: When I looked into myself, Seneca, some of my vices appeared clearly on the surface, so that I could lay my hand on them; some were more hidden away in the depths; some were not there all the time but return at intervals. These last I would say are the most troublesome: they are like prowling enemies who pounce on you when occasion offers, and allow you neither to be at the ready as in war nor at ease as in peace. However, the state I most find myself in (for why should I not admit the truth to you as to a doctor?) is that I am not really free of the vices which I feared and hated, though not, on the other hand, subject to them: this puts me in a condition which is not the worst, but an extremely peevish and quarrelsome one – I am neither ill nor well.

Seneca (4 BCE–65 CE)[1]

12

Qí Jīng Bā Mài/Eight Extraordinary Vessels

The Qí Jīng Bā Mài are a fascinating part of Chinese medicine and treatment. There is so much to learn about them, and even an entire book written about the Eight Extraordinary Vessels will only touch the surface.

This chapter is designed to give you a small taste of the Eight Extraordinary Vessels treatment potential. This will be done via two treatments per vessel. One will be a vessel/channel activator and the other will be a Heart Shén-based point combination.

I'm sure our friend Serenus (in the quotation above) could have benefited from some Eight Extraordinary Vessel treatment!

1. Definition of the Qí Jīng Bā Mài

Qí = extraordinary.

Jīng = vessel or channel.

Bā = eight.

Mài = a vessel that 'fills', 'empties' and/or 'stores'.

2. Brief history of the Qí Jīng Bā Mài

The Eight Extraordinary Vessels have been part of the Chinese medicine landscape since *The Spiritual Pivot* (Líng Shū/靈樞) was written over 2000 years ago. Other famous texts and authors have continued the evolution of the Eight Extraordinary Vessels. Some of these include:

- *The Classic of Difficulties* (*Canon of the Yellow Emperor's Eighty-One Difficult Issues*/Huáng Dì Bā Shí Yī Nán Jīng/黃帝八十一難經) written somewhere around 0–200 CE.

- *The Pulse Classic* (Mài Jīng/脈經) written by Wang Shu He in 280 CE.

- *The Systematic Classic of Acupuncture and Moxibustion* (Zhēn Jiǔ Jiá Yǐ Jīng/針灸甲乙經) written by Huang Fu Mi in 282 CE.

- *The Guide to the Classic of Acupuncture* (Zhēn Jīng Zhǐ Nán/針經指南) written by Dou Han Qing somewhere between 1196 and 1295 CE.

- *The Glorious Anthology of Acupuncture and Moxibustion* (Zhēn Jiǔ Jù Yīng/針灸聚英) written by Gao Wu in 1529 CE.

- *An Exposition on the Eight Extraordinary Vessels* (Qí Jīng Bā Mài Kǎo/奇經八脉考) written by Li Shi Zhen in 1578 CE.

- *The Great Compendium of Acupuncture and Moxibustion/Zhēn Jiǔ Dà Chéng/針灸大成)* by Yang Jizhou in 1601 CE.

- *Methods of Acupuncture and Moxibustion from the Golden Mirror of Medicine* (Yī Zōng Jīn Jiàn Cì Jiǔ Xīn Fǎ/醫宗金鑑刺灸心法) written by Wu Qian in 1742 CE.

3. Overview of the Qí Jīng Bā Mài

The Eight Extraordinary Vessels are a fascinating and important part of the channel system in Chinese medicine. No matter how much one researches them, there is always a new aspect emerging, a new understanding, a new angle. (Maciocia 2006, p.371)

There are a range of differences between the twelve main channels and the Eight Extraordinary Vessels, as shown in Table 12.1.

Table 12.1 Comparison between the twelve main channels and the Eight Extraordinary Vessels[2]

Overview	Twelve main channels	Eight Extraordinary Vessels
Yīn Yáng partners	All have Yīn Yáng partners	Don't have Yīn Yáng partners; have an effect on all the Yīn channels or all the Yáng channels or all together
Organ relationship	Have a direct organ relationship based, in a large part, on the channel name	They do have a relationship with different organs but not in the same way the twelve main channels do
Depth in the body	Travel close to the surface of the body	Travel very deeply in the body
Points on the channel	Each of the channels has its own points	The Rèn Mài and Dū Mài have their own points but the other six borrow points from the twelve main channels
Special point categories	Have a wide range of different special point categories on their channels	The 'opening' point and 'coupled' points are exclusive to these channels. Collectively, they are also termed 'confluent' points

4. Functions of the Qí Jīng Bā Mài

The Eight Extraordinary Vessels have a wide range of functions, some of which are described below.[3]

Provide additional links between the twelve main channels

The Eight Extraordinary Vessels strengthen the association among the channels. They are responsible for controlling, joining, storing and regulating the Vital Substances (Qì, Xuè, Jīn Yè and Jīng) of each channel.

Act as a dam or reservoir for the Vital Substances

When there is a surplus of Vital Substances in the body, this is stored in the Eight Extraordinary Vessels. In this way they act like a dam or reservoir that is filling up with water. Then when the body needs some of this stored energy, the Eight Extraordinary Vessels release it back into the twelve main channels, similar to a dam releasing water when it is full or when the water supply downstream is low.

Inherently linked to the Kidneys

The Rèn Mài, Dū Mài, Chōng Mài and, to a lesser extent, the Dài Mài are the first channels made after conception and all originate in the Dān Tián, the space between the Kidneys. Therefore, they derive their energy from the Kidneys and are inherently linked to the Jīng, Original/Yuán Qì and the basic constitution of the individual.

Provide some support to the Defensive/Wèi Qì

When there is a surplus of Vital Substances in the body, this is transported to the Eight Extraordinary Vessels. Before it gets to the vessels, the Vital Substances travel through the space between the skin and muscles and give the entire area a boost of energy. This is where the Wèi Qì resides and circulates; as a result, it gets a boost (or support) from these Vital Substances.

Connect the main organs and channels with the six extraordinary organs

The six extraordinary organs are the Gall Bladder (it's part of the main organ structure as well), brain, blood vessels, marrow, bones and the uterus. These six extraordinary organs are connected with the Eight Extraordinary Vessels, which then link through into the main organ and channel system of the body.

Are involved with the seven-year cycles of women and eight-year cycles of men

In simple terms, it refers to male and female energies moving at different speeds and decline throughout a lifetime; an ebb and flow if you like. Women operate on seven-year cycles and men operate on eight, which is one of the reasons that women will generally go through puberty earlier than men. This also explains why women will typically go through their change of life earlier than men.

Help to balance the flow of Vital Substances left and right, up and down, anterior and posterior, interior and exterior

The Eight Extraordinary Vessels are a crucial part of Vital Substance flow, not just from the internal to the external parts of the body either. Based on their pathways throughout the body, they all have some involvement in the movement of Vital Substances in every other conceivable direction.

Access the opening and coupled (confluent) points

Each of the Eight Extraordinary Vessels has an opening and coupled point. These are sometimes referred to as confluent points. These points are used to activate the vessels.

Have the potential to treat genetic diseases

The link with the Dān Tián and Kidney Jīng allows these vessels to treat genetic diseases.

> The Eight Extraordinary Vessels are at a deeper level in the energetic strata of the human body...and all can treat the Root. (Matsumoto and Birch 1986, pp.13, 15)

> All of the Eight Extraordinary Vessels give access to primordial energy and each has its special key for the unlocking of stores of memory lodged in the Heart, in the cells, and in the muscles. (Carey and De Muynck 2007, pp.102–103)

Not only can the Eight Extraordinary Vessels potentially treat genetic diseases, but they can also, in theory, treat inherited memory. These genetic memories can be just as damaging to the body (and mind) as genetic diseases are. These locked memories can be guided out and released from the body via the use of the Eight Extraordinary Vessels.

Work on the Three Ancestries[4]

The first ancestry is related to our prenatal and early postnatal period and is governed by the Rèn Mài, Dū Mài and Chōng Mài.

The second ancestry is related to our past, present and future selves and is governed by the Yáng Wéi Mài and the Yīn Wéi Mài.

The third ancestry is related to our view of self. This includes how we view ourselves (self-esteem) as well as how we perceive what others (family, friends, acquaintances, work colleagues, strangers) think of us. This is governed by the Dài Mài, Yáng Qiāo Mài and Yīn Qiāo Mài.

5. When to use the Qí Jīng Bā Mài[5]

There are a range of different times when you might consider using the Eight Extraordinary Vessels. Some of the more common uses include:

- mental and emotional problems

- problems of more than one of the twelve main channels or organs

- complicated, chronic or confusing conditions

- neurological conditions

- elite athletic/sports performance – including musculoskeletal complaints.

6. How to use the Qí Jīng Bā Mài[6]

> When treatments for the extraordinary vessels were described in the old books [classics], there were, unfortunately, few descriptions of the needle or moxa techniques recommended. (Matsumoto and Birch 1986, p.71)

It hasn't been until more recent times that practitioners and authors have started to discuss how to use the Eight Extraordinary Vessels. There is no hard and fast rule here. For me, I generally treat the Eight Extraordinary Vessels in the following manner:

- First I needle the opening point bilaterally.

- Then I needle the coupled point bilaterally.

- After that I use one (or more) points on the chosen vessel.

- I finish off my needling with any other non-vessel points.

- Upon removal of the needles, I take them out in reverse order, ensuring that the last needles removed are the opening points.

As stated earlier, however, there are plenty of other ways you can use the Eight Extraordinary Vessels. In the end, you have to be happy with how you use them and have an understanding of the way that you treat the Eight Extraordinary Vessels.

You will notice that with my treatments described below. They are one way of treating, but not the only way.

7. Opening and coupled pairings of the Qí Jīng Bā Mài

Each of the Eight Extraordinary Vessels has an opening and coupled point – sometimes referred to as confluent points. These points are used to activate the vessels. Coincidentally, each of the eight opening points are also coupled points for another Qí Jīng Bā Mài. The pairings are listed in Table 12.2.

What this effectively means is that it's pretty difficult to treat just one of the Qí Jīng Bā Mài at a time. There is almost definitely going to be some secondary effect from the coupled vessel. But this is not a bad thing as it's often a good strategy to work on more than one channel/vessel/system in the body anyway, as it makes for a more holistic treatment.

Table 12.2 Qí Jīng Bā Mài channel pairings[7]

Main vessel	Opening point	Coupled point	Paired vessel
Rèn Mài	LU 7	KI 6	Yīn Qiāo Mài
Dū Mài	SI 3	BL 62	Yáng Qiāo Mài
Chōng Mài	SP 4	PC 6	Yīn Wéi Mài
Dài Mài	GB 41	TE 5	Yáng Wéi Mài
Yáng Qiāo Mài	BL 62	SI 3	Dū Mài
Yīn Qiāo Mài	KI 6	LU 7	Rèn Mài
Yáng Wéi Mài	TE 5	GB 41	Dài Mài
Yīn Wéi Mài	PC 6	SP 4	Chōng Mài

8. The Qí Jīng Bā Mài
Rèn Mài

It is said at conception the spirit [Shén] of man has the purpose of his life whispered into his ear as he passes through the heavenly gateway into life. As our life unfolds, it is this secret that gives life its purpose… The Ren Mai…governs this inner resource. (Kaatz 2005, p.33)

Opening point = LU 7.

Coupled point = KI 6.

The Rèn Mài is often translated as Conception Vessel, Central Vessel or Directing Vessel. It is also considered to be the 'Sea of Yīn channels', which means that it is responsible for regulating all of the Yīn channels on the body, and all of the Yīn in the body.

The Rèn Mài also binds up the anterior of the body, ensuring that all channels on the front of the body are flowing smoothly and in harmony with all the other channels at the anterior. The Rèn Mài also:[8]

- regulates the reproductive systems of men and women

- regulates Qì in the Lower Jiāo

- aids in the Lung–Kidney respiration dynamic

- aids the Spleen and Kidneys in transforming and transporting (T & T) the Jīn Yè

- helps the bonding between a new-born child and parents – it is part of the first ancestry.

The meaning [of the character for Rèn] is to endure, to bear, to take the burden of something…to bear the burden of being human, which is, for instance, to be able to take charge and cope at each level of human life. (Larre and Rochat De La Vallee 1997, pp.85–86)

Opening point – LU 7 (Liè Quē)

Liè = sequence.

Quē = incomplete, imperfect, broken.

Liè Quē = broken sequence.[9]

The meaning of broken sequence is twofold. One meaning is that the Lung channel deviates at LU 7, which breaks the sequence of Lung channel points that were in a straight line (LU 5, LU 6, LU 8 and LU 9).

The other meaning is that LU 7 can be used to break the sequence/cycle of something that is no longer self-serving. For example, you have a patient that wants help with anger issues. Needle LU 7 and then LR 2 (possibly the best point to treat anger) with the intent from both you and your patient that anger is no longer an emotion that will be the ruling power it once was.[10]

At Lie Que is a place of separation where that which we need can be reorganised and that which we no longer need is let go. (Kaatz 2005, p.408)

Rèn Mài point combination – general

There are plenty of different treatment approaches for the Eight Extraordinary Vessels. I will be offering a general treatment for the Rèn Mài (Table 12.3) plus a Shén-based point combination. These are my own personal choice of points and have therefore not been referenced. There are other points on the vessel that you may prefer to use.

Table 12.3 Rèn Mài point combination – general

Location of point	Point	Reasoning
Trunk (front)	CV 1[11] CV 4 CV 6 CV 12 CV 14 CV 17 CV 21	Accesses the Dān Tián Lower Jiāo plus Xuè and Yīn Lower Jiāo plus Qì and Yáng Middle Jiāo plus Qì and Yáng Middle Jiāo plus Xuè and Yīn Upper Jiāo plus Qì and Xuè Upper Jiāo – crowns the treatment[12]
Arms/hands	LU 7	Opening point
Legs/feet	KI 6	Coupled point
Total points needled		11 needles used bilaterally

Rèn Mài point combination – Heart Shén

All of the points in Table 12.4 can calm the Heart Shén, but not all of the points chosen are on the Rèn Mài. They have been selected because of their affinity for combining with other points in the treatment.

Table 12.4 Rèn Mài point combination – Heart Shén

Location of point	Point	
Head/face/neck	GV 20	M-HN-3 (Yìn Táng)
Trunk (front)	CV 4 CV 12 CV 14	CV 15 CV 17 CV 21
Arms/hands	LU 7	HT 7
Legs/feet	KI 6	SP 6
Total points needled	16 needles used bilaterally	

Although this particular combination has the capacity to treat a large amount of Heart Shén imbalance, I like this treatment for a Heart Shén reset. This is because it targets all the organs locally and distally and has a particularly strong emphasis on the Heart locally as well as the brain.

This reset allows the patient to feel more balanced and in control of their life for a day (or several) before they typically progress back to their usual emotional patterning. What this treatment does do, however, is highlight the key mental issues that they need to deal with moving forward. And this is essentially a green-light moment, thereby allowing a much more dramatic effect on their Heart Shén into future treatments.

If a patient is able to isolate the key areas of concern, they are much more likely to get better results moving forward.

Dū Mài

> The Du Mai…is like the Emperor's governor watching over the kingdom…directed from the wisdom and love of the Emperor's Heart… The Du Mai…directs the activities of the mind, body and spirit [Shén] with pure forceful, dynamic, vital, Yang Qi. (Kaatz 2005, p.59)

Opening point = SI 3.

Coupled point = BL 62.

The Dū Mài is often translated as Governing Vessel and is considered to be the 'Sea of Yáng Channels', which means that it is responsible for regulating all of the Yáng channels on the body, and all of the Yáng in the body.

The Dū Mài also binds up the posterior of the body, ensuring that all channels on the back of the body are flowing smoothly and in harmony with all the other channels at the posterior. The Dū Mài also:[13]

- regulates the Heart Shén via the Heart organ and the brain

- regulates the reproductive systems of men and women, particularly in cases where the patient is Qì Xū or Yáng Xū

- strengthens the back and spine

- nourishes marrow (which helps strengthen the spine and brain)

- clears External and/or Internal Wind

- helps the bonding between a new-born child and parents – it is part of the first ancestry.

> [The Dū Mài] is a relative who keeps an eye on what is going on. In this way the family interests are looked after. This is done with skill and authority to achieve correct action… It is the Du Mai that directs life. (Kaatz 2005, p.59)

Opening point - SI 3 (Hòu Xī)

Hòu = back, a push from behind.

Xī = ravine, creek or mountain stream.

Hòu Xī = back ravine.[14]

SI 3 is the Wood point of the Small Intestine channel. Wood points are great to connect us with our Hún/Ethereal Soul, which is where new ideas, inspiration, insight and our grandest dreams reside.

According to Maciocia (2015, pp.202–203), the Small Intestine organ is in charge of separating and clarifying thoughts into 'Dirty and Clean' or 'Pure and Impure'. In other words, the Small Intestine allows us to determine the difference between right and wrong.[15] Therefore SI 3 assists us with clear judgement and decision making.

> As we experience, grow, and transform, our innate intelligence guides the Du to seek experiences that support our spirit. (Twicken 2013, p.65)

Dū Mài point combination - general

There are plenty of different treatment approaches for the Eight Extraordinary Vessels. I will be offering a general treatment for the Dū Mài (Table 12.5) plus a Shén-based point combination. These are my own personal choice of points and have therefore not been referenced. There are other points on the vessel that you may prefer to use.

Table 12.5 Dū Mài point combination - general

Location of point	Point	Reasoning
Head/face/neck	GV 20	Crowns the treatment[16]
Trunk (front)	GV 4 GV 7 GV 9 GV 11 GV 14	Lower Jiāo – specifically Kidneys Middle Jiāo – specifically Liver and Gall Bladder Middle Jiāo – specifically Spleen and Stomach Upper Jiāo plus Qì and Xuè Regulates Yáng
Arms/hands	SI 3	Opening point
Legs/feet	BL 62	Coupled point
Total points needled		10 needles used bilaterally

Dū Mài point combination - Heart Shén

All of the points in Table 12.6 can calm the Heart Shén, but not all of the points chosen are on the Dū Mài. They have been selected because of their affinity for combining with other points in the treatment.

Table 12.6 Dū Mài point combination - Heart Shén

Location of point	Point	
Head/face/neck	GV 16 GV 20	GV 24
Trunk (back)	GV 1[17] GV 4	GV 10 GV 11
Arms/hands	SI 3	
Legs/feet	BL 62	
Total points needled	11 needles used bilaterally	

I like this particular point combination for treating singular or multiple emotional imbalances. These can be partly known and/or unknown by the patient.

That's what's great about Chinese medicine. It helps the body heal itself, so even if the patient isn't completely aware of what's going on in their emotional space, Chinese medicine can still help.

Chōng Mài - Shén Mén Spirit Gate points

> The *Chong Mai* is an intercommunication with all that is important so we can move forward along a straight pathway…by joining all routes along the way and by gathering together the experiences that come… It is responsible for the pattern of the development of life. (Kaatz 2005, p.89)

Opening point = SP 4.

Coupled point = PC 6.

The Chōng Mài is often translated as Thoroughfare Vessel, Penetrating Vessel or Thrusting Vessel, and is considered to be the 'Sea of the Twelve Main Channels'. This means that it's responsible for regulating all of the Yīn and Yáng channels on the body.

The Chōng Mài also binds up the center of the body, ensuring that all of the twelve main channels are flowing smoothly in and out of the trunk into the five extremities, and that they are in harmony with all the other channels. The Chōng Mài also:[18]

- regulates the uterus, prostate and the Kidneys. This makes it effective in gynecological disorders, in particular fertility and menstruation. By connecting to the Kidneys, it also distributes Jīng all over the body

- links the Pre-Heaven Qì and Post-Heaven Qì, as it's the center of the energetic vortex that connects the Kidneys Pre-Heaven Qì with the Stomach Post-Heaven Qì

- can improve circulation to the legs and feet for problems such as coldness, numbness and tingling

- is sometimes termed the 'Sea of Xuè' channel because it is related to the blood in the uterus and because it controls all the blood vessels (veins, arteries and capillaries). It is particularly effective for Xuè Stasis in the Uterus and Lower Jiāo

- helps the bonding between a new-born child and parents – it is part of the first ancestry.

Chong energetic properties can access our primordial nature, the capacity to become anything, to take any shape or form. This includes having an open and free mind. (Twicken 2013, p.48)

Opening point – SP 4 (Gōng Sūn)

Gōng = grandfather, gentleman, a person of nobility.

Sūn = grandson, grandchild, descendant.

Gōng Sūn = grandfather's grandchild.[19]

Gōng Sūn was also the family name of Huáng Dì (Yellow Emperor),[20] who ruled China from 2697 to 2597 BCE. This period in Chinese history is supposedly the equivalent to Periclean Athens – the perfect race ruled by perfect people. Confucius (Kǒng Zǐ) would sometimes refer to this time period when discussing his concept of Jūn Zǐ (Gentleman – Perfect Person). According to Confucius, this time period was the one you needed to refer back to when aspiring to be perfect.[21] All Chinese were descendants of this perfect race; therefore, by needling Gōng Sūn, we can tweak that perfect part inside ourselves.

SP 4 is also particularly effective at treating intergenerational imprinting. This could consist of genetic diseases that are passed on from generation to generation, including diseases of the body, but also of the mind (Shén). In short, my clinical experience has shown that treating the Chōng Mài (along with the other Qí Jīng Bā Mài) can have a profound effect on a patient's genetic diseases, both physical and mental.

> The Chong Mai is effective to treat mental restlessness and anxiety associated with Rebellious Qi. (Maciocia 2006, p.404)

Chōng Mài point combination – general

There are plenty of different treatment approaches for the Eight Extraordinary Vessels. I will be offering a general treatment for the Chōng Mài (Table 12.7) plus a Shén-based point combination. These are my own personal choice of points and have therefore not been referenced. There are other points on the vessel that you may prefer to use.

Table 12.7 Chōng Mài point combination – general

Location of point	Point	Reasoning
Head/face/neck	CV 23	Regulates the higher portion of the Chōng Mài
Trunk (front)	KI 19 KI 27 ST 30	Middle Jiāo – and middle-trunk portions of the Chōng Mài Upper Jiāo – and higher-trunk portions of the Chōng Mài Lower Jiāo – and lower-trunk portions of the Chōng Mài
Arms/hands	PC 6	Coupled point
Legs/feet	SP 4 SP 6 ST 37	Opening point Regulates the Chōng Mài Sea of Xuè – regulates the Chōng Mài (All three leg points regulate the lower portion of the Chōng Mài)
Total points needled		15 needles used bilaterally

Chōng Mài point combination - Heart Shén

All of the points in Table 12.8 can calm the Heart Shén, but not all of the points chosen are on the Chōng Mài. They have been selected because of their affinity for combining with other points in the treatment.

Table 12.8 Chōng Mài point combination - Heart Shén

Location of point	Point	
Head/face/neck	GV 20	M-HN-3 (Yìn Táng)
Trunk (front)	KI 13 KI 16	KI 21
Arms/hands	PC 6	TE 4
Legs/feet	SP 4	KI 3
Total points needled	16 needles used bilaterally	

I like this particular point combination for treating emotional intergenerational imprinting. These are emotions that have been passed down from generation to generation because nobody in the hereditary line was willing (or even aware enough) to have them treated. These locked-in emotions can be just as damaging to the body as physical blocks.

The Chōng Mài can also be used for emotional imprinting that has happened to you in your lifetime. Again, these could be known or unknown. Regardless, this imprinting can be extremely toxic on the body and the Chōng Mài can help to remove them.

There are a few treatment strategies that can be employed with treating emotional imprinting:

- You can be gentle and gradual. In this case, you only treat the Chōng Mài with the Yīn Wéi Mài. These are the opening and coupled pairings.

- You can be moderately aggressive. Here, you treat the Chōng Mài, Yīn Wéi Mài and two other vessels of the Qí Jīng Bā Mài. Make sure that the other two that you choose are opening and coupled pairings.

- You can be extremely aggressive. If this is the treatment plan, then you open all of the Qí Jīng Bā Mài, not just the Chōng Mài.

Regardless of your treatment preference, you need to be very aware that the Qí Jīng Bā Mài have the potential to be extremely powerful in their effect. This is because they work on the deepest layer of your being. Therefore, they can help to lift/push out the diseases/disorders that are very chronic and innermost in the body.

This poses a potential patient body/mind backlash when that deep/chronic disorder works its way to the surface. From experience, this is never pretty and rocks the patient, as well as everyone close to them. It's very important, therefore, to warn the patient of this probability; and for them to warn their close associates.

The more aggressive you are with the number of Qí Jīng Bā Mài that you open, the more this warning needs to be applied.

You may be asking yourself, why would you be so aggressive with your treatment? Basically, the more aggressive you are, the more likely it will be that you can clear out the chronic mess that is inside the patient. Although there will probably be some short-term pain, there will be long-term gain.

Finally, I have never seen the Qí Jīng Bā Mài create a significant emotional release faster than six months after the prescribed treatment. It has always been in the range of 6–10 months. This may be different for your patients, and I can only go by my clinical experience, especially as the literature is limited on this particular topic.

Make sure you are there for your patient during this time and ease them gently through this experience. Don't try to suppress their emotions because that won't work. Help them work their way through the emotions instead. This is much healthier, and is the reason why you did the treatment in the first place.

> When we allow the natural expression of our prenatal energetic properties in postnatal life, we are living our quest. This process is a type of alchemy. This cultivation influences the way we can change and transform. (Twicken 2013, p.49)

Chōng Mài Spirit Gate/Shén Mén points

The Chōng Mài is an interesting vessel because it has so many probable pathways. One of these travels through the special point group called the Spirit Gate/Shén Mén points.

The Spirit Gate/Shén Mén points are a special point group that work on a patient's Wǔ Shén (Five Spirits), which are:[22]

- Hún – Ethereal/Heavenly/Dream-Big Soul

- Shén – Spirit

- Yì – Thought/Post-Heaven Intellect

- Pò – Corporeal/Grounded/Earthly/Do-Big-Be-Big Soul

- Zhì – Willpower/Pre-Heaven Intellect.

These Chōng Mài points can therefore work on every part of your Wǔ Shén or inherent spirit.

The Spirit Gate/Shén Mén point group is a loaded topic. Most people I have spoken with have strong opposing views about whether these points actually even treat the Wǔ Shén.

Personally, I have had significant successes using these points, sometimes on their own and sometimes as a point combination using other points. Obviously, it's a little harder to judge their ability when they are being used with other points, but I have seen some impressive results using just a small selection of the Spirit Gate points, sometimes using only two needles!

How do you use the Spirit Gate/Shén Mén points?

There are two main strategies/options.

Option one is to choose the point based on its functions and connections with the different organs, elements and Wǔ Shén. Each of the point's individual functions are discussed below.

Option two is to choose the point based on palpation of each of the Spirit Gate points from KI 22 to KI 27. Start at either end and press on the point bilaterally. Press firmly until the patient tells you it is hard enough. I call this a 'hurts good' pain and is right on the edge of being too much for the patient to handle. Move on to the next point and repeat. Do this for all the points and adjust your pressure where necessary so that when you have completed all of the points you have established the perfect 'hurts good' pressure.

Move through all of the Spirit Gate points a second time. This time you are asking the patient to tell you when there is a point that is particularly painful, or one that makes them feel funny (butterflies) in the tummy. Or one that makes them feel yucky or weird. The patient shouldn't spend any time analyzing it; there should be an immediate response. You then need to ask them if it's both points you are pressing bilaterally or only on one side. Establish if it's one or both and make a little mark on the skin with a highlighter.

Repeat this process all the way through the Spirit Gate points. When you are finished, count how many marks you have made on their skin. There will typically be between one and five, and if that's the case, I needle them and explain to the patient what each point represents from a Wǔ Shén perspective.

If there are more than five marks, I tend to go back to the marks and push them again, one at a time, to see if any of them aren't as bad as the others. This almost always reduces the number of points needed to needle. I do this because the Spirit Gate points are a specific treatment approach and I don't want to dilute the important information that I am trying to get to their Wǔ Shén.

On rare occasions, the patient says that all (or almost all) of the Spirit Gate points are super-sensitive or, the opposite, that they feel none of them. In this situation it's likely that the patient's rational brain has become involved, but we were doing this technique to bypass that part of the brain. If this occurs, I choose a different point combination for the patient.

I usually choose option two when using the Spirit Gate points. I prefer this option because I get to see inside the person's body where there are no masks to hide the real truth. To be fair, this truth may also be hidden from the patient.

Therefore, this method bypasses any masks (as well as the patient's rational mind) and isolates the organs, along with their Wǔ Shén that are crying out for help.

The Spirit Gate/Shén Mén points are listed in Table 12.9.

Table 12.9 Spirit Gate/Shén Mén

Points	Treats
KI 22 (Bù Láng) – Veranda/Corridor Walk	Water and Fire elements
KI 23 (Shén Fēng) – Spirit Seal	Earth element
KI 24 (Líng Xū) – Spirit Burial Ground	Metal element
KI 25 (Shén Cáng) – Spirit Storehouse	Fire element
KI 26 (Yù Zhōng) – Lively Center	Wood element
KI 27 (Shū Fǔ) – Palace Treasury Transporter	Water and Metal element

KI 22 (Bù Láng) – Veranda/Corridor Walk[23]

The Water element (Yīn) loves serenity and security, and the home is where we often feel safest. The Fire element (Yáng) loves getting among it in the world and being around lots of people. A veranda is that middle ground between the security of one's house and the big wide world. It's a place of moderation, where the Fire and Water elements feel equally valued and nourished.

KI 22 can treat the Water and Fire elements.[24] See Table 12.10 for two acupuncture point combinations.

Table 12.10 KI 22 (Bù Láng) – Veranda/Corridor Walk

Location of point	Water element point combination[25]		Fire element point combination[26]	
Trunk (front)	KI 22	CV 3	KI 22	CV 14
Trunk (back)	BL 23		N/A	
Arms/hands	N/A		TE 6 SI 5	HT 8
Legs/feet	KI 10	BL 66	N/A	
Total points needled	9 needles used bilaterally		9 needles used bilaterally	

KI 23 (Shén Fēng) – Spirit Seal[27]

This is where we identify with our true spiritual identity. Similar to a Chinese emperor stamping his wax seal on important documents, this point has access to where we have stamped our spirit.

Often this point is effective when a person feels they have lost their way in life, either via a sense of direction or a sense of self.

The Earth element, being in the center, is directly responsible for the balancing of all things. It thrives on the 'Knowing' even if we don't know that we know. Therefore, KI 23 can treat the Earth element.[28] See Table 12.11 for a point combination.

Table 12.11 KI 23 (Shén Fēng) – Spirit Seal

Earth element point combination[29]		
Location of point	Point	
Trunk (front)	KI 23	CV 12
Trunk (back)	BL 20	
Legs/feet	ST 36	SP 3
Total points needled	9 needles used bilaterally	

KI 24 (LÍNG XŪ) – SPIRIT BURIAL GROUND[30]

The point name refers to the deliberate removal of something old that is no longer self-serving, or the impending forced death of something. Therefore, we are looking at two different processes. The first suggests that the person has made an active effort to clear some clutter but has reached an impasse. The second suggests that the person's spirit is about to force the ending (death) of something. Regardless, the old waste has to be buried to make way for the new seedlings or young wood.

Therefore, KI 24 can treat the Metal element. This is because the Pò is housed in the Metal element and the Pò is our grounded soul. When we can bury the old, it makes way for the new. Therefore, KI 24 can also be used, to a lesser extent, for the Wood element.[31]

See Table 12.12 for a point combination for the Metal element.

Table 12.12 KI 24 (Líng Xū) – Spirit Burial Ground

Metal element point combination[32]		
Location of point	Point	
Trunk (front)	KI 24	ST 25
Trunk (back)	BL 13	
Arms/hands	LU 8	LI 1
Total points needled	10 needles used bilaterally	

KI 25 (SHÉN CÁNG) – SPIRIT STOREHOUSE[33]

The spirit or Shén is responsible for every emotion, regardless of whether it is anger, joy, pensiveness, worry, sadness, fear or shock. The Shén is also responsible for every Wǔ Shén, be it the Hún, Pò, Yì or Zhì. Granted, these are all stored in different organs, but the primary organ that controls them all is the Heart Shén.

At KI 25 the Heart Shén can access our stored emotions and Wǔ Shén to encourage emotional health and wellbeing. Therefore, KI 25 can treat the Fire element.[34] See Table 12.13 for a point combination.

> It is perhaps the point of choice in situations when the intensity of feelings of rejection and loneliness have devastated the stability and strength of a person's *shen*. (Hicks *et al.* 2010, p.324)

Table 12.13 KI 25 (Shén Cáng) – Spirit Storehouse

Fire element point combination[35]		
Location of point	**Point**	
Trunk (front)	KI 25	CV 14
Arms/hands	TE 6 SI 5	HT 8
Total points needled	9 needles used bilaterally	

KI 26 (Yù Zhōng) – Lively Center[36]

This is where we can reconnect with our Hún, which is commonly referred to as our 'Heavenly/Ethereal/Artistic/Dream-Big' Soul. The Hún is creative Yáng and is our Lively Center.

KI 26 helps us strengthen our Hún, thereby allowing us access to our grandest dreams, our greatest potential and our unlimited realities. Therefore, KI 26 can treat the Wood element.[37] See Table 12.14 for a point combination.

Table 12.14 KI 26 (Yù Zhōng) – Lively Center

Wood element point combination[38]		
Location of point	**Point**	
Trunk (front)	KI 26	LR 14
Trunk (back)	BL 19	
Legs/feet	GB 41	LR 1
Total points needled	10 needles used bilaterally	

KI 27 (Shū Fǔ) – Palace Treasury Transporter[39]

The Kidneys (Water element) are the site for our Original/Yuán Qì, and the Lungs (Metal element) are the site for our True/Zhēn Qì.

Original/Yuán Qì is considered 'Pre-Heaven', and True/Zhēn Qì is considered 'Post-Heaven'. Both are our life reserves (treasuries) in their own right.

KI 27 is used when we want to ensure good connection between the Pre-Heaven and Post-Heaven Qì. In terms of emotional balance, we are referring to a solid Pò and Zhì relationship.

KI 27 can treat the Water and Metal elements.[40] See Table 12.15 for two acupuncture point combinations.

Table 12.15 KI 27 (Shū Fǔ) – Palace Treasury Transporter

Location of point	Water element point combination[41]		Metal element point combination[42]	
Trunk (front)	KI 22 KI 27	CV 3	KI 24 KI 27	ST 25
Trunk (back)	BL 23		BL 13	

Arms/hands	N/A		LU 8	LI 1
Legs/feet	KI 10	BL 66	N/A	
Total points needled	11 needles used bilaterally		12 needles used bilaterally	

The acupuncture point combinations that I have provided in Tables 12.10–12.15 aren't an exact science. Different authors have alternative views on how to go about using the Spirit Gate/Shén Mén points.

When there are differing views in Chinese medicine – and let's be fair, this occurs regularly – we need to use a trial-and-error approach. These points are perfect for exactly that.

In the end, we need to be able to find our own Chinese medicine identity because with it comes a belief in ourselves and in our medicine, and I can guarantee you that there is not much else more powerful.

Dài Mài

> It [Dài Mài] is a guiding ship from the origins of life itself, uniting and moving our vital circulations as we pilot our course in the great sea of the *Tao* [Dào]. (Kaatz 2005, p.107)

> Opening point = GB 41.

> Coupled point = TE 5.

The Dài Mài is often translated as the Belt Vessel or Girdle Vessel and, similar to the Chōng Mài, binds up all of the Yīn and Yáng channels on the body.

Think of the Dài Mài as splitting the body clean in half. It's the only vessel/ channel that travels horizontally, thereby connecting all the channels in the body, including the twelve main channels and each of the Qí Jīng Bā Mài. Because it cuts the body in half, it also absorbs Vital Substances from the anterior through to the posterior of the body (and vice versa), enriching every organ in its path, namely the Kidneys and uterus in the Lower Jiāo, and the Liver and Gall Bladder in the Middle Jiāo.

The Dài Mài also connects the upper and lower parts of the body, ensuring that all of the twelve main channels are flowing smoothly in and out of the trunk into the five extremities, and that they are in harmony with all the other channels. As a result, the Dài Mài can improve circulation of Vital Substances to/from the legs/feet, arms/hands and head/face. This might be for problems associated with coldness, numbness, tingling, burning and/or color changes, to name just a few.

In addition, the Dài Mài:[43]

- stimulates the smooth flow of Vital Substances through the body via its connection to the channels, but also via its close relationship to the Liver and Gall Bladder organs

- assists in the production of Post-Heaven Qì

- is closely related to the Kidneys, uterus and prostate, thereby assisting in the production of Pre-Heaven Qì and Jīng

- regulates Dampness in the Lower Jiāo. A few Western disorders associated with this diagnosis might be thrush, polycystic ovarian syndrome and endometriosis

- is very effective for hip problems

- treats patients who are stuck in frustration. They might describe the feeling as 'trying to break through but not quite getting there'. The Dài Mài can accelerate mobility to move through the stagnation by opening to the frustration so that it can be released and reformatted[44]

- is part of the third ancestry, thereby making it a vessel to help release past or future anxieties that are affecting the patient in the present moment.

The third ancestry includes the Qiao and Dai channels... When there is a crisis or an acute influence, with its root in a past experience, or thoughts or pressures of the future, consider the Qiao or Dai channels to release them. (Twicken 2013, p.36)

Opening point – GB 41 (Zú Lín Qì)

Zú = foot.

Lín = overlooking, arrive at, above, near to, growing out of.

Qì = tears, weeping.

Zú Lín Qì = foot overlooking tears.[45]

Apart from the obvious effect of regulating eye fluid, GB 41 is also good at balancing the Hún (Ethereal/Heavenly/Dream-Big Soul) and Pò (Corporeal/Grounded/Earthly/Do-Big-Be-Big Soul) relationship. This is because GB 41 can be used to help a patient enhance their planning/processing, decision-making and decisive action skills. All these skills are crucial for a strong Hún/Pò relationship, and GB 41 is the pivot point between thoughts (Hún) and actions (Pò).

When someone is stuck in their Hún, they are always 'off with the fairies'. They never get anything done because they are always dreaming. When someone is stuck in their Pò, they are too grounded/structured. Their life becomes too programmed because they have forgotten how to dream. GB 41 allows us to rest again at the pivot point, happily balanced between our Hún and Pò.

> Accumulations in the Dai channel can prevent us from growing, developing, and being creative. The accumulations slow our response to life experiences. (Twicken 2013, p.138)

Dài Mài point combination - general

There are plenty of different treatment approaches for the Eight Extraordinary Vessels. I will be offering a general treatment for the Dài Mài (Table 12.16) plus a Shén-based point combination. These are my own personal choice of points and have therefore not been referenced. There are other points on the vessel that you may prefer to use.

Table 12.16 Dài Mài point combination – general

Location of point	Point	Reasoning
Trunk (front)	LR 13 GB 26 CV 3 CV 4	All front-of-trunk points listed regulate the anterior portion of the Dài Mài[46]
Trunk (back)	BL 23 GV 4	Both points regulate the posterior portion of the Dài Mài[47]
Arms/hands	TE 5	Coupled point
Legs/feet	GB 41	Opening point
Total points needled		13 needles used bilaterally

Dài Mài point combination - Heart Shén

All of the points in Table 12.17 can calm the Heart Shén, but not all of the points chosen are on the Dài Mài. They have been selected because of their affinity for combining with other points in the treatment.

Table 12.17 Dài Mài point combination – Heart Shén

Location of point	Point	
Head/face/neck	GV 20	
Trunk (front)	LR 13 GB 26 (for women) or GB 27 (for men) or GB 26 and GB 27 for Yīn Yáng balance	
Trunk (back)	BL 52	
Arms/hands	TE 5	
Legs/feet	GB 41	KI 1
Total points needled	13–15 needles used bilaterally	

This is quite a rare point combination in this book because it has a choice of points based on whether you are treating a female or male patient. The use of specific points for female (GB 26) or male (GB 27) is obviously target-specific, but if you don't want to treat that way, then use both GB 26 and GB 27.

The Dài Mài point combination helps to regulate our Hún and Pò energies so that we are making better life decisions that align with our inherited source.

> The Dai channel is a means of releasing excesses and intensities, and is often used in initial treatments to release or let go. (Twicken 2013, p.38)

Qiāo Mài

> The Yang and Yin Qiao channels relate to our stance in life…[including how we] relate to the internal (self-esteem) or the external world (society). (Twicken 2013, p.37)

The Yīn and Yáng Qiāo Mài directly influence who we are as a person, both from a pure inward self-esteem view and the external societal view of us. It is here that we filter these external and internal opinions, thereby giving us our sense of self. This is then the self we live with in the present moment.

However, it's rarely that simple, and the Qiāo Mài are also affected (positively and negatively) by how the past and future are affecting us. We are living in the present but we are allowing old patterning to intrude on our present existence and/or allowing the future to interfere with how we are living right now.

> These [channels] are about the current moment. They offer the possibility of releasing or diminishing current intensities influencing our life… The Qiao channels can release pathology from the past that is being experienced in the present. They can also release stresses about the future that are affecting the present moment. (Twicken 2013, pp.37, 119)

Yáng Qiāo Mài

> [T]rauma or chronic emotional stresses that are not resolved, and not let go, can be deposited in the Qiao channels. (Twicken 2013, p.120)

Opening point = BL 62.

Coupled point = SI 3.

Xì Cleft point = BL 59.

The Yáng Qiāo Mài is often translated as the Yáng Heel, Yáng Stepping or Yáng Motility Vessel. It binds up the right and left sides of the body.

In addition, the Yáng Qiāo Mài:[48]

- regulates motion in the lower limbs, thereby ensuring strong muscle tone. This also makes it a great vessel to treat muscle atrophy in the legs

- absorbs excess Yáng that is traveling into the head. Signs and symptoms of this might include pounding headaches, mania, anger, red eyes, rosacea, insomnia and heartburn

- removes External/Internal Wind invading the head. Signs and symptoms of this might include stiff neck, severe headache, stroke, aphasia, facial tics/ twitches/spasms, numbness and Bell's palsy (facial paralysis)

- is effective for most eye disorders

- regulates sleeping – either too much (somnolence) or not enough (insomnia)

- helps with low back/hip pain with unilateral sciatica

- helps to slow down the Shén (Spirit). When the Shén is slow, the body will follow

- helps us when we are too busy looking at our external environment – that is, looking 'outside' ourselves and the way we carry ourselves in everyday relationships. The Yáng Qiāo Mài helps to bring us back into the middle space between external and internal, creating a more harmonious balance. Alternatively, it can be used when no more energy can be taken in, when cellular information cannot be assimilated and integrated, and when the nervous system is overcharged from life changes and psycho-spiritual evolution. The Yáng Qiāo Mài acts as an external pivot regulating energy in and out of the body/mind[49]

- treats what's haunting us (known or unknown). The Yáng Qiāo Mài allows us to release it back into our Shén (Spirit) so it can be dealt with.[50]

In some classical Chinese texts, the Yáng Qiāo Mài is indicated in cases of 'excessive interest/dabbling in the occult', or 'excessive grieving over a dead relative'.[51]

It is part of the third ancestry, thereby making it a vessel to help release past or future anxieties that are affecting the patient in the present moment. The Yáng Qiāo Mài is more inclined towards the future affecting the present, but can be used to release the past as well.[52]

OPENING POINT – BL 62 (SHĒN MÀI)

Shēn = extend, stretch out, to give orders, to notify, to report.

Mài = vessel, pulse, Vital Substances.

Shēn Mài = extending vessel.[53]

BL 62 orders our Vital Substances to do their jobs to the best of their ability. In the context of the Heart Shén, BL 62 has a calming effect on the patient who is too over-excited/hyped-up. It can also be used for sleep disturbances such as insomnia or narcolepsy. BL 62 is also effective to treat a patient who is dazed, confused and unable to concentrate.[54]

Yáng Qiāo Mài point combination – general

There are plenty of different treatment approaches for the Eight Extraordinary Vessels. I will be offering a general treatment for the Yáng Qiāo Mài (Table 12.18) plus a Shén-based point combination. These are my own personal choice of points and have therefore not been referenced. There are other points on the vessel that you may prefer to use.

Table 12.18 Yáng Qiāo Mài point combination – general

Location of point	Point	Reasoning
Head/face/neck	BL 1 GB 20 ST 9	All the head/face/neck points listed regulate the higher portion of the Yáng Qiāo Mài
Trunk (front)	GB 29	Regulates the middle portion of the Yáng Qiāo Mài
Arms/hands	SI 3	Coupled point
Legs/feet	BL 59 BL 62	Xì Cleft point Opening point
Total points needled		14 needles used bilaterally

Yáng Qiāo Mài point combination – Heart Shén

All of the points in Table 12.19 can calm the Heart Shén, but not all of the points chosen are on the Yáng Qiāo Mài. They have been selected because of their affinity for combining with other points in the treatment.

Table 12.19 Yáng Qiāo Mài point combination – Heart Shén

Location of point	Point	
Head/face/neck	GV 20 GB 20	ST 2
Trunk (front)	CV 14 CV 15	CV 17 GB 29
Trunk (back)	BL 52	
Arms/hands	SI 3	LI 15
Legs/feet	BL 62	
Total points needled	18 needles used bilaterally	

This particular treatment is for what's haunting us (known or unknown). The Yáng Qiāo Mài allows us to release it back into our Shén (Spirit) so it can be dealt with.

As you can imagine with this type of treatment, there could be some significant backlash in the coming weeks or months as this internal fear/phobia comes to the surface. It's very important to keep treating the patient during this time to help them process and assimilate the fear/phobia more easily.

Yīn Qiāo Mài

> If you can't accept yourself in the current moment, or don't feel good about yourself, consider treating the Yin Qiao channels. (Twicken 2013, p.121)

> Opening point = KI 6.

> Coupled point = LU 7.

> Xì Cleft point = KI 8.

The Yīn Qiāo Mài is often translated as the Yīn Heel, Yīn Stepping or Yīn Motility Vessel. It binds up the right and left sides of the body.
In addition, the Yīn Qiāo Mài:[55]

- regulates motion in the lower limbs, thereby ensuring strong muscle tone. This also makes it a great vessel to treat muscle atrophy in the legs

- treats abdominal pain associated with distension, masses, lumps or swellings. It can also be used post-pregnancy for a woman who has had a difficult delivery or a retained placenta. The Yīn Qiāo Mài can also treat adhesions following abdominal surgery

- is effective for most eye disorders

- regulates sleeping – either too much (somnolence) or not enough (insomnia)

- helps us when we are too busy looking at our internal environment – that is, looking 'inside' ourselves, our view of self, or self-esteem. The Yīn Qiāo Mài helps to bring us back into the middle space between external and internal, creating a more harmonious balance. It also helps us with our ability to flow with the natural course of events, to be in the (known) unknown – some might call that our 'destiny'. It enhances our inner strength and faith-in-self.

The Yīn Qiāo Mài acts as an internal pivot, regulating energy in and out of the body/mind.[56]
It is part of the third ancestry, thereby making it a vessel to help release past or future anxieties that are affecting the patient in the present moment. The Yīn Qiāo Mài is more inclined towards the past affecting the present, but can be used to release the future as well.[57]

Opening point – KI 6 (Zhào Hǎi)

Zhào = shine, reflect.

Hǎi = sea.

Zhào Hǎi = shining sea.[58]

KI 6 is a point that allows us to rediscover our inner beauty, thereby assisting in enhancing our self-esteem and self-worth. Looking deep inside ourselves and seeing this treasure allows us to shine on the outside.[59]

Yīn Qiāo Mài point combination – general

There are plenty of different treatment approaches for the Eight Extraordinary Vessels. I will be offering a general treatment for the Yīn Qiāo Mài (Table 12.20) plus a Shén-based point combination. These are my own personal choice of points and have therefore not been referenced. There are other points on the vessel that you may prefer to use.

Table 12.20 Yīn Qiāo Mài point combination – general

Location of point	Point	Reasoning
Head/face/neck	BL 1 ST 9	Both the head/face/neck points regulate the higher portion of the Yīn Qiāo Mài
Trunk (front)	ST 12	Regulates the middle portion of the Yīn Qiāo Mài
Arms/hands	LU 7	Coupled point
Legs/feet	KI 2 KI 6 KI 8	Regulates the lower portion of the Yīn Qiāo Mài, along with KI 6 and KI 8 Opening point Xì Cleft point
Total points needled		14 needles used bilaterally

Yīn Qiāo Mài point combination – Heart Shén

All of the points in Table 12.21 can calm the Heart Shén, but not all of the points chosen are on the Yīn Qiāo Mài. They have been selected because of their affinity for combining with other points in the treatment.

Table 12.21 Yīn Qiāo Mài point combination – Heart Shén

Location of point	Point	
Head/face/neck	GV 20	
Trunk (front)	ST 12 LR 14	GB 24
Trunk (back)	BL 18	BL 19
Arms/hands	LU 7	
Legs/feet	KI 6	KI 8
Total points needled	17 needles used bilaterally	

This particular treatment is for patients who seek treatment for alcoholism, especially if it's a genetic/familial trait. The process here is to ease the patient through the withdrawal phase and to help them deal more effectively with the cravings that will inevitably arise. This treatment is also designed to help the patient's Shén, which should help with emotion balancing and hormone regulation.

Wéi Mài

> The *Wei Mai* are like a fine net of heaven that…covers everything…giving harmony to the constant changes… Here everything is kept at a good level to keep life in balanced harmony. (Kaatz 2005, p.137)

The Yīn and Yáng Wéi Mài link our present self with our past and future self. This is both within our own life and ancestrally.

Although it is ideal to live our life in the present moment as much as possible, we can use the past and future to help define who we are as a person. For example, we do something really stupid, so we reflect (go into the past) on the event to learn from it and limit the likelihood of doing it again. The future can also help us with our present self. For example, you might have a very difficult decision to make in the coming days. If you use that to strengthen your resolve in the present moment, it could allow you the opportunity to plan a strategy/attack, so that when you get to that future event, it is nowhere near as difficult as it might otherwise have been.

The Yīn and Yáng Wéi Mài also link us to our past and future ancestors. If we draw from the experiences of our former ancestors, we can access our Pre-Heaven Intellect.

If we acknowledge that we can positively (or negatively) impact on our future offspring, then we may be inclined to strive to be a better person. This would certainly be important if you were yet to have children because you could improve your Jīng.

> The Yang Wei and Yin Wei channels link different transitions or milestones in our life. People can invest their qi, blood, and essence (Jing) in reliving past moments or living a fantasy of the future. Being out of the present moment can be draining. The Wei channels can assist in releasing these attachments. (Twicken 2013, p.37)

Yáng Wéi Mài

> Yang Wei reflects our activities, actions, and movements. If we have difficulties with what we do and how we do it, including our work, consider treating the Yang Wei channel. (Twicken 2013, p.98)

Opening point = TE 5.

Coupled point = GB 41.

Xì Cleft point = GB 35.

The Yáng Wéi Mài is often translated as the Yáng Linking, Yáng Regulating or Yáng Tie Vessel. It binds up the interior and exterior of the body. The Yáng Wéi Mài is also connected to all the other Yáng channels.

In addition, the Yáng Wéi Mài:[60]

- expels External Wind from the exterior of the body. Signs and symptoms of this might include shivering and aversion to cold. The Yáng Wéi Mài can be used for either Wind Cold or Wind Heat invasions

- can treat the Shào Yáng division in both a physical and spiritual perspective

  - Physically it can be used for patients who always seem to be getting sick or coming down with something, or those who can't seem to get over a cold/flu, especially if accompanied by alternating chills and fevers.

  - Spiritually, it can be someone who is caught up in inaction/indecision. It could also be someone who refuses to let go of something that is hurting them spiritually, not letting what is dead die so that there is energy to bring something new forth – someone who isn't listening to the inner guidance of their Heart Shén.[61]

- can treat painful obstruction syndrome/Bì of the lateral aspect of the body

- treats headaches, ear disorders and neck and back pain

- is part of the second ancestry. Helps us when we are too busy looking into the future. The Yáng Wéi Mài helps to bring us back into the present moment, creating a more harmonious balance.[62]

Opening point - TE 5 (Wài Guān)

Wài = outer, outside, exterior.

Guān = pass, gate, close, shut.

Wài Guān = outer pass.[63]

TE 5 can be used when our internal world doesn't match our external façade. This works particularly well if your patient doesn't have a high opinion of themselves yet throws on a mask of happiness and confidence when around others. This is also relevant for people with suicidal tendencies.

TE 5 can also be used when we feel disconnected with the external world. This could be with people close to you or far away. Or perhaps the external world is hurting you with all its deaths, wars, injustices?

TE 5 is also particularly effective for people who have unfair expectations of themselves, and especially for those around them.

TE 5 is a trek up the Kūn Lún mountain where we reach a mountain/frontier pass and on the other side we can gain access to our strength and resolve, our hopes and dreams for ourselves and those that inhabit the planet with us.

YÁNG WÉI MÀI POINT COMBINATION – GENERAL

There are plenty of different treatment approaches for the Eight Extraordinary Vessels. I will be offering a general treatment for the Yáng Wéi Mài (Table 12.22) plus a Shén-based point combination. These are my own personal choice of points and have therefore not been referenced. There are other points on the vessel that you may prefer to use.

Table 12.22 Yáng Wéi Mài point combination – general

Location of point	Point	Reasoning
Head/face/neck	GB 15 GB 20	Both the head/face/neck points listed regulate the higher portion of the Yáng Wéi Mài
Trunk (side)	GB 29	Regulates the middle portion of the Yáng Wéi Mài
Arms/hands	TE 5 LI 14	Opening point Regulates the arm portion of the Yáng Wéi Mài along with TE 5
Legs/feet	GB 35 GB 41	Xì Cleft point Coupled point
Total points needled		14 needles used bilaterally

YÁNG WÉI MÀI POINT COMBINATION – HEART SHÉN

All of the points in Table 12.23 can calm the Heart Shén, but not all of the points chosen are on the Yáng Wéi Mài. They have been selected because of their affinity for combining with other points in the treatment.

Table 12.23 Yáng Wéi Mài point combination – Heart Shén

Location of point	Point	
Head/face/neck	GV 20	GB 20
Trunk (back)	TE 15	GB 21
Arms/hands	TE 5	TE 13
Legs/feet	GB 35 GB 41	BL 63
Total points needled	17 needles used bilaterally	

This treatment is for someone who is caught up in inaction/indecision. It could also be used for someone who refuses to let go of something that is hurting them spiritually, not letting what is dead die so that there is energy to bring something new forth.

In particular, this treatment is good for someone who isn't listening to the inner guidance of their Heart Shén.

Yīn Wéi Mài

Yin Wei energetic properties include how we respond to changes in our…body shape, form, and appearance… This includes how we feel about the way we look physically. If there are difficulties in this area, consider treating the Yin Wei channel. (Twicken 2013, p.98)

Opening point = PC 6.

Coupled point = SP 4.

Xì Cleft point = KI 9.

The Yīn Wéi Mài is often translated as the Yīn Linking, Yīn Regulating or Yīn Tie Vessel. It binds up the interior and exterior of the body. The Yīn Wéi Mài is also connected to all the other Yīn channels.

In addition, the Yīn Wéi Mài:[64]

- regulates Yīn and Xuè by regulating the Heart

- regulates the Heart Shén – good for anxiety, depression, fear, worry, sadness, hysteria and insomnia

- is good for someone who has issues with personal relationships, especially when they have trust issues

- can help people open up when they are shut down/emotionally detached, due to relationships in which they were abused[65]

- treats the chest and hypochondriac regions

- can treat painful obstruction syndrome/Bì of the medial aspect of the legs

- treats headaches and neck pain

- is part of the second ancestry. Helps us when we are too busy looking into the past. The Yīn Wéi Mài helps to bring us back into the present moment, creating a more harmonious balance.[66]

Opening point – PC 6 (Nèi Guān)

Nèi = inner, inside, to enter.

Guān = pass, gate, close, shut.

Nèi Guān = inner pass.[67]

PC 6 can be used when we want to deal with internal issues, either known or unknown. Needling PC 6 not only gives us insight into our internal environment, but also strengthens our resolve that it will be okay and we will work through it.

PC 6 also works on our inherent Pre-Heaven Intellect, which is housed in the Kidneys. This intellect is 'all-knowing', because it was programmed by the Universe before we were born into this world. This intellect knows all the answers because our journey has already been mapped out for us. PC 6 gives us insight into this 'knowing'.

You may not always like what you find, but it was never meant to be easy. PC 6 is a trek up the Kūn Lún mountain where we reach a mountain/frontier pass and on the other side we gain access to our Pre-Heaven Intellect.

YĪN WÉI MÀI POINT COMBINATION – GENERAL

There are plenty of different treatment approaches for the Eight Extraordinary Vessels. I will be offering a general treatment for the Yīn Wéi Mài (Table 12.24) plus a Shén-based point combination. These are my own personal choice of points and have therefore not been referenced. There are other points on the vessel that you may prefer to use.

Table 12.24 Yīn Wéi Mài point combination – general

Location of point	Point	Reasoning
Head/face/neck	CV 22 CV 23	Both the head/face/neck points listed regulate the higher portion of the Yīn Wéi Mài
Trunk (front)	SP 15 LR 14	Both points regulate the middle portion of the Yīn Wéi Mài
Arms/hands	PC 6	Opening point
Legs/feet	KI 9 SP 4	Xì Cleft point Coupled point
Total points needled		12 needles used bilaterally

YĪN WÉI MÀI POINT COMBINATION – HEART SHÉN

All of the points in Table 12.25 can calm the Heart Shén, but not all of the points chosen are on the Yīn Wéi Mài. They have been selected because of their affinity for combining with other points in the treatment.

Table 12.25 Yīn Wéi Mài point combination – Heart Shén

Location of point	Point	
Head/face/neck	GV 20	CV 22
Trunk (front)	SP 15	LR 14
Arms/hands	PC 6	HT 7
Legs/feet	SP 4	KI 9
Total points needled	14 needles used bilaterally	

This point combination helps to align with our true way or Dào. If we feel that we have lost our way, or maybe didn't feel as if we had a way to begin with, this point combination can help.

In particular, this treatment is good for someone who isn't listening to the inner guidance of their Heart Shén.

Notes

1   Seneca 1997, p.68. The original text was written somewhere between 30 and 65 CE. Seneca (4 BCE–65 CE) is, currently, my favorite Western philosopher ever. His ideas, thoughts and actions were unforgettable. The battles he had with the Goddess Fortune were, though quite unorthodox, simply breathtaking. I actually don't agree with a fair chunk of what he wrote, but that doesn't make him any less amazing in my eyes. For example, he preferred to focus on the worst possible outcome in any given situation, whereas I prefer to focus on the best possible outcome. Regardless, he is the King of Western philosophy!

2   Maciocia 2006.

3   Li 2010, pp.93–96; Maciocia 2006, pp.375–385; Matsumoto and Birch 1986, pp.13–18; Ross 1995, pp.102–104.

4   Twicken 2013, pp.35–36.

5   Maciocia 2006, pp.403–405; Ross 1995, pp.108–116.

6   Maciocia 2006, pp.395–402; Matsumoto and Birch 1986, pp.60–61; Ross 1995, pp.116–123.

7   Maciocia 2006, p.393.

8   Ibid., pp.450–465; Matsumoto and Birch 1986, pp.74–84; Ross 1995, pp.111–112.

9   Ellis et al. 1989, pp.30–31; Kaatz 2005, p.408.

10 Kaatz 2005, p.408.

11 If you don't use CV 1, then it can be left out. It doesn't need to be replaced with any other point as the rest of the point combination will still be very effective without it.

12 CV 21 is an excellent point to help all the other Rèn Mài points work better.

13 Maciocia 2006, pp.417–434; Matsumoto and Birch 1986, pp.92–96; Ross 1995, pp.109–111.

14 Ellis et al. 1989, p.130.

15 It is worth noting that this statement from Maciocia has divided opinion. Some scholars of ancient Chinese medicine texts can't find anything in the literature that suggests this is a valid function of the Small Intestine. On the other hand, some practitioners agree with what he says. Personally, I appreciate what the scholars say, but I also believe that organ diseases have the potential to create emotional imbalance in the same way that emotional imbalances can create organ disease. I also have the view that an organ's jobs have a physical and spiritual element to them. I think we can all agree that the Small Intestine is charged with separating pure and impure liquids and solids. This is a legitimate physical task that the organ does a great job of doing. But, as is common with Chinese medicine, there is typically a spiritual/mental response that can be attached to a physical task. Therefore, is it really such a leap to apply the same concept of separating the pure and impure physical to the pure and impure spiritual/mental? I don't

believe that it is, so I am quite comfortable with what Maciocia says in this instance.

16 GV 20 is the highest point on the Dū Mài and therefore it crowns the treatment. Further, it can regulate the flow of Vital Substances up and down the body.

17 If you don't use GV 1, then it can be left out. It doesn't need to be replaced with any other point as the rest of the point combination will still be very effective without it.

18 Maciocia 2006, pp.491–515; Matsumoto and Birch 1986, pp.85–92; Ross 1995, pp.113–115.

19 Ellis et al. 1989, p.103; Kaatz 2005, p.373.

20 Ellis et al. 1989, p.103.

21 Mou 2009, pp.107–132.

22 Hicks et al. 2010, pp.295–296, 323–324; Kaatz 2009, pp.208–211.

23 Ellis et al. 1989, pp.217–218.

24 Hicks et al. 2010, p.323.

25 Hartmann 2009, p.170.

26 Ibid., p.64.

27 Ellis et al. 1989, p.218.

28 Twicken 2013, p.61.

29 Hartmann 2009, p.56.

30 Maciocia 2015, p.1075.

31 Twicken 2013, p.61.

32 Hartmann 2009, p.102.

33 Deadman et al. 2007, p.361.

34 Twicken 2013, p.61.

35 Hartmann 2009, p.64.

36 Ellis et al. 1989, p.220.

37 Kaatz 2005, p.541.

38 Hartmann 2009, p.172.

39 Ibid., p.542.

40 Farrell 2016, p.72. She suggests that KI 27 treats all of the Wŭ Shén and not just the Water and Metal elements.

41 Hartmann 2009, p.170.

42 Ibid., p.102.

43 Maciocia 2006, pp.534–541; Matsumoto and Birch 1986, pp.96–101; Ross 1995, pp.112–113.

44 Carey and De Muynck 2007, p.116.

45 Ellis et al. 1989, pp.286–287; Kaatz 2005, p.212.

46 There is some debate as to which points are actually on the Dài Mài, in particular those that are inside/medial to the generally accepted points of LR 13, GB 26, GB 27 and GB 28. If you consider that the Dài Mài doesn't just disappear as it cuts through the anterior portion of the body, then there have to be some other channels and points that it passes through on the way to the anterior midline. There are four more channels anterior to the Liver and Gall Bladder channel points, which are the Spleen, Stomach and Kidney channels as well as the Rèn Mài. The Dài Mài appears to cut through these channels roughly 1.5 cùn above the pubic symphysis, so it doesn't line up directly with any points on these channels and is between points. Therefore, in my mind you could needle any of these channels in that 1.5 cùn superior

vicinity, and I have done just that from time to time.

47 Similar to the anterior Dài Mài points, there is further debate about the points that may/may not be on the posterior aspect of the body. Most of what I have read suggests the Dài Mài passes through at the level of BL 23, which also happens to line up with BL 52 and GV 4. So even though these points aren't classically referred to when discussing the Dài Mài pathway, they are almost certainly points you could choose to balance the posterior aspect of the Dài Mài.

48 Maciocia 2006, pp.569–576; Matsumoto and Birch 1986, pp.101–106, 110–111; Ross 1995, pp.109–111.

49 Carey and De Muynck 2007, p.107.

50 Ibid.

51 Maciocia 2006, p.572.

52 Twicken 2013, pp.35–36.

53 Ellis *et al.* 1989, pp.190–191; Kaatz 2005, p.507.

54 Lian *et al.* 2000, p.164; Matsumoto and Birch 1986, pp.238–240, 243.

55 Maciocia 2006, pp.551–558; Matsumoto and Birch 1986, pp.101–110; Ross 1995, pp.111–112.

56 Carey and De Muynck 2007, p.107.

57 Twicken 2013, pp.35–36.

58 Ellis *et al.* 1989, pp.201–202; Kaatz 2005, p.521.

59 Kaatz 2005, p.521.

60 Maciocia 2006, pp.621–627; Matsumoto and Birch 1986, pp.111–121; Ross 1995, pp.112–113.

61 Carey and De Muynck 2007, pp.101, 117.

62 Twicken 2013, pp.35–36.

63 Ellis *et al.* 1989, p.235; Kaatz 2005, p.292.

64 Maciocia 2006, pp.603–611; Matsumoto and Birch 1986, pp.111–121; Ross 1995, pp.113–115.

65 Carey and De Muynck 2007, p.115.

66 Twicken 2013, pp.35–36.

67 Ellis *et al.* 1989, pp.227–228; Kaatz 2005, p.281.

That as you ought not to attempt to cure the eyes without the head, or the head without the body, so neither ought you to attempt to cure the body without the soul…for the part can never be well unless the whole is well… [For this] is the great error of our day in the treatment of the human body, that physicians separate the soul from the body.

Plato (428–347 BCE)[1]

In spite of a clouded memory, the mind seeks its own good, though like a drunkard it cannot find the path home.

Boethius (480–524 CE)[2]

13

Wǔ Shén/Five Spirits

The Wǔ Shén or Five Spirits are a collective of five different parts of our soul that are inherent in all of us. They are linked to the Wǔ Xíng/Five Elements, which indicates that we have these five parts within us at all times because they are part of our spirit. You can't have one (Wǔ Shén) without the others, in the same way that everything in the Universe is divided up into five equal parts within the Wǔ Xíng philosophical system.

> The viscera [Yīn organs] store and are the abode of a person's spirit qi. The liver stores the hun [or Ethereal Soul]. The lungs store the po [or Corporeal Soul]. The heart stores the spirit [Shén]. The spleen stores ideas and intelligence [Yì]. And the kidneys store the essence and will [Zhì]. (Flaws 2004, p.72 – 34th difficulty)[3]

The Wǔ Shén, their English meaning and Wǔ Xíng partner are shown in Table 13.1.

Table 13.1 Wǔ Shén/Five Spirits

Wǔ Shén/Five Spirits	Translated meaning	Wǔ Xíng
Hún	Ethereal/Heavenly/Dream-Big Soul	Wood element
Shén	Spirit	Fire element
Yì	Thought/Post-Heaven Intellect	Earth element
Pò	Corporeal/Grounded/Earthly/Do-Big-Be-Big Soul	Metal element
Zhì	Willpower/Pre-Heaven Intellect	Water element

Each of the Wǔ Shén is slightly different, and collectively they define who we are as a person.

Theoretically, each of the Wǔ Shén should be equally balanced in the body, but that is rarely the case. In most people who I spend time with, including myself, there tends to be one or two Wǔ Shén that dominate over the others, with one or two hidden away and rarely accessed.

This a crucial concept to grasp – that is, we *all* tend to have an imbalance in our Wǔ Shén. This occurs because of how we live our life and how that gears in with Universal Qì.

What I mean is this: as we live our daily lives, we tend to get pushed and pulled in different directions, and it's how we react to these factors that defines who we are. The way that we live will invariably drive some of our Wǔ Shén into Excess/Shí and some into Deficiency/Xū.

Dominant and submissive relationships with family members, bosses, friends and/or acquaintances can also activate and deactivate some of the Wǔ Shén. This can lead to an imbalance in our spirit/soul that has a negative impact on our future development.

There are a variety of ways that you can realign or reset the Wǔ Shén in treatments. Some of these will be discussed as we progress through this chapter. There is also a great point combination called the 'Figure Eight' method (see Chapter 7) which is designed to reset all of the Wǔ Shén in one treatment.

Before we discuss each of the Wǔ Shén and provide a point combination, there are two final concepts to grasp – that of 'Pre and Post-Heaven Intellect' and 'destiny versus desires'.

1. Further concepts to grasp
Pre-Heaven and Post-Heaven Intellect

Pre-Heaven Intellect is the stuff we know without ever having remembered that we learned it in the first place. In other words, it's knowledge about the world that has been passed on to us at conception. The two main organs associated with Pre-Heaven Intellect are the Kidneys and Heart. Therefore, the Wǔ Shén of Zhì and Shén are linked with Pre-Heaven Intellect.[4]

Our Post-Heaven Intellect is the stuff we learn once we are born. It relies heavily on our senses to help take in this new information, plus our brain and Heart Shén to store this new knowledge. The two main organs associated with Post-Heaven Intellect are the Liver and Heart. Therefore, the Wǔ Shén of Hún and Shén are linked with Post-Heaven Intellect.[5]

The Spleen and Lungs use a mix of Pre-Heaven Intellect and Post-Heaven Intellect. Therefore, the Wǔ Shén of Yì and Pò are linked with both.[6]

Destiny versus desires
Destiny

Question: There are criminals who become kings and ministers who starve to death, men who fall from high rank and men who rise from low rank; are all such things destiny?

Answer: 'Everything is destiny.' It is because of what is called the destiny that there are such inequalities of fortune. There is nothing strange about it. (Chéng Yí/程颐 1033–1107 CE)[7]

Our destiny is the life that we were meant to live. We have been born into our bodies to live a certain life. If we are born into a farming family, then we should be the best farmer we can be. If we are born into a healing family, then we should be the best healer we can be. Our life has already been planned out for us because this is our destiny.

Destiny provides us with a full brain, which is our Pre-Heaven Intellect. Our senses and experiences just remind us of what we already inherently knew and this drives our destiny.

If this theory is correct, then it suggests that we have no free will.

Desires

> Desire is the very essence of man. (Baruch Spinoza 1632–1677 CE)[8]

Our desires are the things that we think (or feel) that we want. If our desires are strong enough, then we go out and get that thing we want. A desire can be substantial or non-substantial. A substantial desire might be a chocolate bar or a hamburger. A non-substantial desire might be a feeling of joy or contentment.

Having desires suggests that we have free will to choose what we want, when we want it, and uses our Post-Heaven Intellect. Our senses are active with our desires and Post-Heaven Intellect.

Having desires suggests that destiny isn't/can't be real.

Interestingly, quite a number of Chinese, and Western, philosophies believe that we were born with our life already laid out for us (destiny), but that we can, to some degree, alter how we live our pre-planned life. The Figure Eight method (see Chapter 7) offers a template for how that might work.

I brought this topic up because each of the Wŭ Shén has some involvement in destiny and desires. Additional debate is outside the scope of this book. Suffice to say that I believe we have a destiny, but we have desires as well.

Therefore, we have a brain that is already full of knowledge (Pre-Heaven Intellect), and we use our senses (Post-Heaven Intellect) to access this knowledge; but we also use our senses to create new knowledge.

> OUR knowledge springs from two fundamental sources of the mind; the first is the capacity of receiving representations (receptivity for impressions), the second is the power of knowing an object through these representations (spontaneity [in the production] of concepts). (Immanuel Kant 1724–1804 CE)[9]

Each of the Wŭ Shén will now be discussed below.

2. Wǔ Shén/Five Spirits
Hún[10]

> [The Hún endows] us with the ability to discern our path, stay clear on our direction, imagine possibilities, move forward toward our goals and take a stand for what we believe is right. (Dechar 2006, p.196)

In a basic sense the Hún is our:

- Ethereal Soul
- Heavenly Soul
- 'Dream-Big' Soul.

But the Hún is also associated with our:[11]

- sleeping and dreaming
- emotional balance
- decision making and planning
- courage
- vision and imagination
- eyes and sight.

The Hún is our creative, artistic, poetic, imaginative soul. Up here (Hún) anything is possible, therefore dream your grandest dreams. Be playful, fun, energetic and inspired.

The Hún doesn't have limits or boundaries. It's like the Universe or Heaven where there is no beginning or end.

The Hún is also where we plan, process, filter, discriminate, organize, set goals and prepare for action.

The Hún is our senses in overdrive. It operates best via the senses, which is why the Hún uses our Post-Heaven Intellect. In this way, the Hún is also linked to the Yì.

Our Hún isn't tied to the Earth via gravity, but it is tied to the Earth in a different way: via our Pò. Our Pò is our 'Grounded/Earthly Soul' and is the Hún's dreams put into action. Whereas the Hún is our 'Dream-Big' Soul, the Pò is our 'Do-Big' and 'Be-Big' Soul (see the section 'Pò' below). They are linked together just like Yīn Yáng. Hún is our Yáng Soul, and the Pò is our Yīn Soul; just like Yīn Yáng, our Hún and Pò can occasionally tilt excessively in favor of one or the other. There is never a complete severing of Hún and Pò, as this only happens when we die.

Hún Shí/Excess[12]
This is when we have tilted in favor of Hún. Therefore:

- We will still 'dream big' but no longer will we 'do big' or 'be big'.

- We come up with heaps of ideas but we never finish what we start. Or we just threaten to get stuff done – all talk and no action!

- We will have a 'glass half full' attitude.[13]

- Our friends might say we are 'off with the fairies', 'too flighty' or 'on another planet'. If our name was Cara, this place might be called 'Cara Land'.

I'm sure we all know of someone who is Hún Shí. When you visit their house, they have something partly completed in every room, and their garden will be the only one on the street that looks as if it's either half finished or half started.

Hún Xū/Deficiency[14]
This is when we have tilted in favor of Pò. Therefore:

- We will 'do big' but no longer will we 'dream big'. We will also most definitely not 'be big' (Wŭ Wèi).

- Because we have lost our ability to dream, forward plan and create, we structure our lives mercilessly.

- We become too rigid and are no longer open to change because change is now scary.

- We will be obsessed with ensuring everything in our life is planned down to the minutest detail. Nothing can change; everything has to stay the same.

- We will feel stuck in our life, in our rigidity, in our systems. But because we don't dream anymore, we don't know how to break out.

- Not surprisingly, we will have a 'glass half empty' attitude.

In ancient times the Chinese believed that the Hún left your body when you slept to travel the Heavens and the Earth. Upon waking, the Hún descended to the eyes. Most modern views on this are different and suggest that at rest the Hún travels to the Liver; upon waking the Hún ascends to the eyes.[15]

That meant a part of you was missing, thereby allowing another entity to invade your body while you slept. This entity was essentially maleficent and could be a demon or another sleeping person's Hún.[16] In order to protect a sleeping person from invasion, the Chinese used moxibustion (*Artemisia vulgaris*) smudging.[17] Another option was to sprinkle pepper seeds around a sleeping person.[18]

Hinrichs and Barnes (2013, p.27) suggest: 'Valuable items (such as jades, cowries, and precious stones) or clothing items (such as gowns cut certain ways and caps with hanging strings) were also used for protection.'

Hún-regulating point combination treatment
There are quite a few points that can be used to regulate the Hún. In effect, they can treat either Hún Shí or Hún Xū.

The Hún is housed in the Wood element, and therefore the Liver and Gall Bladder are key organs to treat when regulating the Hún. Further, the Hún is the Heavenly, or higher, part of our spirit; therefore, points higher up the body can also be effective for regulating the Hún.

The Hún is located in the Liver (and Heart[19]), so points located on the face/head and over the chest, abdomen and upper and mid-back will also be effective for regulating the Hún, as would points on the Liver, Gall Bladder and Heart channels.

Tables 13.2 and 13.3 have a face-up treatment and a face-down treatment for regulating the Hún.

Table 13.2 Hún-regulating point combination: Session 1 – face up[20]

Location of points	Points	Point's specialty
Head/face/neck	GV 20	Highest point on the body; Heavenly
Trunk (front)	LR 14 CV 4	Front Mù Collecting point of the Liver Anchors the Hún in the Liver
Arms/hands	PC 6	Moves Liver Qì; calms the Shén
Legs/feet	LR 3 LR 8 GB 40 KI 1	Yuán Source point of the Liver Anchors the Hún in the Liver Stimulates Hún movement Regulates the flow of Qì up and down the body; calms the Shén and Hún
Total points needled		14 needles used bilaterally

Table 13.3 Hún-regulating point combination: Session 2 – face down[21]

Location of points	Points	Point's specialty
Head/face/neck	GV 20	Highest point on the body; Heavenly
Trunk (back)	BL 18 BL 47	Back Shù Transporting point of the Liver Gate of the Hún – see below
Arms/hands	PC 6	Moves Liver Qì; calms the Shén
Legs/feet	LR 3 SP 6 GB 40 KI 1	Yuán Source point of the Liver Anchors the Hún in the Liver Stimulates Hún movement Regulates the flow of Qì up and down the body; calms the Shén and Hún
Total points needled		15 needles used bilaterally

Likely Hún Zàng Fǔ patterns[22]

Perhaps you would prefer to treat your patient using the Zàng Fǔ patterns that are causing the Hún Shí or Hún Xū? The following lists provide the more common presenting patterns. The lists are not exhaustive by any means.

HÚN SHÍ/EXCESS ZÀNG FǓ PATTERNS

- Liver Fire Blazing.

- Liver Yáng Rising (Shí on Xū).

- Damp Heat in the Liver and Gall Bladder.

- Liver Qì Stagnation turning into Heat.

- Lung Qì Xū (the Pò becomes deficient, thereby losing connection to the Hún; the Hún then flies up into the Heavens creating a Hún excess).

The Zàng Fŭ patterns are outside the scope of this book, but there are some excellent books available, some of which are in my reference and further reading lists.

HÚN XŪ/DEFICIENCY OR ZHÌ/STAGNANT ZÀNG FŬ PATTERNS

- Liver Xuè Xū.

- Liver Yīn Xū.

- Liver Yáng Rising (Shí on Xū).

- Liver Qì Stagnation.

- Gall Bladder Xū.

- Lung Heat (the Pò becomes excess, thereby losing connection to the Hún; the Pò then drives down into the Earth creating a Hún deficiency).

- Heat in the Large Intestine (the Pò becomes excess, thereby losing connection to the Hún; the Pò then drives down into the Earth creating a Hún deficiency).

In humans, the hun inhabits the vaporous, ever-changing region of our visions, dreams and imagination and is the animating agent of all mental processes. (Dechar 2006, p.194)

Shén[23]

The shen 'gives the orders' that precipitate each human life. But the shen also gives us our 'heavenly mandate'…our individual destiny. (Dechar 2006, p.174)

In a basic sense the Shén is our:

- memory – short-term and long-term

- consciousness – semi-conscious, unconscious

- sleep – insomnia, narcolepsy, dreaming/nightmares

- emotions – all of them; not just joy

- Hún – Ethereal/Heavenly/Dream-Big Soul

- Pò – Corporeal/Grounded/Earthly/Do-Big-Be-Big Soul

- Yì – Thought/Post-Heaven Intellect

- Zhì – Willpower/Pre-Heaven Intellect.

Based on the assumption that we are born with inherent (Pre-Heaven) knowledge about the world, the two main organs involved with that process are the Heart (as the Emperor, he is all-seeing/all-knowing) and the Kidneys (where this inherent or Pre-Heaven knowledge is housed). Therefore, the Shén, which is housed in the Heart, can be used to stimulate the release of that Pre-Heaven knowledge.

Some people like to give that knowledge a name or even describe it as a person.

If we revisit the destiny-versus-desires argument and assume, for the sake of this book, that we are living the life we were meant to live, our life has been planned out for us and this is our destiny. This destiny is housed in the Heart, as is the Shén; therefore, if a patient feels they have lost their way, you could treat the Shén to remind them of their true path. You could also treat the Kidney Zhì because this is also where our Pre-Heaven knowledge is housed.

This would be particularly good if you had a patient who felt there was no point to life or felt that there should be more to life, or felt they weren't living the life they were meant to, or perhaps felt they had no reason for living.

Confucius (Kǒng Zǐ) and Mencius (Mèng Zǐ) also had important things to say about the Heart, destiny and desires.

Mencius suggested that when a person loses their Heart, they lose their sense of purpose and destiny, and their connection to Tiān (Heaven). As a result, they fill that space with desires that are coming from Dì (Earthly), worldly and sensory attractions. This is because we are linked with Heaven and Earth through Tiān Dì Rén (Heaven, Earth, Human).

> He [the gentleman] is not governed by the attractions and repulsions of the senses [desires]; he can engage in moral reflection [destiny]. Mencius speaks of the heart as the organ of thought and of its having the role of a kind of reflective conscience which should govern one's life. (Collinson, Plant and Wilkinson 2000, p.235)

Mencius believed that people are born good and that this 'Goodness' is housed in the Heart. This Goodness is made up of four parts:[24]

- the Heart of Compassion and Pity

- the Heart of Shame

- the Heart of Courtesy and Modesty

- the Heart of Right and Wrong.

From a Chinese medicine perspective, we could treat the Shén not only to stimulate our inherent Goodness, but also to rouse the four ingrained tendencies mentioned above.

Shén Shí/Excess[25]

This is when we have planted ourselves too much in the Shén. Therefore, we might be:

- over-excited

- hypersensitive

- anxious

- confused

- selfish

- agitated

- the life of the party – fun, engaging, over-the-top, extroverted, energetic, loud

- having trouble sleeping – insomnia, nightmares

- having problems with sensory perception – such as seeing things that aren't there

- addicted to stimulants or mind-altering substances

- manic, psychotic, aggressive and very dangerous

- out of synch ethically – without a moral compass.

Shén Shí can really be categorized into two types – the harmless and the dangerous. The harmless will be the life of the party. They will be funny, engaging, energetic, loud, extroverted and keen to ensure everyone has a great time.

The dangerous are manic, aggressive and psychotic, and have a sensory perception issue which gives them wrong information. This wrong information is often detrimental to those around them because it paints everyone in a bad light. This makes them more aggressive and more violent.

They also won't have a moral compass. What most people would consider morally acceptable behavior is not something that will register on their radar. They will treat others poorly. They will take what they want. They won't consider other people's livelihoods.

Shén Xū/Deficiency[26]

This is when we have fallen away from our Shén. Therefore, we might be:

- easily startled

- mute and quiet

- gullible, naïve, innocent

- dazed, confused, disoriented

- depressed, unhappy, disheartened

- lost

- panicky

- nervously exhausted

- having trouble sleeping – insomnia or over-sleeping

- apathetic, lethargic, disinterested

- addicted to stimulants or mind-altering substances

- semi-conscious

- (quietly) dangerous.

Shén Xū people will be very quiet and withdrawn individuals. Don't confuse that with a lack of intelligence or assume that they are naturally shy people. Chances are, they used to be very energetic and excitable people who enjoyed life and had fun. Their deficiency has dragged them into unfamiliar territory and they want to get out.

Shén-regulating point combination treatment

There are quite a few points that can be used to regulate the Shén. In effect, they can treat either Shén Shí or Shén Xū.

The Shén is housed in the Fire element, and therefore the Heart, Pericardium, Small Intestine and Sān Jiāo are key organs to treat when regulating the Shén. Furthermore, the Shén is located in the Heart, but also in the brain,[27] so points located on the face/head and over the chest and upper back will also be effective for regulating the Shén, as would points on the Heart, Pericardium, Small Intestine and Sān Jiāo channels.

There are also points with Shén in their Pīn Yīn name. A lot of these points can also be used to regulate the Shén (see Chapter 4).

Tables 13.4 and 13.5 have a face-up treatment and a face-down treatment for regulating the Shén.

Table 13.4 Shén-regulating point combination: Session 1 – face up[28]

Location of points	Points	Point's specialty
Head/face/neck	GV 20 GV 24 M-HN-3 (Yìn Táng)	Calms the Shén Calms the Shén Calms the Shén
Trunk (front)	CV 14 CV 15	Front Mù Collecting point of the Heart Calms the Shén
Arms/hands	PC 6 HT 3 HT 5 HT 7	Calms the Shén Calms the Shén Calms the Shén Yuán Source point of the Heart
Total points needled		13 needles used bilaterally

Table 13.5 Shén-regulating Point Combination: Session 2 – face down[29]

Location of points	Points	Point's specialty
Head/face/neck	GV 20 GB 20 BL 10	Calms the Shén Calms the Shén Calms the Shén
Trunk (back)	BL 15 BL 44	Back Shù Transporting point of the Heart Temple of the Shén – see below
Arms/hands	PC 6 HT 5 HT 7	Calms the Shén Calms the Shén Yuán Source point of the Heart
Total points needled		15 needles used bilaterally

Likely Shén Zàng Fǔ patterns[30]

Perhaps you would prefer to treat your patient using the Zàng Fǔ patterns that are causing the Shén Shí or Shén Xū? The following lists provide the more common presenting patterns. The lists are not exhaustive by any means.

SHÉN SHÍ/EXCESS ZÀNG FǓ PATTERNS

- Heart Fire Blazing.

- Phlegm Fire Harassing the Heart.

- Phlegm Misting the Heart Shén.

- Full Heat in the Small Intestine (Fire Blazing).

SHÉN XŪ/DEFICIENCY ZÀNG FǓ PATTERNS

- Heart Qì Xū.

- Heart Xuè Xū.

- Heart Yīn Xū.

- Heart Yáng Xū.

- Small Intestine Xū and Cold (Yáng Xū).

Most of all, the presence of healthy shen results in a life that is uniquely suited to the individual and a person whose actions make sense within the context of the surrounding environment. (Dechar 2006, p.171)

Yì[31]

The yi holds the center. It is the connecting link between the hun and po souls. (Dechar 2006, p.230)

In a basic sense the Yì is our:

- thought

- intellect – Post-Heaven (but some Pre-Heaven)

- balance/pivot between the Hún and Pò

- balance/pivot between the Shén and Zhì

- dreams (Hún) being filtered to decide which of them become our reality (Pò).

But it is also associated with our:[32]

- intent

- memory

- ideas

- studying, focusing and concentrating

- integrity

- devotion.

The Yì gives us the ability to study, concentrate, memorize and recall learned facts via clear, fast and accurate thinking.

The Yì takes the Hún dreams and plants them into the Pò, thereby ensuring dreams become reality. The Yì can also act as a filter of truth because it has the ability to ensure that the dreams we wish to become reality are in fact our own and not someone else's. This will only work, though, if the person is willing to listen to all of the Wǔ Shén and not just the Yì. Thankfully, this is actually very easy. One just has to accept the Wǔ Shén exist and are relevant to our story. It's that simple!

Even though all the Wǔ Shén are involved with ensuring we follow our destiny, the Yì is in a unique position – that of the middle. This allows the Yì to understand and appreciate how the other four Shén operate and function. This is because the Yì has a little piece of the other four Shén within it. See Diagram 13.1.

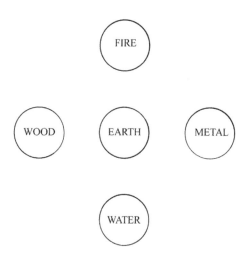

Diagram 13.1 Wŭ Xíng/Wŭ Shén Earth Central

This means that the Yì can function for our greatest good by using the Pre-Heaven Intellect and/or the Post-Heaven Intellect. This will ensure that we aren't distracted by false truths and can therefore follow our one true path. The Yì operates in the middle of the 'Known' and 'Unknown' and uses the knowledge of all the Wŭ Shén to create a system of connection and balance.

The Yì also ensures we remain true to the belief that the world can be saved by integrity and altruism.

Yì Shí/Excess[33]

This is when we have planted ourselves too much in the Yì. Therefore, we might be:

- overprotective, overbearing – can overcrowd

- meddlesome

- likely to take unnecessary risks

- suffering from poor memory – we could be a slow learner, have scattered thoughts or be pensive (plunged in thought)

- excessively worried about everything and everyone

- obsessive

- a candidate for overextending or overreaching

- so worried about the future that we become obsessed by it and therefore live in the future

- resentful of other people's sympathetic advances.

Yì Xū/Deficiency[34]

This is when we have fallen away from our Yì. Therefore, we might be:

- unmotivated, stuck, can't be bothered – 'It's all too hard'

- vague and suffering from poor memory

- too tired to study or concentrate

- a slow learner – can't retain information

- a procrastinator

- melancholic

- excessively worried about everything and everyone

- obsessive

- sloppy

- obsequious, servile, submissive, conforming

- reflecting obsessively about the past so that we live in the past

- a craver of sympathy from others – we may even manufacture signs/symptoms/diseases in order to receive more sympathy

- in a 'shame of self' poor self-esteem cycle, accompanied by grief, sadness, worry and fear.

Yì-regulating point combination treatment

There are quite a few points that can be used to regulate the Yì. In effect, they can treat either Yì Shí or Yì Xū.

The Yì is housed in the Earth element, and therefore the Spleen and Stomach are key organs to treat when regulating the Yì. Further, the Yì is located in the Spleen (and Heart[35]), so points located on the face/head and over the chest, abdomen and upper and mid-back will also be effective for regulating the Yì, as would points on the Heart, Spleen and Stomach channels.

Tables 13.6 and 13.7 have a face-up treatment and a face-down treatment for regulating the Yì.

Table 13.6 Yì-regulating point combination: Session 1 – face up[36]

Location of points	Points	Point's specialty
Head/face/neck	GV 20 M-HN-3 (Yìn Táng) ST 8	Calms the Shén and Yì Calms the Shén and Yì Calms the Shén and Yì
Trunk (front)	LR 13 CV 12	Front Mù Collecting point of the Spleen Front Mù Collecting point of the Stomach
Arms/hands	PC 6 HT 7	Calms the Shén and Yì Calms the Shén and Yì
Legs/feet	ST 36 SP 3 SP 6	Horary point (Earth of Earth) of Stomach Yuán Source point of the Spleen Regulates the Spleen and Yì
Total points needled		17 needles used bilaterally

Table 13.7 Yì-regulating point combination: Session 2 – face down[37]

Location of points	Points	Point's specialty
Head/face/neck	GB 20 BL 10	Calms the Shén and Yì Calms the Shén and Yì
Trunk (back)	BL 20 BL 21 BL 49	Back Shù Transporting point of the Spleen Back Shù Transporting point of the Stomach Abode of the Yì – see below
Arms/hands	HT 7	Calms the Shén and Yì
Legs/feet	ST 36 SP 3	Horary point (Earth of Earth) Yuán Source point of the Spleen
Total points needled		16 needles used bilaterally

Likely Yì Zàng Fŭ patterns[38]

Perhaps you would prefer to treat your patient using the Zàng Fŭ patterns that are causing the Yì Shí or Yì Xū? The following lists provide the more common presenting patterns. The lists are not exhaustive by any means.

YÌ SHÍ/EXCESS ZÀNG FŬ PATTERNS

- Stomach Fire Blazing.

- Stomach Phlegm Fire Blazing.

- Damp Heat in the Spleen.

- Cold Damp in the Spleen.

YÌ XŪ/DEFICIENCY OR ZHÌ/STAGNANT ZÀNG FŬ PATTERNS

- Stomach Qì Xū.

- Stomach Yáng Xū.

- Stomach Yīn Xū.

- Stomach Qì Stagnation.

- Spleen Qì Xū.

- Spleen Yáng Xū.

- Spleen Qì Sinking.

- Spleen Xuè Xū.

[The Yì] lets the world know that we mean to stand by our dreams. (Dechar 2006, p.216)

Pò[39]

Deep below the level of our conscious ability to articulate in words what we think about a person, place or situation, the po spirits already know – and, whether or not we realise it, our body has begun to respond by contracting or expanding, hardening or softening. (Dechar 2006, p.239)

In a basic sense the Pò is our:

- Corporeal Soul

- Earthly Soul

- Grounded Soul

- 'Do-Big/Action' Soul

- 'Be-Big/Non-Action/Wǔ Wèi' Soul

- dreams-in-action

- systems, patterns, habits, goals and processes.

The Pò is our action, forward movement and unlimited applied force. It ensures that the dreams from the Hún become reality. But this requires systems, patterns, habits, goals and processes to ensure success, which is what the Pò thrives on.

The Pò plays a part in our sensation, breathing, balance, correct muscle/tendon function, feeling, sight and hearing. It also has a minor role in certain organ functions, namely the Lungs and Large Intestine.

Down here (Pò) any dream can become reality. Stay focused, committed and driven. But know also that everything that is meant to be will be; therefore, never 'force the issue'. So, although the Pò is your 'doing-big' soul, also practice the art of 'being big' too. After all, we are human beings, not human doings. This art of 'just being' is called Wǔ Wèi.

The Pò is our inherent knowing in overdrive. It operates best via this inner trust and faith; therefore, the Pò uses what's called Pre-Heaven Intellect. In this way, the Pò is also linked to the Zhì and the Shén.

In fact, the Pò is created from our parents' Kidney Jīng at conception.

Even though the Pò uses this Pre-Heaven Intellect to great effect, it also needs the use of the senses (eyes, ears, nose and mouth), which is part of our Post-Heaven Intellect. In this way, the Pò ensures that two things happen:

- Dreams become reality via action and the use of the senses.

- Our inherent knowing is validated and actioned.

Our Pò is tied to Heaven via the Hún. The Pò needs this ethereal anchor because, without it, the Pò will tunnel underground. Whereas the Hún is our 'dream-big' soul (see the section 'Hún' above), the Pò is our 'do-big' and 'be-big' soul. They are linked together just like Yīn Yáng. Hún is our Yáng Soul, and the Pò is our Yīn Soul; just like Yīn Yáng, our Hún and Pò can occasionally tilt excessively in favor of one or the other. There is never a complete severing of Hún and Pò, as this only happens when we die.

Pò Shí/Excess[40]

This is when we have tilted in favor of Pò. Therefore:

- We will 'do big' but no longer will we 'dream big'. We will also most definitely not 'be big' (Wŭ Wèi).

- Because we have lost our ability to dream, forward plan and create, we structure our lives mercilessly.

- We become too rigid and are no longer open to change because change is now scary.

- We will be obsessed with ensuring everything in our life is planned down to the minutest detail. Nothing can change; everything has to stay the same.

- We will feel stuck in our life, in our rigidity, in our systems. But because we don't dream anymore, we don't know how to break out.

- Not surprisingly, we will have a 'glass half empty' attitude.

Pò Xū/Deficiency[41]

This is when we have tilted in favor of Hún. Therefore:

- We will still 'dream big' but no longer will we 'do big' or 'be big'.

- We come up with heaps of ideas but we never finish what we start. Or we just threaten to get stuff done – all talk and no action!

- We will have a 'glass half full' attitude.

- Our friends might say we are 'off with the fairies', 'too flighty' or 'on another planet'. If our name was Cara, this place might be called 'Cara Land'.

Pò-regulating point combination treatment

There are quite a few points that can be used to regulate the Pò. In effect, they can treat either Pò Shí or Pò Xū.

The Pò is housed in the Metal element, and therefore the Lungs and Large Intestine are key organs to treat when regulating the Pò. Further, the Pò is located in the Lungs (and Heart[42]), so points located on the face/head and over the chest and upper back will also be effective for regulating the Pò, as would points on the Heart, Lung and Large Intestine channels.

Tables 13.8 and 13.9 have a face-up treatment and a face-down treatment for regulating the Pò.

Table 13.8 Pò-regulating point combination: Session 1 – face up[43]

Location of points	Points	Point's specialty
Head/face/neck	GV 20	Calms the Shén and Pò
Trunk (front)	LU 1 CV 17	Front Mù Collecting point of the Lungs Calms the Shén and Pò
Arms/hands	LU 3 LU 7 LU 9	Anchors the Pò in the Lungs Calms the Shén and Pò Yuán Source point of the Lungs
Legs/feet	KI 1	Regulates the flow of Qì up and down the body; calms the Shén and Pò
Total points needled		12 needles used bilaterally

Table 13.9 Pò-regulating point combination: Session 2 – face down[44]

Location of points	Points	Point's specialty
Head/face/neck	GV 20	Calms the Shén and Pò
Trunk (back)	BL 13 BL 42 BL 44	Back Shù Transporting point of the Lungs Corporeal Soul Door – see below Calms the Shén and Pò
Arms/hands	HT 7 LI 4	Calms the Shén and Pò Calms the Shén and Pò
Legs/feet	KI 1	Regulates the flow of Qì up and down the body; calms the Shén and Pò
Total points needled		13 needles used bilaterally

Likely Pò Zàng Fǔ patterns[45]

Perhaps you would prefer to treat your patient using the Zàng Fǔ patterns that are causing the Pò Shí or Pò Xū? The following lists provide the more common presenting patterns. The lists are not exhaustive by any means.

Pò Shí/Excess Zàng Fŭ patterns

- Lung Heat.

- Phlegm Heat Obstructing the Lungs.

- Heat in the Large Intestine.

- Damp Heat in the Large Intestine.

- Liver Xuè Xū (the Hún becomes deficient, thereby losing connection to the Pò; the Pò then drives down into the Earth creating a Pò excess).

- Gall Bladder Xū (the Hún becomes deficient, thereby losing connection to the Pò; the Pò then drives down into the Earth creating a Pò excess).

Pò Xū/Deficiency Zàng Fŭ patterns

- Lung Qì Xū.

- Lung Yīn Xū.

- Lung Dryness.

- Large Intestine Dry.

- Liver Fire Blazing (the Hún becomes excess, thereby losing connection to the Pò; the Hún then flies up into the Heaven, causing a Pò deficiency).

- Damp Heat in the Liver and Gall Bladder (the Hún becomes excess, thereby losing connection to the Pò; the Hún then flies up into the Heaven, causing a Pò deficiency).

The Po are our embodied knowing, our animal wit, our street smarts, the part of us that can sniff out what's right or wrong, good or bad, safe or unsafe. (Dechar 2006, p.239)

Zhì[46]

Clarity of purpose, direction and a strong sense of identity…are the things that are needed in order for the zhi to unfold along its destined path. (Dechar 2006, p.285)

In a basic sense the Zhì is our:[47]

- Willpower

- Pre-Heaven Intellect

- instinctual power

- courage.

The Willpower of Zhì is a lot more than we might think. It encompasses things such as:

- Courage – it can be tough to take a stand in order to live in our truth. The Zhì gives us the pluck/mettle to succeed.

- Fortification – our Zhì keeps us committed and focused to stay the right and proper course.

- Strength – our Zhì gives us the power to say no to people, and to feel good about the decision we made.

- Truth – our Zhì allows us to stand in our truth. Here we can't be bullied, threatened, pressured or convinced to change our mind.

The Zhì is inexorably linked to the Pre-Heaven Intellect. A strong Zhì ensures a strong connection with our Pre-Heaven Intellect, and vice versa.

The Zhì is housed in the Kidneys, and this gives it access to our 'fight, flight, freeze' (FFF) associated with the adrenal glands. As you are probably aware, this is our automatic response to danger – and involves us either fighting, fleeing or freezing. This has both a positive and a negative component:

- Positive – because the Zhì inherently knows the correct path to take; when the Zhì is functioning well, the FFF will react instinctively in our best interests.

- Negative – if we are Zhì Shí, then we may choose to fight when in fact to flee was the correct response; on the other hand, if we are Zhì Xū, we may freeze when to fight was the correct response. That lack of connection between the Zhì and FFF can get us into a lot of trouble.

When the Zhì is balanced, there is no such thing as phobias. This is because we will operate on an even keel that doesn't allow us to move into extremes of anything. We will, however, still get fearful from time to time because that is a balanced response to certain environmental triggers.

The Zhì also gives us courage to take on challenging tasks with the added benefit of feeling incredibly amazing when we complete the difficult task. This will drive us on to the next challenge. The Zhì uses Pre-Heaven Intellect to weigh up challenges and therefore we inherently know if the next decision is going to be successful or reckless. These correct decisions allow us to operate in a balanced manner that doesn't function in the realm of phobias.

Zhì Shí/Excess[48]

This is when we have planted ourselves too much in the Zhì. Therefore, we might be:

- extremely critical, cynical, blunt, sarcastic, pessimistic, tactless, rash

- someone who never shares anything

- cagey, suspicious (of everyone and everything)

- unforgiving

- dishonest

- superficial

- anxious

- forgetful

- preoccupied (or appear to be to others)

- fussy, precious, trivial

- constantly getting distracted from a task via 'anxiety and fear of failure'.

We might also:

- rarely finish what we start – fall in an exhausted heap if we go to the trouble of finishing the task

- quit when afraid

- harbor non-specific feelings of dread and foreboding.

Zhì Xū/Deficiency[49]

This is when we have fallen away from our Zhì. Therefore, we might:

- lock ourselves away from the world

- constantly get distracted from a task by giving up before it gets too hard

- be dishonest

- be soft/spineless

- easily become discouraged – give up – never complete anything

- be dull, stupid, dim-witted, forgetful

- have a phobia of some description, such as agoraphobia

- lack stamina

- be thrifty, frugal, miserly

- feel useless

- be suspicious of everyone and everything

- harbor non-specific feelings of dread and foreboding.

Zhì-regulating point combination treatment

There are quite a few points that can be used to regulate the Zhì. In effect, they can treat either Zhì Shí or Zhì Xū.

The Zhì is housed in the Water element, and therefore the Kidneys and Urinary Bladder are key organs to treat when regulating the Zhì. Further, the Zhì is located in the Kidneys (and Heart[50]), so points located on the head/face and over the chest, lower abdomen and upper/lower back will also be effective for regulating the Zhì, as would points on the Heart, Kidney and Urinary Bladder channels.

Tables 13.10 and 13.11 have a face-up treatment and a face-down treatment for regulating the Zhì.

Table 13.10 Zhì-regulating point combination: Session 1 – face up[51]

Location of points	Points	Point's specialty
Head/face/neck	GV 20	Calms the Shén and Zhì
Trunk (front)	CV 4	Local Kidney point to calm the Zhì
	CV 6	Local Kidney point to calm the Zhì
	GB 25	Front Mù Collecting point of the Kidneys
Arms/hands	SI 3	Calms the Shén and Zhì; regulates the Dū Mài/Governing Vessel[52]
Legs/feet	BL 62	Calms the Shén and Zhì; regulates the Dū Mài/Governing Vessel[53]
	KI 1	Regulates the flow of Qì up and down the body; calms the Shén and Zhì
	SP 6	Calms the Shén and Zhì
Total points needled		13 needles used bilaterally

Table 13.11 Zhì-regulating point combination: Session 2 – face down[54]

Location of points	Points	Point's specialty
Head/face/neck	GV 20	Calms the Shén and Zhì
	GV 16	Calms the Shén and Zhì
Trunk (back)	BL 23	Back Shù Transporting point of the Kidneys
	BL 52	Willpower Room – see below
Legs/feet	BL 58	Luò Connecting point of the Urinary Bladder
	KI 1	Regulates the flow of Qì up and down the body; calms the Shén and Zhì
	KI 3	Yuán Source point of the Kidneys
	KI 6	Calms the Shén and Zhì
Total points needled		14 needles used bilaterally

Likely Zhì Zàng Fǔ patterns[55]

Perhaps you would prefer to treat your patient using the Zàng Fǔ patterns that are causing the Zhì Shí or Zhì Xū? The following lists provide the more common presenting patterns. The lists are not exhaustive by any means.

ZHÌ SHÍ/EXCESS ZÀNG FŬ PATTERNS

- Kidney Yáng Xū with Damp Accumulation.[56]

- Kidney Yīn Xū with Fire Blazing.[57]

- Damp Heat in the Urinary Bladder.

- Cold Damp in the Urinary Bladder.

ZHÌ XŪ/DEFICIENCY ZÀNG FŬ PATTERNS

- Kidney Yīn Xū.

- Kidney Yáng Xū.

- Kidney Jīng Xū.

- Urinary Bladder Xū and Cold.

The realm of the zhi spirits is the…karma, the realm of the unconscious forces and collective energy threads that determine the course of our lives. (Dechar 2006, p.275)

3. Urinary Bladder Wŭ Shén/Five Spirits points

This category of special points is a loaded topic. Most people I have spoken with have strong opposing views about whether these points actually treat the Wŭ Shén that they are named after.

Regardless of your personal view, there is no denying that each of these points is named after a different Wŭ Shén.[58] See Table 13.12 for the full list of points.

Table 13.12 Urinary Bladder Wŭ Shén/Five Spirits points

Wŭ Shén/Five Spirits	Urinary Bladder channel points
Pò	BL 42 (Pò Hù) – Corporeal/Grounded Soul Door
Shén	BL 44 (Shén Táng) – Spirit Hall
Hún	BL 47 (Hún Mén) – Ethereal/Heavenly Soul Gate
Yì	BL 49 (Yì Shè) – Thought Abode
Zhì	BL 52 (Zhì Shì) – Willpower Residence

Each of the Urinary Bladder Wŭ Shén points will be briefly discussed below. In my personal view, these points do treat their respective Wŭ Shén.

BL 47 (Hún Mén)[59]

Hún = Ethereal Soul.

Mén = Gate.

BL 47 is an excellent point to regulate the Ethereal Soul (Hún).

Hun Men [BL 47] is the gateway to our inner core, our spiritual source and our beautiful soul. (Kaatz 2005, p.487)

BL 44 (Shén Táng)[60]

Shén = Spirit.

Táng = Temple or Hall.

BL 44 is an excellent point to regulate the Spirit (Shén).

When we are struggling and feel down, this point [BL 44] can take us to a quiet resting place where our spirit can be recharged, replenished and inspired. (Kaatz 2005, p.484)

BL 49 (Yì Shè)[61]

Yì = Thought.

Shè = Abode.

BL 49 is an excellent point to regulate the Thought (Yì).

This point [BL 49] puts us back into sympathy and communion with life. We are no longer alone or struggling. (Kaatz 2005, p.489)

BL 42 (Pò Hù)[62]

Pò = Corporeal Soul.

Hù = Door.

BL 42 is an excellent point to regulate the Corporeal Soul (Pò).

Here [BL 42] with each breath our soul is filled with the beauty of nature giving us clarity, brightness and inspiration. (Kaatz 2005, p.482)

BL 52 (Zhì Shì)[63]

Zhì = Will/Willpower.

Shì = Room/Residence/Chamber.[64]

BL 52 is an excellent point to regulate the Willpower (Zhì).

This point [BL 52] stirs the fires of our soul purpose and revitalizes our ambition, will, and determination. Here we can find our path and rekindle our desires and enthusiasm for life. (Kaatz 2005, p.492)

Notes

1 Plato (428–347 BCE) was a philosophical marvel who is considered to be one of the most significant Western philosophers of all time. Personally, I loved his dialogues with Socrates as his figurehead, helping to inspire change in the young Athenians of the time. What strikes me as quite ironic, however, is that Socrates and Plato were attempting positive change, but the issues they were trying to resolve are still issues we have today.

This quotation is from Plato's dialogue titled *Charmides* (or *Temperance*), which was originally written around 380 BCE. The quotation was retrieved from http://classics.mit.edu/Plato/charmides.html.

2 Boethius 1999, p.49. Anicius Boethius (480–524 CE) wrote *The Consolation of Philosophy* in 524 CE while in prison awaiting execution for conspiracy against his king. The quotation in question is part of that incredible text.

3 *The Classic of Difficulties* (*Canon of the Yellow Emperor's Eighty-One Difficult Issues*/Huáng Dì Bā Shí Yī Nán Jīng) was originally written between 0 and 200 CE.

4 Maciocia 2009, pp.63–64.

5 Ibid.

6 Dechar 2006, pp.216–217, 224, 230, 239; Maciocia 2009, pp.47–66.

The idea here is that the Earth element and Yì resides in the middle, thereby drawing from the other four elements. In that way it can draw on Pre-Heaven and Post-Heaven Intellect.

The Metal element and Pò are linked to our Pre-Heaven via the Kidneys (the Pò is created from our parents' Jīng at conception) and our Post-Heaven via its relationship with the Hún and Shén.

7 Liang 1996, p.78. Chéng Yí (1033–1107 CE) was, together with his brother, Chéng Hào (1032–1085 CE), considered a forefather of Neo-Confucian thought. They are easily two of the more famous Chinese philosophers from that era.

8 Spinoza 2006, p.93. Baruch Spinoza (1632–1677 CE) was a hugely influential rationalist philosopher who laid the groundwork for the Age of Enlightenment. His philosophy encouraged us to monitor/learn to control our passions, which would lead us to virtue and happiness. It all sounds good in theory, but I'm a Fire archetype, so I associate happiness with passions. Sorry, Spinoza!

This quotation is from Baruch Spinoza's book *Ethics* (or *Ethica: Ordine Geometrico demonstrata*), which was written between 1664 and 1665 and published in 1677.

9 Immanuel Kant (1724–1804 CE) is, in some circles, considered to be the greatest philosopher of all time (Eastern or Western, Ancient or Modern). I find this a bit of a stretch myself. There is no denying the incredible impact he has had on philosophical thinking, but he is just so hard to read and understand. My favorite part of his philosophy is the idea that we should *never* ever lie.

This quotation is from Immanuel Kant's book *The Critique of Pure Reason* (or *Kritik der reinen Vernunft*), originally published in 1781, and was retrieved from http://web.mnstate.edu/gracyk/courses/web%20publishing/Critique1.htm.

10 Dechar 2006, pp.193–213; Maciocia 2009, pp.25–46.

11 Dechar 2006, pp.196–197; Maciocia 2009, pp.25–46.

12 Dechar 2006, pp.200–202.

13 The Hún is an inherently positive part of our soul. Therefore, even if we have lost access to some of the other Wŭ Shén, the Hún will remain forever positive.

14   Dechar 2006, pp.200–202.
15   Maciocia 2015, pp.29–30.
16   Unschuld 1985, pp.34–45.
17   Maleficent demonic beings were considered anthropomorphic. Therefore, it was important to smudge your room with moxa so that the demon couldn't see its way through the smog. The demon was also repulsed by the smell of moxa.
18   Hinrichs and Barnes 2013, p.27.
19   All of the Wǔ Shén are governed by the Heart because the Heart is the Emperor – all seeing, all knowing!
20   Hartmann 2009, p.59; Maciocia 2009, pp.29–30, 34–35, 44.
21   As previous note.
22   Some of the Zàng Fǔ patterns listed can be referenced, but others cannot; suffice to say, most Liver, Gall Bladder, Lung and Large Intestine Zàng Fǔ patterns can injure the Hún. This is obviously the case for the Liver and Gall Bladder because they house the Hún. The Lungs and Large Intestine can damage the Hún because of the Pò. As stated above, the Hún and Pò are linked. When one is injured, the other usually follows. To a lesser extent, the Heart can also injure the Hún because the Heart governs all of the Wǔ Shén.
23   Dechar 2006, pp.169–192; Maciocia 2009, pp.15–24.
24   Collinson et al. 2000, pp.233–240.
25   Dechar 2006, pp.179–189; Maciocia 2009, pp.18–22.
26   As previous note.
27   Maciocia 2015, p.112.
28   Hartmann 2009, pp.3, 139; Maciocia 2009, pp.18, 20, 23–24.
29   As previous note.
30   Some of the Zàng Fǔ patterns listed can be referenced, but others cannot; suffice to say, most Heart and Small Intestine Zàng Fǔ patterns (the Pericardium and Sān Jiāo don't really have Zàng Fǔ patterns) can injure the Shén.
31   Dechar 2006, pp.215–235; Maciocia 2009, pp.63–66.
32   As previous note.
33   Dechar 2006, pp.224–225.
34   Ibid.
35   All of the Wǔ Shén are governed by the Heart because the Heart is the Emperor – all seeing, all knowing!
36   Hartmann 2009, pp.17, 19, 156; Maciocia 2009, p.65.
37   As previous note.
38   Some of the Zàng Fǔ patterns listed can be referenced, but others cannot; suffice to say, most Spleen and Stomach Zàng Fǔ patterns can injure the Yì. To a lesser extent, the Heart can

also injure the Yì because the Heart governs all of the Wǔ Shén.
39   Dechar 2006, pp.237–272; Maciocia 2009, pp.47–61.
40   Dechar 2006, pp.246–248.
41   Ibid.
42   All of the Wǔ Shén are governed by the Heart because the Heart is the Emperor – all seeing, all knowing!
43   Hartmann 2009, p.45; Maciocia 2009, p.60.
44   As previous note.
45   Some of the Zàng Fǔ patterns listed can be referenced, but others cannot; suffice to say, most Lung, Large Intestine, Liver and Gall Bladder Zàng Fǔ patterns can injure the Pò. This is obviously the case for the Lungs and Large Intestine because they house the Pò. The Liver and Gall Bladder can damage the Pò because of the Hún. As stated above, the Pò and Hún are linked. When one gets injured, the other usually follows. To a lesser extent, the Heart can also injure the Pò because the Heart governs all of the Wǔ Shén.
46   Dechar 2006, pp.273–293; Maciocia 2009, pp.67–69.
47   Dechar 2006, p.273.
48   Ibid., pp.278–279, 285–286, 292–293.
49   Ibid.
50   All of the Wǔ Shén are governed by the Heart because the Heart is the Emperor – all seeing, all knowing!
51   Hartmann 2009, p.171; Maciocia 2009, p.67.
52   According to Maciocia (2009, p.67), it is important to tonify the Dū Mài/Governing Vessel when treating the Zhì. Therefore, use the opening and coupled points of the Dū Mài, which are SI 3 and BL 62.
53   See previous note.
54   Hartmann 2009, p.171; Maciocia 2009, p.67.
55   Some of the Zàng Fǔ patterns listed can be referenced, but others cannot; suffice to say, most Kidney and Urinary Bladder Zàng Fǔ patterns can injure the Zhì. To a lesser extent, the Heart can also injure the Zhì because the Heart governs all of the Wǔ Shén.
56   The Kidneys cannot become excess according to the Zàng Fǔ patterns diagnostic model. However, when the Kidneys become deficient, other organs can be damaged. Alternatively, the opposite can occur, with a different organ becoming diseased, which then injures the Kidneys. In either case, the Zhì can be damaged, and in all likelihood, another Wǔ Shén will too.
57   See previous note.
58   Ellis et al. 1989, pp.173–175, 177–180.
59   Maciocia 2009, p.258.
60   Ellis et al. 1989, p.175.
61   Deadman et al. 2007, p.308.
62   Maciocia 2009, pp.53–55, 256–257.

63   Deadman *et al.* 2007, p.310; Ellis *et al.* 1989,
     p.180; Maciocia 2009, p.259.
64   The Pīn Yīn for BL 52 is Zhì Shì. This Shì
     translates as room, residence or chamber. It is
     obviously different to the other Shí that I have
     been using in this chapter, which translates as
     excess.

The soul is dyed the color of its thoughts. Think only on those things that are in line with your principles and can bear the light of day. The content of your character is your choice. Day by day, what you choose, what you think, and what you do is who you become. Your integrity is your destiny... [I]t is the light that guides your way.

Heraclitus (540–480 BCE)[1]

The Master [Confucius] said, 'In his errors a man is true to type. Observe the errors and you will know the man.'

Confucius/Kǒng Zǐ/孔子 (551–479 BCE)[2]

14

Wǔ Xíng/Five Element Archetypes

The Wǔ Xíng archetypes are a fascinating component of Chinese medicine and philosophy. It is a blending of ancient Chinese ideas with more modern/recent Chinese and Western thinking.

The system looks at every individual as being unique, but this uniqueness is still housed within one of the five archetypes, in the same way that everything in the Universe is housed within one of the Wǔ Xíng/Five Elements.

An individual's strengths, weaknesses, loves, fears and difficulties are all factored in, with the end result being that you belong to a particular archetype.

Like every archetype system ever written, the Wǔ Xíng archetypes don't work for everyone. Sometimes a person is an equal amount of two, three or even all five. This will be discussed in more detail throughout this chapter. Suffice to say that, because of our individuality, I am perfectly comfortable with this scenario.

1. Definition[3]

Wǔ - five.

Xíng = to walk, to travel, to step, movement.

Commonly referred to as the Five Elements or Five Phases, even though this isn't the best English translation.

The Wǔ Xíng refer to five categories in the natural world that all correspond to one another, namely Wood, Fire, Earth, Metal and Water. They are in a state of constant motion and change.

Each of the Wǔ Xíng generates (Shēng) and controls (Kè) another element and is generated and controlled by a different element. Even though they are different, they are also complementary and cannot exist without the others.

2. Brief history/overview

The theory of the Wǔ Xíng was first formed in China at about the time of the Shāng and Zhōu dynasties (1600–221 BCE).[4] Historically, it derives from observations of the Universe by the Chinese people in their day-to-day lives. Wood, Fire, Earth, Metal and Water were considered to be the five materials required for the maintenance of life, as well as representing five important states that initiated normal changes in the Universe. The Chinese were therefore convinced that this external Universe mirrored their internal Universe.

Although having different characteristics, the Wǔ Xíng depend on each other and are inseparable. Therefore, in ancient times, people took these mutual relationships to explain all phenomena in the natural world.

As Unschuld (2009, p.16) states:

> This is the origin of the doctrines of yin-yang and the five agents [Wǔ Xíng]. The latter was initially conceived of expressly – and the sources are very clear about this – to explain social and political change. Only in a second step was the doctrine of the five agents expanded to explain all kinds of change.

From about 600 BCE onwards, the Greeks also became fascinated by the elements. Through this process they came to the conclusion that Delta Rhizomata, or Four Roots/Elements, governed everything in the Universe. These were called Aer (Air), Pur (Fire), Ge (Earth) and Hudor (Water).[5]

Interestingly, a fifth element was proposed, firstly by Anaximander (610–546 BCE) and then by Aristotle (384–322 BCE). Anaximander called it Apeiron, which essentially meant an unlimited, infinite or indefinite substance.[6] Aristotle called it Aether, which was an unchangeable and Heavenly quintessence/substance.[7] After this time, some historians started referring to the Epsilon Stoicheion, or Five Elements.

For a more thorough analysis of the Wǔ Xíng/Five Elements, along with acupuncture point combinations, please refer to Chapters 8–10.

3. Archetype relationships with the emotions and Wǔ Shén/Five Spirits

Each of the Wǔ Xíng archetypes has a love–hate relationship with a range of different emotions and spirits.

Every single emotion is an important reaction to an event where that emotion is most appropriate. When that emotion is displayed appropriately, this refers to a love relationship between emotion and archetype. For example, we bang our thumb with a hammer and we yell and scream and complain.

However, when the emotion is displayed outside of an appropriate response, then this is a hate relationship between emotion and archetype. For example, becoming inconsolable because your shoelace snapped.

Alternatively, rather than an excessive emotional response, the patient never displays the appropriate emotion – ever again! This is also a hate relationship between emotion and archetype. For example, not showing sadness and grief when a loved one dies.

Let's use a real-life example. While reading, decide how you would likely react. Zeno (334–262 BCE), the founder of the Stoic philosophy school, was given terrible news one day that all his belongings (which were being transported by sea) had sunk to the bottom of the Mediterranean Sea.

If that had happened to me, I probably would have lost my bundle. There would likely have been swearing, rage and anger. There could have been the 'Why me?' and I may even have shaken my fists at the sky.

How did Zeno react? Well, instead of responding the way I might have, Zeno calmly said: 'Fortune [Goddess] bids me to be a less encumbered philosopher' (De Botton 2000, p.108).

Now, don't get me wrong, because I take my hat off to him for his calm demeanor (which just so happens to be one of the stoic traits), but the appropriate emotional response would likely be any number of possibilities from anger, to rage or sorrow, to name just a few. Zeno's response was highly unusual, unorthodox and, in Chinese medicine theory, probably unhealthy.

A list of the more common archetype and emotions/spirits relationships are in Table 14.1.

Table 14.1 Archetype relationships with the emotions and Wŭ Shén/Five Spirits[8]

Wŭ Xíng archetype	Emotions[9]	Wŭ Shén/Five Spirits
Wood	Anger Depression Frustration Stress	Hún
Fire	Joy Mania Shock Sadness Depression Anxiety Stress Manic depression Every other emotion[10]	Shén
Earth	Pensiveness Sympathy Worry	Yì
Metal	Sadness Depression Grief Worry	Pò
Water	Fear Shock	Zhì

For a more thorough discussion on the Wŭ Shén/Five Spirits, please refer to Chapter 13.

4. What are the archetypes?

According to www.dictionary.com, an archetype refers to 'The original pattern or model from which all things of the same kind are copied or on which they are based; A model or first form; Prototype'.

What about the Wǔ Xíng archetypes?

- They are a collective of everything that has come before on the Wǔ Xíng.

- It is not a system that has stayed the same in ancient China through to modern times, nor is it a system that originated in our modern Western world.

- It is a collective of ideas that started in ancient China and then evolved over the millennia via different authors/philosophers/poets. It has then been merged with modern Western ideas as a result of archetype pioneers such as Carl Jung, along with countless Chinese medicine advancers.

What can you expect with the Wǔ Xíng archetypes?

There is not one single rule when it applies to the archetypes. In fact, there are a range of different theories out there to posit what archetype a person belongs to. The three main ones I have seen written, as well as witnessed with patients, students, family members, friends, acquaintances and otherwise, are:[11]

- One of the Wǔ Xíng will be your archetype. Franglen (2014, pp.21–23) calls it our 'Guardian Element'. This may, or may not, align with your Chinese astrological animal and element.[12]

- You will be a fairly equal measure of all the Wǔ Xíng without much change throughout your entire life.

- You will cycle through each of the Wǔ Xíng throughout your life, spending roughly 12 years on each one. This suggests that by the time you reach 60 years of age you have evolved through all five of the archetypes. For the remainder of your life you will then display equal parts of each of the Wǔ Xíng.

From the three possibilities listed above, the one that gets the most coverage is the first one: that is, you have one overriding guardian element. In that instance there are a few more thoughts that are also very important to understand.

You are highly unlikely to be 100% of what is listed for that guardian archetype

We are all unique individuals, and, using myself as an example, every archetype system I have seen (Eastern or Western) has never had me agreeing with what was written 100% of the time. Typically, my main archetypes define me around 70–80%. Most other people I speak with have had the same experience.

You will almost certainly have a second element that is your support act

In our day-to-day lives, it's hard to do everything ourselves, and the element archetypes operate in the same manner. It's like a marriage of sorts, but with one element being dominant over the other. This dominant element will use its support element in a really harmonious manner, recognizing its skills where necessary and applying them to our daily lives. This is similar to the Yīn Yáng principle where you can't have one without the other.

You are likely to be somewhere around 40–60% of what is listed for this support element.

You will always be a small amount of the remaining three element archetypes

This is because the Wŭ Xíng are five parts in the macrocosmic Universe, and this is mirrored in our microcosmic Universe.

> People of different elements have a tendency to approach things in different ways, to act in different ways, to make decisions in different ways, even to dress in different ways. (Franglen 2014, p.55)

Destiny versus desires

Assuming we each have a guardian element archetype, then this poses the question about destiny versus desires. Put another way, you might refer to it as no free will or free will. This is discussed in more detail in Chapter 13.

A guardian element archetype does suggest that we have been born into our bodies to live a particular life, which would be classed as our destiny. But what happens if our guardian archetype is operating in an excess or deficient manner? Does that then mean we start operating at a level where desires take over? Regardless of which one is right, or whether, in fact, both are right, the Wŭ Xíng archetype treatments listed below can help.

5. What is discussed for each archetype

Each of the Wŭ Xíng archetypes is discussed in a fair amount of detail. Therefore, I have split each section up into different headings to make it easier to follow. The headings for each of the Wŭ Xíng archetypes are:

- Yīn Yáng organ relationship
- Emotions and Wŭ Shén/Five Spirits relationship
- Archetype characteristics

- Archetype loves and fears

- What the archetype has difficulty with

- Archetype diagnosis – Shí/Excess and Xū/Deficiency signs and symptoms

- How to communicate to the archetype

- Archetype treatments – general, Shí/Excess and Xū/Deficiency.

Each of the Wǔ Xíng archetypes will now be discussed in more detail. Please be aware that the references given next to each of the element archetypes are designed to cover the entire archetype section. There will be situations where I include more references within the section, and these are designed to offer you further reading on those topics that were referenced.

6. The archetypes
Wood archetype[13]

Also known as: The Adventurer.

The Wood archetype has other titles including pioneer, founder, forerunner, innovator, inventor, creator, developer, discoverer, forger or explorer.

> Like a locomotive that gathers momentum and speed as it hurtles down the track, the *Pioneer* [Wood archetype] steers an awesome power. (Beinfield and Korngold 1991, p.161)

Yīn Yáng organ relationship

Yīn organ = Liver.

Yáng organ = Gall Bladder.

The 8th chapter of *The Yellow Emperor's Classic* (*Inner Canon of the Yellow Emperor/* Huáng Dì Nèi Jīng/黃帝內經) discusses the two organs in terms of their official capacity. These are quoted below.

LIVER

> The liver is like the [army] general, courageous and smart. (Ni 1995, p.34)

GALL BLADDER

> The gallbladder is like a judge for its power of discernment. (Ni 1995, p.34)

Emotions and Wŭ Shén/Five Spirits relationship

The key emotions and spirit that the Wood archetype has a love–hate relationship with are:

- Emotions – anger, depression, frustration, stress.
- Spirit – Hún (Ethereal/Heavenly/Dream-Big Soul).[14]

Wood archetype characteristics

A wide range of different characteristics define a Wood archetype. Typically, they will:

- be creative, dynamic, expansive, full of vitality
- show initiative
- be flexible in their approach, and therefore adaptable to change
- be decisive, direct and committed
- show solid clarity, judgement and foresight
- be appropriately assertive
- be confident yet prudent, courageous, bold, brave and ambitious
- desire purpose
- be compelled to win
- be fiercely independent and must have freedom; they also like to be in groups where they are the leader and the center of attention
- make the rules but then like to break them/better them
- be balanced between their Hún (Ethereal/Heavenly/Dream-Big Soul) and Pò (Corporeal/Grounded/Earthly/Do-Big-Be-Big Soul)
- briefly weigh up 'risk versus reward'.[15]

Infatuated with what is new, curious about what is untried, she is eager to innovate, reform and revolutionise. (Beinfield and Korngold 1991, p.161)

What a Wood archetype loves and fears

Every archetype system has perceived positives and negatives associated with it. They also have perceived strengths and weaknesses. Table 14.2 lists the Wood archetype's loves and fears.

Table 14.2 Wood archetype – loves and fears

Loves	Fears
Setting and achieving goals	The same/constancy
Problem solving – finding solutions to problems	Powerlessness, dependency, helplessness
Intense competitive pressure	Feeling vulnerable, or having the belief that other people hold that view of them
Thrives on challenges and fast pace – when action is required, they kick into gear	Losing control or a loss of control
Pushing to the absolute limits, and beyond	Confinement/bondage
Showing a willingness to take surprisingly bold yet calculated risks (audacious)	
Winning – strive to be the best and to beat their personal best	
Battling adversity – love the fight/struggle	
Staying busy	
The road less traveled; they might even build new roads[16]	

What a Wood archetype has difficulty with

As with any archetype system, each element has areas in which they need to grow/evolve and mature as they progress through their lives. Some of the difficulties displayed by a Wood archetype include:

- intensity, restraint, equality, sharing and cooperation

- consistency

- hypocrisy, double standards

- anger, irritability

- conflicting purposes, choices, impulses – they don't like it when they have too many things on at exactly the same time

- can miss the companionship of equals – this is partly because they don't believe they have any equals; if it turns out they have an equal or a superior, they will make it their mission to supersede them

- substance abuse – stimulants and/or sedatives

- can slip into Hún Shí – becomes too 'off with the fairies', dreaming up the next big thing; may fail to come back to earth and therefore never gets anything done but just dreams big

- can slip into Hún Xū – becomes too grounded, too structured, not open to change.

Wood archetype diagnosis

Every one of the Wǔ Xíng archetypes will, from time to time, become excess or deficient. In rare circumstances, they can be excess and deficient at the same time. Table 14.3 outlines some of the more commonly seen signs and symptoms for a Wood archetype excess or deficiency. The signs and symptoms that are likely to be the same for excess and deficiency are at the bottom of the table in the merged rows.

Table 14.3 Wood archetype – Excess/Shí and Deficiency/Xū signs and symptoms

Excess signs and symptoms	Deficiency signs and symptoms
Overbearing, overconfident, dominant, aggressive, intolerant, stupid and dangerous	Slow, clumsy, vague, unclear, compromises, submits, follows orders, stupid and dangerous
Arrogant, aggressive, reckless, driven, antagonistic, tyrannical, confrontational, compulsive, impulsive	Compressed, confined, passive, timid
Subject to uncontrollable impulses	Habit-bound with a rigid approach; hates change because change is scary
Outwardly volatile emotions – particularly favors getting angry and frustrated	Inwardly volatile emotions – particularly favors feeling overwhelmed, stressed, depressed, powerless, frustrated, resentful and suspicious of others
Self-indulgent	Self-punishing – very low self-esteem with a total lack of confidence
Intolerant, impatient, makes hasty decisions	Indecisive
Poor judgement due to arrogance	Poor judgement due to people pleasing
Pretentious, pompous, fake, erratic, premature, contrary, ineffectual, devious, fickle, ambivalent	
Plans poorly (either through no planning or over-planning) and then blames others when they fail	

How to communicate with a Wood archetype

Regardless of the archetype, if you can speak their language, they will be much more amenable to you as a patient. A Wood archetype would like you to:

- discuss the treatment in a way that makes them think they are going on a wonderful new adventure – one that no other patient you have had has ever been on

- explain that you know what to do because you have treated patients similar to them but not quite like them

- assure them of your conviction in the treatment

- make them feel that they are heavily involved in the successful outcome of the treatment

- explain what your hopes/goals are with the treatment and then ask them how they will achieve those goals when they leave.

Wood archetype treatment

I have listed a general treatment (Table 14.4) as well as ones specifically for an excess or deficient patient (Tables 14.5 and 14.6). These are just some of the many ways you can treat the Wood archetype. In the end, it's up to you how you choose to treat your patient.

The general treatment is designed to regulate/balance the archetype. It will also act in a subtler, less intense manner, which can be a very good approach for some patients.

Table 14.4 Wood archetype point combination – general[17]

Location of point	Point name	Reasoning
Trunk (front)	KI 26 LR 14 GB 24	Wood point on the Kidney Spirit Gate Front Mù Collecting point of the Liver Front Mù Collecting point of the Gall Bladder
Trunk (back)	BL 18 BL 19	Back Shù Transporting point of the Liver Back Shù Transporting point of the Gall Bladder
Legs/feet	LR 1 LR 3 GB 41	Horary point (Wood on Wood) Yuán Source point of the Liver Horary point (Wood on Wood)
Total points needled		16 points used bilaterally

Table 14.5 Wood archetype point combination – excess[18]

Location of point	Point name	Reasoning
Head/face/neck	GB 20	Clears excess from the head, Shén and Hún
Trunk (front)	LR 14 GB 24	Front Mù Collecting point of the Liver Front Mù Collecting point of the Gall Bladder
Legs/feet	LR 1 LR 2 GB 38 GB 41	Horary point (Wood on Wood) Child (sedating) point on the Liver channel Child (sedating) point on the Gall Bladder channel Horary point (Wood on Wood)
Total points needled		14 points used bilaterally

Table 14.6 Wood archetype point combination – deficiency[19]

Location of point	Point name	Reasoning
Trunk (back)	BL 18 BL 19	Back Shù Transporting point of the Liver Back Shù Transporting point of the Gall Bladder
Legs/feet	LR 1 LR 8 GB 41 GB 43	Horary point (Wood on Wood) Mother (tonifying) point on the Liver channel Horary point (Wood on Wood) Mother (tonifying) point on the Gall Bladder channel
Total points needled		12 points used bilaterally

Fire archetype[20]

Also known as: The Magician.

The Fire archetype has other titles including salesperson, wizard, shaman, conjurer, prodigy, sorcerer/sorceress, warlock/witch or witchdoctor.

> Enchanting and persuasive, the *Wizard* [Fire archetype] is a natural salesman, selling not so much the product itself as the experience of possessing an instrument of magic, a veritable talisman, that endows us with the power to transcend our ordinary existence. The magic, however, is in the *Wizard*, not in the merchandise. (Beinfield and Korngold 1991, p.177)

Yīn Yáng organ relationship

Yīn organs = Heart and Pericardium.

Yáng organs = Small Intestine and Sān Jiāo.

The 8th chapter of *The Yellow Emperor's Classic* (*Inner Canon of the Yellow Emperor/ Huáng Dì Nèi Jīng/*黃帝內經) discusses each of the four organs in terms of their official capacity. These are quoted below.

HEART

> The heart is the sovereign of all organs and represents the consciousness of one's being. It is responsible for intelligence, wisdom, and spiritual transformation. (Ni 1995, p.34)

PERICARDIUM

> The pericardium is like the court jester who makes the king laugh, bringing forth joy. (Ni 1995, p.34)

SMALL INTESTINE

> The small intestine receives the food that has been digested by the spleen and stomach and further extracts, absorbs, and distributes it throughout the body, all the while separating the pure from the turbid. (Ni 1995, p.34)

SĀN JIĀO

> The sanjiao, or the three visceral cavities, promotes the transformation and transportation of water and fluids throughout the body. (Ni 1995, p.34)

Emotions and Wŭ Shén/Five Spirits relationship

The key emotions and spirit that the Fire archetype has a love–hate relationship with are:

- Emotions – joy, mania, shock, sadness, depression, anxiety, stress, manic depression (Diān Kuáng). Any other emotion.[21]

- Spirit – Shén.[22]

Fire archetype characteristics

A wide range of different characteristics define a Fire archetype. Typically, they will:

- be excited, lively, enthusiastic

- be devoted, enchanting, charismatic, seductive, flirtatious, intimate, tender, passionate – seeks the perfect lover

- be persuasive

- be alert, mentally clear, aware, well oriented, focused, intuitive

- be happy and hearty

- be emotionally balanced

- have a strong Shén – memory, consciousness, sleeping, thinking and emotions

- take pleasure in the achievements of their goals

- enjoy life's ups but not the downs

- be a talented communicator

- be an eternal optimist, sanguine

- be spontaneous

- be compassionate, empathetic

- perceive gratification as the end goal of any situation

- saturate 'normal' with 'phenomenal'.

His excitement and enthusiasm generate…fusion…[and] with this tremendous catalytic energy, he brings the transforming power of light, love, and awareness into the world. (Beinfield and Korngold 1991, p.177)

What a Fire archetype loves and fears

Every archetype system has perceived positives and negatives associated with it. They also have perceived strengths and weaknesses. Table 14.7 lists the Fire archetype's loves and fears.

Table 14.7 Fire archetype – loves and fears

Loves	Fears
Pleasure, intimacy, romance, being in love	Separation, boredom, dullness, pain
Seeking excitement and joy	Inactivity or 'down' time
Performing for others	To be cut off from others, dissolution
Touch, sensation, feeling	Being overwhelmed by intensity
Living in the 'now'	Dread of what the future might hold
To say 'yes'	The conservative
Grandiosity	The ordinary/mundane
Drama	Boundaries
Adrenaline	Confusion
Seeking the Divine	The unknown

What a Fire archetype has difficulty with

As with any archetype system, each element has areas in which they need to grow/ evolve and mature as they progress through their lives. Some of the difficulties displayed by a Fire archetype include:

- can be preoccupied with self-stimulation
- conflicting needs, desires, attractions
- solitude – but does need it on occasion to recharge
- saying 'no'
- sleeping
- shutting down
- boundaries, giving others space
- separation from loved ones
- might perceive gratification as the end goal of any situation
- stimulant addiction, including gambling.

Fire archetype diagnosis

Every one of the Wŭ Xíng archetypes will, from time to time, become excess or deficient. In rare circumstances, they can be excess and deficient at the same time. Table 14.8 outlines some of the more commonly seen signs and symptoms for a Fire archetype excess or deficiency. The signs and symptoms that are likely to be the same for excess and deficiency are at the bottom of the table in the merged rows.

Table 14.8 Fire archetype – Excess/Shí and Deficiency/Xū signs and symptoms

Excess signs and symptoms	Deficiency signs and symptoms
Over-excited	Easily startled
Hypersensitive	Gullible, naïve, innocent
Long-winded	Panicked
Anxious, agitated	Depressed, unhappy, disheartened
Manic, psychotic, aggressive and very dangerous	Mute, quiet, but still dangerous
Confused	Dazed, confused, disoriented, semi-conscious, apathetic, lethargic, disinterested
Selfish	Lost
Sensory perception issues – such as seeing things that aren't there	Nervously exhausted
Insomniac	
Abuse of mind-altering substances	
Addicted to stimulants	

How to communicate with a Fire archetype

Regardless of the archetype, if you can speak their language, they will be much more amenable to you as a patient. A Fire archetype would like you to:

- explain to them that Chinese medicine is not a 'normal' medicine; it is a phenomenal medicine that is already treating them at this very moment, and will continue to for a considerable amount of time afterwards

- use grand sweeping arm movements to describe Chinese medicine; change the volume and pitch of your voice

- be enthusiastic and lively, and remain optimistic throughout

- try to include some Tuī Ná in your treatment because they love touch

- sell them the medicine!

Fire archetype treatment[23]

I have listed a general treatment (Table 14.9) as well as ones specifically for an excess or deficient patient (Tables 14.10 and 14.11). These are just some of the many ways you can treat the Wǔ Xíng archetypes. In the end, it's up to you how you choose to treat your patient.

The general treatment is designed to regulate/balance the archetype. It will also act in a subtler, less intense manner, which can be a very good approach for some patients.

Table 14.9 Fire archetype point combination – general[24]

Location of point	Point name	Reasoning
Trunk (front)	KI 22 KI 25 CV 14 CV 17	Fire point on the Kidney Spirit Gate Fire point on the Kidney Spirit Gate Front Mù Collecting point of the Heart Front Mù Collecting point of the Pericardium
Arms/hands	HT 8 SI 5 TE 6	Horary point (Fire on Fire) Horary point (Fire on Fire) Horary point (Fire on Fire)
Legs/feet	BL 39 ST 39	Lower Hé (Uniting) Sea point of the Sān Jiāo Lower Hé (Uniting) Sea point of the Small Intestine
Total points needled		16 points used bilaterally

Table 14.10 Fire archetype point combination – excess[25]

Location of point	Point name	Reasoning
Head/face/neck	GV 20	Drives excess down from the head and Shén
Trunk (front)	CV 14 CV 4	Front Mù Collecting point of the Heart Front Mù Collecting point of the Small Intestine
Arms/hands	HT 7 HT 8 SI 5 SI 8	Child (sedating) point on the Heart channel Horary point (Fire on Fire) Horary point (Fire on Fire) Child (sedating) point on the Small Intestine channel
Legs/feet	KI 1	Draws excess away from the head and Shén
Total points needled		13 points used bilaterally

Table 14.11 Fire archetype point combination – deficiency[26]

Location of point	Point name	Reasoning
Head/face/neck	GV 20	Draws Vital Substances up into the head and Shén
Trunk (back)	BL 14 BL 22	Back Shù Transporting point of the Pericardium Back Shù Transporting point of the Sān Jiāo
Arms/hands	PC 8 PC 9 TE 3 TE 6	Horary point (Fire on Fire) Mother (tonifying) point on the Pericardium channel Mother (tonifying) point on the Sān Jiāo channel Horary point (Fire on Fire)
Legs/feet	KI 1	Drives Vital Substances up into the head and Shén
Total points needled		15 points used bilaterally

Earth archetype[27]

Also known as: The Saviour.

The Earth archetype has other titles including negotiator, mediator, peacemaker, diplomat, arbitrator, intermediary, go-between, appeaser, pacifier or balancer.

The *Peacemaker* [Earth archetype] embodies sympathy and caring, a ready advocate for those in greatest need – of friendship, sustenance, and recognition. Negotiating peace for its own sake, she tirelessly serves humanity as the great balancer and equaliser, the preserver of families and societies. (Beinfield and Korngold 1991, p.191)

Yīn Yáng organ relationship

Yīn organ = Spleen.

Yáng organ = Stomach.

The 8th chapter of *The Yellow Emperor's Classic* (*Inner Canon of the Yellow Emperor/ Huáng Dì Nèi Jīng*/黃帝內經) discusses the two organs in terms of their official capacity. These are quoted below.

SPLEEN AND STOMACH

The stomach and spleen are like warehouses where one stores all the food and essences. They digest, absorb, and extract the food and nutrients. (Ni 1995, p.34)

Emotions and Wǔ Shén/Five Spirits relationship

The key emotions and spirit that the Earth archetype has a love–hate relationship with are:

- Emotions – pensiveness, sympathy, worry.
- Spirit – Yì (Thought, Post-Heaven Intellect).[28]

Earth archetype characteristics

A wide range of different characteristics define an Earth archetype. Typically, they will:

- be a negotiator or peacemaker
- be stable, poised, composed, moderate
- be sociable
- be nurturing, supportive
- be sympathetic, considerate, attentive
- be agreeable
- be loyal
- be self-aware
- have a focused intent

- be intelligent – using Post-Heaven Intellect (knowledge you learn via the senses)

- have exceptional memory, be a quick learner, remember things with minimal study, have good concentration

- be a constructive thinker

- reflect on past events (successes and failures) and productively learns from them.

[The Earth archetype] can assume and enhance the attributes of those around her, putting people at ease in an environment of trust. (Beinfield and Korngold 1991, p.191)

What an Earth archetype loves and fears

Every archetype system has perceived positives and negatives associated with it. They also have perceived strengths and weaknesses. Table 14.12 lists the Earth archetype's loves and fears.

Table 14.12 Earth archetype – loves and fears

Loves	Fears
Unification	Conflicting roles/loyalties/frames of reference/ value system
Harmony, serenity, security, predictability	Obstruction, stagnation, sluggishness
Details	Other people being disloyal, treacherous, unfaithful, untrustworthy; a 'snake in the grass'
Seeking comfort	Change
Feeling needed	Conflict in general
Family	To feel lost, isolated, separated, displaced, independent of their wider community
Stable relationships for themselves and the people close to them	Insecurity
Sharing	Self-doubt
Being involved in everything	That things are not going according to plan
Being the negotiator, during which they need to be the 'go to' person	Not feeling valued for their negotiation skills
Being well organized	
Living in the 'now'	

What an Earth archetype has difficulty with

As with any archetype system, each element has areas in which they need to grow/ evolve and mature as they progress through their lives. Some of the difficulties displayed by an Earth archetype include:

- interfering/meddling where they are not wanted or not needed
- manipulating situations to make them fit what they believe is best for everyone – what would they know? How can they know with absolute certainty what is right?
- self-sacrifice, pleasing others
- being everything to everyone
- unrealistic expectations of another person's behavior and/or how the world should operate
- feeling extreme disappointment if people fall below the lofty standards they set
- melancholy
- independence.

According to Beinfield and Korngold (1991, p.136), Earth archetypes 'may be so concerned with establishing balance and harmony that the dynamic tension essential for movement and change is neutralised'.

Earth archetype diagnosis

Every one of the Wǔ Xíng archetypes will, from time to time, become excess or deficient. In rare circumstances, they can be excess and deficient at the same time. Table 14.13 outlines some of the more commonly seen signs and symptoms for an Earth archetype excess or deficiency. The signs and symptoms that are likely to be the same for excess and deficiency are at the bottom of the table in the merged rows.

Table 14.13 Earth archetype – Excess/Shí and Deficiency/Xū signs and symptoms

Excess signs and symptoms	Deficiency signs and symptoms
Overprotective, can overcrowd; overbearing	Unmotivated, stuck, can't be bothered – 'it's all too hard'
Meddlesome	Conforming
Takes unnecessary risks	Sloppy
Poor memory, slow learner; scattered thought or pensive (plunged in thought)	Poor memory – too tired to study; slow learner, can't concentrate or retain information, vague, procrastinates
Obsessive	Melancholic
Over-extends/over-reaches	Lethargic, tired, sleeps all the time, exhausted
Can worry so much about the future that they become obsessed with it; therefore, they live in the 'future'	Reflect excessively on the past; therefore, they live in the 'past'
Can reject other people's sympathetic advances	Craves sympathy from others; may manufacture signs and symptoms, even diseases, in order to receive more sympathy

Narcissistic – this is a mask, rather than an inherent love of oneself	Poor self-esteem with a real 'shame-for-self' cycle with accompanying grief, sadness, worry, fear
Excessively worries about everyone and everything	
Can become obsessed (cling/attach themselves) towards a particular person to the point of displaying psychotic behavior	

How to communicate with an Earth archetype

Regardless of the archetype, if you can speak their language, they will be much more amenable to you as a patient. An Earth archetype would like you to:

- show a real focused intent during the treatment – they are your 'entire world' for the time you have with them

- not look distracted or disinterested – don't yawn and don't appear vague or uncommitted; and definitely don't get up to answer the clinic phone if it rings

- talk about how the treatment will provide harmony and balance

- make them feel comforted and needed; that you care that they came to you for treatment

- understand that they are also extremely intelligent people, so don't treat them like children.

Earth archetype treatment

I have listed a general treatment (Table 14.14) as well as ones specifically for an excess or deficient patient (Tables 14.15 and 14.16). These are just some of the many ways you can treat the Earth archetypes. In the end, it's up to you how you choose to treat your patient.

The general treatment is designed to regulate/balance the archetype. It will also act in a subtler, less intense manner, which can be a very good approach for some patients.

Table 14.14 Earth archetype point combination – general[29]

Location of point	Point name	Reasoning
Trunk (front)	KI 23 CV 12 LR 13	Earth point on the Kidney Spirit Gate Front Mù Collecting point of the Stomach Front Mù Collecting point of the Spleen
Trunk (back)	BL 20 BL 21	Back Shù Transporting point of the Spleen Back Shù Transporting point of the Stomach
Legs/feet	ST 36 SP 3	Lower Hé (Uniting) Sea point of the Stomach Yuán Source point of the Spleen
Total points needled		13 points used bilaterally

Table 14.15 Earth archetype point combination – excess[30]

Location of point	Point name	Reasoning
Head/face/neck	ST 8	Clears excess from the head, Shén and Yì
Trunk (back)	BL 20 BL 21	Back Shù Transporting point of the Spleen Back Shù Transporting point of the Stomach
Legs/feet	SP 3 SP 5 ST 36 ST 45	Horary point (Earth on Earth) Child (sedating) point on the Spleen channel Horary point (Earth on Earth) Child (sedating) point on the Stomach channel
Total points needled		14 points used bilaterally

Table 14.16 Earth archetype point combination – deficiency[31]

Location of point	Point name	Reasoning
Head/face/neck	GV 20	Draws Vital Substances up into the head, Shén and Yì
Trunk (front)	CV 12 LR 13	Front Mù Collecting point of the Stomach Front Mù Collecting point of the Spleen
Legs/feet	SP 2 SP 3 ST 36 ST 41	Mother (tonifying) point on the Spleen channel Horary point (Earth on Earth) Horary point (Earth on Earth) Mother (tonifying) point on the Stomach channel
Total points needled		12 points used bilaterally

When the vicissitudes [fluctuations] of our lives threaten to overturn or deflect us from our path, our *Earth* aspect returns us to an even keel. (Beinfield and Korngold 1991, p.136)

Metal archetype[32]

Also known as: The Alchemist.

The Metal archetype has other titles including modifier, transformer, experimenter, hermetic, converter or pseudoscientist.

Like an abbot ensconced in his sanctuary, serene, detached, unflappable, he instructs us in the meaning of ritual and doctrine, providing the structure that enables people to apply the metaphysical to the mundane. (Beinfield and Korngold 1991, p.205)

Yīn Yáng organ relationship

Yīn organ = Lungs.

Yáng organ = Large Intestine.

The 8th chapter of *The Yellow Emperor's Classic* (*Inner Canon of the Yellow Emperor/* Huáng Dì Nèi Jīng/黃帝內經) discusses the two organs in terms of their official capacity. These are quoted below.

Lungs

The lung is the advisor. It helps the heart in regulating the body's qi. (Ni 1995, p.34)

Large Intestine

The large intestine is responsible for transportation of all turbidity. All waste products go through this organ. (Ni 1995, p.34)

Emotions and Wŭ Shén/Five Spirits relationship

The key emotions and spirit that the Metal archetype has a love–hate relationship with are:

- Emotions – sadness, depression, grief, worry.

- Spirit – Pò (Corporeal/Grounded/Earthly/Do-Big-Be-Big Soul).[33]

Metal archetype characteristics

A wide range of different characteristics define a Metal archetype. Typically, they will:

- be able to discriminate

- be calm, stoic, patient

- be very precise, methodical

- find the beauty in things

- be very ethical people

- stay the level/moderate course; reserved

- be emotionally balanced

- be neat and tidy

- set high standards for themselves, and subsequently the rest of humanity

- be optimistic

- be intrepid and adventurous – if they feel safe

- be adaptable to change – if given time

- throw out the old to make way for the new

- have strong sensation, feeling, hearing and sight

- be able to spot liars from a mile away

- be able to recognize, isolate and then extract the 'pure' from the 'impure'.[34]

When we let go of old habits and values to prepare for a new stage of our life, the power of *Metal* enables us to sigh deeply and release. (Beinfield and Korngold 1991, p.136)

What a Metal archetype loves and fears

Every archetype system has perceived positives and negatives associated with it. They also have perceived strengths and weaknesses. Table 14.17 lists the Metal archetype's loves and fears.

Table 14.17 Metal archetype – loves and fears

Loves	Fears
Definition, structure, discipline	Being overcrowded
Organizing everything, systems	Conflicting principles/standards
Precision	Differences
Control	Spontaneity
Ethics, moral values, standards, righteousness, correctness	To become corrupted
Finding the beauty in things, purity	Intimacy
Authoritarian role models/peers – as viewed using their own 'world view' filter[35]	Things that can't be made sense of
Digging out order from the disorder/chaos	Lack of order, things falling into disrepair, chaos
	Particularly complex problems
	Immoral people/immoral planet

What a Metal archetype has difficulty with

As with any archetype system, each element has areas in which they need to grow/evolve and mature as they progress through their lives. Some of the difficulties displayed by a Metal archetype include:

- constantly striving for perfection and order in all things

- being too judgemental of others; prejudiced

- always being right

- close relationships – want to be close to others but must be given their distance

- will fight to stay the 'moderate' and 'safe' course

- disappointment in everyone and everything; not meeting the high standards they set

- expressing emotions

- intimacy

- authority – if they view the authority figure as inferior

- can slip into Pò Xū – becomes too 'off with the fairies'; dreaming up the next big thing; may fail to come back to earth and therefore never gets anything done; just dreams big

- can slip into Pò Shí – becomes too grounded, too structured, not open to change.

According to Beinfield and Korngold (1991, p.136): '*Metal* adheres to rules and protocols even when these have become a hindrance [ritualistic].'

Metal archetype diagnosis

Every one of the Wŭ Xíng archetypes will, from time to time, become excess or deficient. In rare circumstances, they can be excess and deficient at the same time. Table 14.18 outlines some of the more commonly seen signs and symptoms for a Metal archetype excess or deficiency. The signs and symptoms that are likely to be the same for excess and deficiency are at the bottom of the table in the merged rows.

Table 14.18 Metal archetype – Excess/Shí and Deficiency/Xū signs and symptoms

Excess signs and symptoms	Deficiency signs and symptoms
Overly strict, dogmatic, despotic, autocratic	Can feel constricted, restricted
Self-righteous, sanctimonious, holier-than-thou	Disillusioned, dispirited, resigned to failure, pessimistic
Distant/cool	'Pit' depression; severe suicidal tendencies
Petty	Sloppy
Hypocritical	Compliant, conservative
Scattered/numb sensation, feeling, hearing and sight	Weak sensation, feeling, hearing and sight
	Stays indoors and at home; doesn't usually travel, but if they do, they pack everything
Indifferent	
Hangs on to the past	
Never throws anything away	
Carries emotional baggage	

How to communicate with a Metal archetype

Regardless of the archetype, if you can speak their language, they will be much more amenable to you as a patient. A Metal archetype would like you to:

- be honest in your approach and discuss how clinical trials have shown Chinese medicine to be effective in treating their condition – don't lie to them or try to put one over on them

- methodically outline your personal approach to treatment and why you chose this methodology

- outline a set plan for treatment and book the same appointment time every week – never change their appointment time once it has been agreed upon

- encourage them to research Chinese medicine at home and come back the following session with additional queries

- allow them to be actively involved in their recovery.

Metal archetype treatment

I have listed a general treatment (Table 14.19) as well as ones specifically for an excess or deficient patient (Tables 14.20 and 14.21). These are just some of the many ways you can treat the Metal archetype. In the end, it's up to you how you choose to treat your patient.

The general treatment is designed to regulate/balance the archetype. It will also act in a subtler, less intense manner, which can be a very good approach for some patients.

Table 14.19 Metal archetype point combination – general[36]

Location of point	Point name	Reasoning
Trunk (front)	KI 24 LU 1	Metal point on the Kidney Spirit Gate Front Mù Collecting point of the Lungs
Trunk (back)	BL 13 BL 25	Back Shù Transporting point of the Lungs Back Shù Transporting point of the Large Intestine
Arms/hands	LU 8 LU 9 LI 1	Horary point (Metal on Metal) Yuán Source point of the Lungs Horary point (Metal on Metal)
Legs/feet	ST 37	Lower Hé (Uniting) Sea point of the Large Intestine
Total points needled		16 points used bilaterally

Table 14.20 Metal archetype point combination – excess[37]

Location of point	Point name	Reasoning
Head/face/neck	GV 20	Regulates energy flow up into the head, Shén and Pò[38]
Trunk (back)	BL 13 BL 25	Back Shù Transporting point of the Lungs Back Shù Transporting point of the Large Intestine
Arms/hands	LU 5 LU 8 LI 1 LI 2	Child (sedating) point on the Lung channel Horary point (Metal on Metal) Horary point (Metal on Metal) Child (sedating) point on the Large Intestine channel
Legs/feet	KI 1	Regulates energy flow up into the head, Shén and Pò
Total points needled		15 points used bilaterally

Table 14.21 Metal archetype point combination – deficiency[39]

Location of point	Point name	Reasoning
Trunk (front)	LU 1 ST 25	Front Mù Collecting point of the Lungs Front Mù Collecting point of the Large Intestine
Arms/hands	LU 8 LU 9 LI 1 LI 11	Horary point (Metal on Metal) Mother (tonifying) point on the Lung channel Horary point (Metal on Metal) Mother (tonifying) point on the Large Intestine channel
Legs/feet	ST 37	Lower Hé (Uniting) Sea point of the Large Intestine
Total points needled		14 points used bilaterally

Water archetype[40]

Also known as: The Philosopher.

The Water archetype has other titles including truth-seeker, theorist, thinker, academic, intellectual, logician, scholar or dreamer.

> Revelation propels the *Philosopher* [Water archetype] in her relentless quest for truth. She brings to light that which is hidden, uncovering new knowledge, dispelling mystery, eroding ignorance... The *Philosopher* yearns for meaning that transcends the rudderless meandering of human affairs. (Beinfield and Korngold 1991, p.219)

Yīn Yáng organ relationship

Yīn organ = Kidneys.

Yáng organ = Urinary Bladder.

The 8th chapter of *The Yellow Emperor's Classic* (*Inner Canon of the Yellow Emperor/* Huáng Dì Nèi Jīng/黃帝內經) discusses the two organs in terms of their official capacity. These are quoted below.

Kidneys

> The kidneys store the vitality and mobilize the four extremities. They also aid the memory, willpower, and coordination. (Ni 1995, p.34)

Urinary Bladder

> The bladder is where the water converges and where, after being catalyzed by the qi, it is eliminated. (Ni 1995, p.34)

Emotions and Wŭ Shén/Five Spirits relationship

The key emotions and spirit that the Water archetype has a love–hate relationship with are:

- Emotions – fear, shock.

- Spirit – Zhì (Willpower, Pre-Heaven Intellect).[41]

Water archetype characteristics

A wide range of different characteristics define a Water archetype. Typically, they will:

- be honest

- be self-sufficient, durable, tough, particular

- remember everything

- be intelligent – using Pre-Heaven Intellect (knowledge you are born with)

- get things done

- be sensible, practical, utilitarian

- have incredible imagination/creativity

- have strong willpower and determination

- persevere – despite fear

- be tranquil

- be energetic

- be introspective, contemplative

- be cautious, conservative, careful, watchful

- be extremely modest – almost to a fault

- be curious

- be articulate and well spoken (when they need to be).

When our labours demand that we stop, rest, and take stock of what we have done, and rededicate ourselves to a fresh purpose, our *Water* aspect gives us the renewed vitality and will to carry on. (Beinfield and Korngold 1991, p.136)

What a Water archetype loves and fears

Every archetype system has perceived positives and negatives associated with it. They also have perceived strengths and weaknesses. Table 14.22 lists the Water archetype's loves and fears.

Table 14.22 Water archetype – loves and fears

Loves	Fears
Facts	Distraction
Getting to the truth of the matter	Other people invading their space and time
Uncovering new knowledge or old/obscure knowledge	The ending of something
Always finishing what they start; get a 'super-charge' when they complete difficult tasks	Becoming forgetful
Unlocking the mysteries of the world	Becoming a hypochondriac
Finding a good teacher	Being exposed
Connecting with someone's brain/intellect; not their body/intimacy	Sharing
Privacy	Conforming to the status quo
Remaining anonymous, enigmatic	
'Me' time	

What a Water archetype has difficulty with

As with any archetype system, each element has areas in which they need to grow/evolve and mature as they progress through their lives. Some of the difficulties displayed by a Water archetype include:

- conflicting visions, stories, expectations

- ponders excessively, which may result in missing an opportunity

- tendency to become a hermit, seeks solitude – therefore, they can have difficulty with social gatherings

- confidence around others

- trusting others

- being selfish and mean

- expressing their emotions

- can come across as being very eccentric.

According to Beinfield and Korngold (1991, p.219), a Water archetype is able to 'envision what can be, [and therefore] she is critical of what is by comparison. She discerns the inevitable disparity between apparent and ultimate reality.'

Water archetype diagnosis

Every one of the Wŭ Xíng archetypes will, from time to time, become excess or deficient. In rare circumstances, they can be excess and deficient at the same time. Table 14.23 outlines some of the more commonly seen signs and symptoms for a Water archetype excess or deficiency. The signs and symptoms that are likely to be the same for excess and deficiency are at the bottom of the table in the merged rows.

Table 14.23 Water archetype – Excess/Shí and Deficiency/Xū signs and symptoms

Excess signs and symptoms	Deficiency signs and symptoms
Extremely critical, cynical, blunt, sarcastic, pessimistic, tactless, rash	Locks themselves away from the world
Constantly getting distracted from a task by anxiety and fear of failure	Constantly getting distracted from a task because they feel like giving up
Never shares anything; cagey, suspicious	Obsessively craves protection
Unforgiving	Dull, stupid, dim-witted
Superficial or deep	Thrifty, frugal, miserly
Quits when afraid	Feels abandoned
Anxious	Useless
Rarely finish what they start – likely to fall in an exhausted heap if they go to the trouble of finishing a task; alternatively, they never give up and keep searching, which still results in them rarely finishing what they start	Gives up – never completes anything
Outwardly covets/craves/yearns for what they don't or can't have	Inwardly covets/craves/yearns for what they don't or can't have
Appears preoccupied	Easily discouraged; lacks stamina
Voyeuristic	Soft/spineless
Fussy, precious, trivial	Likely to have a phobia of some kind, such as agoraphobia
Dishonest	
Forgetful	
Suspicious of everyone and everything	
Non-specific feeling of dread and foreboding	

How to communicate with a Water archetype

Regardless of the archetype, if you can speak their language, they will be much more amenable to you as a patient. A Water archetype would like you to:

- discuss the history and philosophy of Chinese medicine – how it came to be, how it's stayed pretty much the same (yet evolved massively) for the past 2000 years – and tweak their inherent curiosity to know more about Chinese medicine

- get them to use their willpower, determination and drive to enhance the success of treatment

- always tell the truth if you don't know the answer to something, as they will respect you more because of their honest nature – they will know if you're lying!

- suggest a few books or websites for them to enhance their knowledge base if they want to know more.

Water archetype treatment

I have listed a general treatment (Table 14.24) as well as ones specifically for an excess or deficient patient (Tables 14.25 and 14.26). These are just some of the many ways you can treat the Water archetype. In the end, it's up to you how you choose to treat your patient.

The general treatment is designed to regulate/balance the archetype. It will also act in a subtler, less intense manner, which can be a very good approach for some patients.

Table 14.24 Water archetype point combination – general[42]

Location of point	Point name	Reasoning
Trunk (front)	KI 22 GB 25 CV 3	Water point on the Kidney Spirit Gate Front Mù Collecting point of the Kidneys Front Mù Collecting point of the Urinary Bladder
Trunk (back)	BL 23 BL 28	Back Shù Transporting point of the Kidneys Back Shù Transporting point of the Urinary Bladder
Legs/feet	KI 3 KI 10 BL 40	Yuán Source point of the Kidneys Horary point (Water on Water) Lower Hé (Uniting) Sea point of the Urinary Bladder
Total points needled		15 points used bilaterally

Table 14.25 Water archetype point combination – excess[43]

Location of point	Point name	Reasoning
Head/face/neck	GV 20	Draws energy up into the head, Shén and Zhì [44]
Trunk (front)	GB 25 CV 3	Front Mù Collecting point of the Kidneys Front Mù Collecting point of the Urinary Bladder
Legs/feet	KI 1 KI 10 BL 65 BL 66	Child (sedating) point on the Kidney channel Horary point (Water on Water) Child (sedating) point on the Urinary Bladder channel Horary point (Water on Water)
Total points needled		12 points used bilaterally

Table 14.26 Water archetype point combination – deficiency[45]

Location of point	Point name	Reasoning
Head/face/neck	GV 20	Drops energy out of the head, Shén and Zhì[46]
Trunk (back)	BL 23 BL 28	Back Shù Transporting point of the Kidneys Back Shù Transporting point of the Urinary Bladder
Legs/feet	KI 7 KI 10 BL 66 BL 67	Mother (tonifying) point on the Kidney channel Horary point (Water on Water) Horary point (Water on Water) Mother (tonifying) point on the Urinary Bladder channel
Total points needled		13 points used bilaterally

Notes

1   Heraclitus (540–480 BCE) was a fascinating Greek philosopher – for the most part, because he refused to side with Greek ideals of the time. He was more than happy to rock the boat by, for example, suggesting that events that had occurred in a linear manner previously wouldn't continue to occur in a linear manner forevermore. He suggested that events were, quite often, cyclical. He was also famous because he thought that he could cure his tuberculosis (consumption) by covering himself in cow dung. It didn't work – he died – and he has been ridiculed ever since. Regardless, I find him an extraordinary philosopher. The quotation was retrieved from www.goodreads.com/author/quotes/77989.Heraclitus.

2   Lau 1979, p.73. Confucius or Kǒng Zǐ (551–479 BCE) has become one of the most famous philosophers of all time, Eastern or Western. He became so popular in Europe in the Middle Ages that Western society latinized his name so they could pronounce it better. His popularity came about because he never proclaimed himself to be a god, and nothing that he said went directly against Christian beliefs in Western countries, where Christianity was still the ruling power of thought. He is, in my view, one of the most remarkable men to have ever lived.

This quotation is from *The Analects*/Lún Yǔ, which was compiled somewhere between 400 and 300 BCE (definitely before the Han dynasty).

3   Ellis *et al.* 1989, pp.400, 403.

4   Although the concept of the Wǔ Xíng/Five Elements did originate somewhere between 1600 and 221 BCE, my research suggests that it wasn't until the Wǔ Xíng philosophical school was founded during the Warring States Period (472–221 BCE) that it was considered to be a legitimately developed theory.

5   Unschuld 2009, p.70.

6   Ibid., pp.23–24.

7   Furley 1999, pp.15–17. In my mind, Apeiron, or Aether, sounds a lot like Qì.

8   Maciocia 2009, pp.115–122. This is an excellent series of pages which looks into the origins/classics of the emotions and Wǔ Shén.

9   The Seven Emotions are traditional emotional states that were attributed to the organs and elements. The list in Table 14.1 includes additional emotions beyond the original seven. Chapter 11 is dedicated to the Seven Emotions.

10   Theoretically, the Heart Shén governs all of the emotions.

11   Beinfield and Korngold 1991, pp.131–159; Franglen 2014, pp.15–28; Hicks *et al.* 2010, pp.44–52.

12   In Chinese astrology, you are assigned an animal that represents the year of your birth. For example, I was born in 1973, which makes me an Ox. Further to that, in every 12-year cycle, the element shifts, so you are an animal plus an element. Using me as the example again, I am a Water Ox (Thompson 2012, pp.44–45). But I am not a Water archetype; my guardian element is Fire. An excellent Chinese Horoscope book is Thompson (2012). See the reference list for the full title.

13   Beinfield and Korngold 1991, pp.140–145, 160–175; Franglen 2014, pp.28–30, 45–46, 115–130, 150–151; Hicks *et al.* 2010, pp.53–77, 205–207, 269–288; Ross 1995, pp.21–24, 33–36.

14   Dechar 2006, pp.193–213.

15   What I mean here is that they make decisions quickly and decisively. They don't spend weeks, days or even hours making most decisions. They are made faster than for any other element archetype. But this doesn't make them impetuous; it just makes them focused and determined. Once they make the decision, they attack it with 100% commitment.

16   Wood archetypes like to be the first to do something. Therefore, if they reach a fork in the road, they will take the one less traveled. But if they think there is a chance that they will be the first to take a new path, then they will likely make a new fork in the road. This is both metaphorically and/or physically.

17   Hartmann 2009, p.172. KI 26 isn't part of the point combination in the reference, but it is still an excellent point to work on Wood element emotional and spiritual aspects. It is part of the Shén Mén Spirit Gate points (see Chapter 12, Section 8).

18   Deadman *et al.* 2007, pp.37–38, 437, 441–442, 455, 460, 473–475, 490–491.

19   Hicks *et al.* 2010, pp.279–280, 284–285.

20   Beinfield and Korngold 1991, pp.140–145, 176–189; Franglen 2014, pp.30–35, 45–46, 115–128, 130–132, 152–154; Hicks *et al.* 2010, pp.78–104, 205–208, 269–288; Ross 1995, pp.21–26.

21   Theoretically, the Heart Shén governs all of the emotions.

22   Dechar 2006, pp.169–192.

23   The Fire element has four channels/organs from which you can construct a baseline treatment. In the three acupuncture point combinations, I have offered a selection of points across the four channels, but these can be changed around quite a bit.

24   Hartmann 2009, p.64. KI 22, KI 25, BL 39 and ST 39 aren't part of the point combination in the reference. Having said that, they are all still very good points to regulate the Fire archetype.

25   Deadman *et al.* 2007, pp.37–38, 219–221, 236, 239, 336, 501, 514, 552–553.

26   Deadman *et al.* 2007, pp.42–43, 336–337, 553; Hicks *et al.* 2010, pp.279–280, 284–285, 321.

27   Beinfield and Korngold 1991, pp.140–145, 190–203; Franglen 2014, pp.35–37, 45–46, 115–128, 132–133, 155–157; Hicks *et al.* 2010,

pp.105–128, 205–206, 208–209, 269–288; Ross 1995, pp.21–24, 26–28.

28 Dechar 2006, pp.215–235.

29 Hartmann 2009, p.56. KI 23 isn't part of the point combination in the reference, but it is still an excellent point to work on Earth element emotional and spiritual aspects. It is part of the Shén Mén Spirit Gate points (see Chapter 12, Section 8).

30 Deadman *et al.* 2007, pp.37–38, 43, 136, 158, 172–173, 184, 188; Ellis *et al.* 1991, p.118.

31 Deadman *et al.* 2007, pp.43–44, 553; Hicks *et al.* 2010, pp.279–280, 284–286.

32 Beinfield and Korngold 1991, pp.140–145, 204–217; Franglen 2014, pp.37–41, 45–46, 115–128, 134–135, 158–160; Hicks *et al.* 2010, pp.129–151, 205–206, 209–210, 269–288; Ross 1995, pp.21–24, 28–31.

33 Dechar 2006, pp.237–272.

34 This is across the physical, mental and spiritual planes.

35 This is referring to someone who has the same views as them in most things they consider important.

36 Hartmann 2009, p.102. KI 24 and LU 1 aren't part of the point combination in the reference. Having said that, they are both still very good points to regulate the Metal archetype.

37 Deadman *et al.* 2007, pp.37–38, 86, 100, 267, 286, 336, 552–553.

38 When the Pò is Excess/Shí, it plummets into the earth as if you are wearing concrete boots. It doesn't rise up into the head as with Wood Shí, Fire Shí or Earth Shí.

39 Deadman *et al.* 2007, pp.43–44; Hicks *et al.* 2010, pp.279–280, 284–286; Ross 1995, pp.68–69.

40 Beinfield and Korngold 1991, pp.140–145, 218–231; Franglen 2014, pp.41–46, 115–128, 135–137, 161–162; Hicks *et al.* 2010, pp.152–177, 205–206, 210–211, 269–288; Ross 1995, pp.21–24, 32–33.

41 Dechar 2006, pp.273–293.

42 Hartmann 2009, p.170. KI 22, GB 25 and BL 40 aren't part of the point combination in the reference. Having said that, they are all still very good points to regulate the Water archetype.

43 Deadman *et al.* 2007, pp.43–44, 552–553; Hicks *et al.* 2010, pp.279–280, 284–286.

44 When the Zhì is Excess/Shí, it plunges into the earth like a high-powered waterfall. It doesn't rise up into the head as with Wood Shí, Fire Shí or Earth Shí.

45 Deadman *et al.* 2007, pp.42–43, 553; Hicks *et al.* 2010, pp.279–280, 284–285.

46 When the Zhì is Deficient/Xū, it rises up into the heavens like a hot-air balloon that is taking off from earth. It doesn't descend as with Wood Xū, Fire Xū or Earth Xū.

Appendix 1

Key Terms – English, Pīn Yīn and Traditional Chinese Characters

Term used in text	English term/name (if different)	Pīn Yīn 拼音 (if different)	Traditional Chinese characters
Ā Shì	Painful point/spot		阿是穴
Acupuncture point combinations		Zhēn Jiǔ Pèi Xué Fǎ	針灸配穴法
An Explanation of the Acupuncture Points		Jīng Xué Jiě	經穴解
Bā Liáo	Eight Crevices		八髎
Back Shù Transporting point			俞穴
Běn	Root		本
Bì	Painful obstruction syndrome		痺
Biāo	Manifestation		表
Blood		Xuè	血
Body fluid		Jīn Yè	津液
Celestial/Heavenly		Tiān	天
Channels and collaterals		Jīng Luò	經絡
Chéng/Overacting cycle			乘
Chǐ Mài	Proximal pulse		尺脈
Chōng Mài	Thoroughfare Vessel		衝脈
Cold Damp		Hán Shī	濕冷
Cold Damp in the Spleen		Pí Hán Shī	脾濕冷
Cold Damp in the Urinary Bladder		Páng Guāng Hán Shī	膀胱濕冷
Conception Vessel		Rèn Mài	任脈
Confucianism			孔子學說

cont.

Term used in text	English term/name (if different)	Pīn Yīn 拼音 (if different)	Traditional Chinese characters
Confucius		Kǒng Zǐ	孔子
Cùn	Inch (measurement)		寸
Cùn Mài	Distal pulse		寸脈
Dài Mài	Girdle Vessel		帶脈
Damp		Shī	濕
Damp Bì		Shī Bì	濕痺
Damp Heat		Shī Rè	濕熱
Damp Heat in the Liver and Gall Bladder		Gān Dǎn Shī Rè	肝膽濕熱
Damp Heat in the Spleen		Pí Shī Rè	脾濕熱
Damp Heat in the Urinary Bladder		Páng Guāng Shī Rè	膀胱濕熱
Dān Tián	Cinnabar Field		丹田
Dào	Path, road or way		道
Daoism			道學
Dé Qì	Obtaining Qì		得氣
Deficiency		Xū	虛
Dì	Earth		地
Diān Kuáng	Manic depression		癲狂
Dū Mài	Governing Vessel		督脈
Earth		Tǔ	土
Earth element		Tǔ Xíng	土行
Earth point		Tǔ Xué	土穴
Eight Extraordinary Vessels		Qí Jīng Bā Mài	奇經八脈
Emotions		Qíng	情
Emotions (Seven)		Qī Qíng	七情
Energizer		Jiāo	焦
Energy		Qì	氣
Essence		Jīng	精
Excess		Shí	实
External Pathogenic Factors	External diseases		
Figure Eight			八俞
Fire		Huǒ	火
Fire element		Huǒ Xíng	火行
Five Elements		Wǔ Xíng	五行
Five Shū/Transporting points		Wǔ Shū Xué	五俞穴

Term used in text	English term/name (if different)	Pīn Yīn 拼音 (if different)	Traditional Chinese characters
Four Gates		Sì Guān	四關
Front Mù Collecting point			募穴
Gall Bladder		Dǎn	膽
Gall Bladder Xū		Dǎn Xū	膽虛
Girdle Vessel		Dài Mài	帶脈
Governing Vessel		Dū Mài	督脈
Guān Mài	Border pulse		關脈
Hé (Uniting) Sea point			合穴
Heart		Xīn	心
Heart Fire Blazing		Xīn Huǒ Shàng Yán	心火上炎
Heart Qì Xū		Xīn Qì Xū	心氣虛
Heart Shén		Xīn Shén	心神
Heart Xuè Xū		Xīn Xuè Xū	心血虛
Heart Yáng Xū		Xīn Yáng Xū	心陽虛
Heart Yīn Xū		Xīn Yīn Xū	心陰虛
Heavenly/Celestial		Tiān	天
Horary point			
Huáng Dì Nèi Jīng	*Inner Canon of the Yellow Emperor*		黃帝內經
Huì Meeting point			會穴
Hún	Ethereal/Heavenly Soul		魂
Jiāo	Energizer		焦
Jiāo Huì Meeting/ Intersecting point			交會穴
Jīn Yè	Body fluid		津液
Jīng	Essence		精
Jīng Luò	Channels and collaterals		經絡
Jīng River point			經穴
Jīng Well point			井穴
Jué Yīn	Terminal Yīn		厥陰
Jūn Zǐ	Perfect person		君子
Kè/Controlling cycle			剋
Kidney Jīng Xū	Kidney Essence deficiency	Shèn Jīng Xū	腎精虛
Kidney Xū		Shèn Xū	腎虛
Kidney Yáng Xū		Shèn Yáng Xū	腎陽虛

cont.

Term used in text	English term/name (if different)	Pīn Yīn 拼音 (if different)	Traditional Chinese characters
Kidney Yīn Xū		Shèn Yīn Xū	腎陰虛
Kidneys		Shèn	腎
Large Intestine		Dà Cháng	大腸
Large Intestine Dry		Dà Cháng Zào	大腸燥
Large Intestine Fire Blazing		Dà Cháng Huǒ Shàng Yán	大腸火上炎
Large Intestine Heat		Dà Cháng Rè	大腸熱
Líng Shū	*The Spiritual Pivot*		靈樞
Liver		Gān	肝
Liver Fire Blazing		Gān Huǒ Shàng Yán	肝火上炎
Liver Heat		Gān Rè	肝熱
Liver Qì Invading the Stomach		Gān Qì Fàn Wèi	肝氣犯胃
Liver Qì Rebellion		Gān Qì Shàng Nì	肝氣上逆
Liver Qì Stagnation		Gān Qì Zhì	肝氣滯
Liver Wind		Gān Fēng	肝風
Liver Xuè Xū	Liver Blood deficiency	Gān Xuè Xū	肝血虛
Liver Yáng Rising		Gān Yáng Shàng Kàng	肝陽上亢
Liver Yīn Xū		Gān Yīn Xū	肝陰虛
Lower Hé (Uniting) Sea point			下合溪穴
Lower Jiāo		Xià Jiāo	下焦
Lung Dryness		Fèi Zào	肺燥
Lung Heat		Fèi Rè	肺熱
Lung Qì Xū		Fèi Qì Xū	肺氣虛
Lung Yīn Xū		Fèi Yīn Xū	肺陰虛
Lungs		Fèi	肺
Luò Connecting point			絡穴
Manic depression		Diān Kuáng	癲狂
Manifestation		Biāo	表
Mencius		Mèng Zǐ	孟子
Metal		Jīn	金
Metal element		Jīn Xíng	金行
Middle Jiāo		Zhōng Jiāo	中焦
Original/Yuán Qì		Yuán Qì	原氣
Painful obstruction syndrome		Bì	痺
Painful Urinary Dysfunction		Lín Zhèng	淋症

Term used in text	English term/name (if different)	Pīn Yīn 拼音 (if different)	Traditional Chinese characters
Pericardium		Xīn Bāo	心包
Phlegm		Tán	痰
Phlegm Accumulation		Tán Jī	痰積
Pīn Yīn			拼音
Plum-stone throat		Méi Hé Qì	梅核氣
Pò	Corporeal/Grounded Soul		魄
Point combinations		Zhēn Jiǔ Pèi Xué Fǎ	針灸配穴法
Post-Heaven		Hòu Tiān	後天
Pre-Heaven		Xiān Tiān	先天
Pre-Heaven Intellect		Xiān Tiān Zhī Yì	先天之意
Primary/Yuán Yáng		Yuán Yáng	原陽
Primary/Yuán Yīn		Yuán Yīn	原陰
Qì	Energy[1]		氣
Qì Gōng	Chinese exercise		氣功
Qí Jīng Bā Mài	Eight Extraordinary Vessels		奇經八脈
Qī Qíng	Seven Emotions		七情
Qì Rebellion		Qì Shàng Nì	氣上逆
Qì Sinking		Qì Xià Xiàn	氣下陷
Qì Stagnation		Qì Zhì	氣滯
Qì Xū			氣虛
Rén	Human being		人
Rèn Mài	Conception Vessel		任脈
Root		Běn	本
Sage		Jūn Zǐ	君子
Sān Jiāo	Triple Energizer		三焦
Sān Jiāo not Communicating			三焦不通
Seven Emotions		Qī Qíng	七情
Shāng Hán Lùn	*Treatise on Cold Injury*		傷寒論
Shào Yáng	Lesser Yáng		少陽
Shào Yīn	Lesser Yīn		少陰
Shén	Spirit/mind		神
Shén Mén/Spirit Gate			神門
Shén points		Shén Xué	神穴
Shēng/Generating cycle			生
Shí	Excess		实

cont.

Term used in text	English term/name (if different)	Pīn Yīn 拼音 (if different)	Traditional Chinese characters
Shù (Transport) Stream point			輸穴
Shū/Transporting points		Shū Xué	俞穴
Six Divisions		Liù Jīng	六經
Small Intestine		Xiǎo Cháng	小腸
Small Intestine Fire Blazing		Xiǎo Cháng Huǒ Shàng Yán	小腸火上炎
Small Intestine Yáng Xū		Xiǎo Cháng Yáng Xū	小腸陽虛
Spirit Gate/Shén Mén			神門
Spleen		Pí	脾
Spleen Damp		Pí Shī	脾濕
Spleen Invaded by Liver Qì		Gān Qì Fàn Pí	肝氣犯脾
Spleen Qì Sinking		Pí Qì Xià Xiàn	脾氣下陷
Spleen Qì Xū		Pí Qì Xū	脾氣虛
Spleen Xuè Xū	Spleen Blood deficiency	Pí Xuè Xū	脾血虛
Spleen Yáng Xū		Pí Yáng Xū	脾陽虛
Spring and Autumn Period			春秋
Stagnation		Zhì	滯
Stomach		Wèi	胃
Stomach Fire Blazing		Wèi Huǒ Shàng Yán	胃火上炎
Stomach Qì Rebellion		Wèi Qì Shàng Nì	胃氣上逆
Stomach Qì Xū		Wèi Qì Xū	胃氣虛
Stomach Yáng Xū		Wèi Yáng Xū	胃陽虛
Stomach Yīn Xū		Wèi Yīn Xū	胃陰虛
Sūn Sī Miǎo Ghost points			孫思邈鬼穴
Tài Jí Quán	Chinese exercise		太極拳
Tài Yáng	Greater Yáng		太陽
Tài Yīn	Greater Yīn		太陰
The Classic of Difficulties	*Canon of the Yellow Emperor's Eighty-One Difficult Issues*	Huáng Dì Bā Shí Yī Nán Jīng	黃帝八十一難經
The Classic of Supporting Life	*The Classic of Supporting Life with Acupuncture and Moxibustion*	Zhēn Jiǔ Zī Shēng Jīng	針灸資生經

Term used in text	English term/name (if different)	Pīn Yīn 拼音 (if different)	Traditional Chinese characters
The Classic of the Jade Dragon	*Bian Que's Spiritual Guide to Acupuncture and Moxibustion, Jade Dragon Classic*	Biǎn Què Shēn Yīng Zhēn Jiǔ Yù Lóng Jīng	扁鵲神應針灸玉龍經
The Great Compendium – Volume V	*The Great Compendium of Acupuncture and Moxibustion*	Zhēn Jiǔ Dà Chéng	針灸大成. 第5卷
The Great Compendium – Volume VIII	*The Great Compendium of Acupuncture and Moxibustion*	Zhēn Jiǔ Dà Chéng	針灸大成. 第8卷
The Spiritual Pivot		Líng Shū	靈樞
The Yellow Emperor's Classic	*Inner Canon of the Yellow Emperor*	Huáng Dì Nèi Jīng	黃帝内經
Thoroughfare Vessel		Chōng Mài	衝脈
Three Powers		Tiān Dì Rén	天地人
Three Regions		Tiān Dì Rén	天地人
Throat Painful Obstruction		Hóu Bì	喉痛
Tiān	Heavenly/Celestial		天
Tiān Dì Rén²	Heaven, Earth, Human		天地人
Tiān Mìng	Heavenly Mandate		天命
Tiān points		Tiān Xué	天穴
Treatise on Cold Injury		Shāng Hán Lùn	傷寒論
Triangle of Power/ Influence		Sān Jiāo Lì	三角影響力
Triple Energizer		Sān Jiāo	三焦
Tuī Ná	Chinese massage		推拿
Upper Jiāo		Shàng Jiāo	上焦
Urinary Bladder		Páng Guāng	膀胱
Visual Dizziness		Mù Xuàn	目眩
Vital Substances			
Warring States Period			戰國
Water		Shuǐ	水
Water element		Shuǐ Xíng	水行
Wèi Qì	Defensive energy		衛氣
Wind		Fēng	風
Wind Cold		Fēng Hán	風濕
Wind Damp		Fēng Shī	風冷
Wind External/ Exterior		Fēng Biǎo	風錶

cont.

Term used in text	English term/name (if different)	Pīn Yīn 拼音 (if different)	Traditional Chinese characters
Wind Heat		Fēng Rè	風熱
Wind Stroke/Wind Strike		Zhōng Fēng	中風
Window of Heaven/Windows of the Sky		Tiān Chuāng	天窗穴
Wood		Mù	木
Wood element		Mù Xíng	木行
Wǔ Shén	Five Spirits		五神
Wǔ Wèi	Non-action		五味
Wǔ Xíng	Five Elements		五行
Wǔ/Insulting cycle			侮
Xì Cleft point			郄穴
Xū	Deficiency		虛
Xuè	Blood		血
Xuè Stasis	Blood stasis	Xuè Yū	血瘀
Xuè Xū	Blood deficiency		血虛
Yáng	Sunny side of a hill		陽
Yáng channels		Yáng Jīng	陽經
Yáng Míng	Bright Yáng		陽明
Yáng Míng Fire Blazing		Yáng Míng Huǒ Shàng Yán	陽明火上炎
Yáng Qiāo Mài	Yáng Heel Vessel		陽蹺脈
Yáng Rising		Yáng Shàng Kàng	陽上亢
Yáng Shí			陽实
Yáng Wéi Mài	Yáng Linking Vessel		陽維脈
Yáng Xū			陽虛
Yì	Thought		意
Yīn	Shady side of a hill		陰
Yīn channels		Yīn Jīng	陰經
Yīn Qiāo Mài	Yīn Heel Vessel		陰蹺脈
Yīn Wéi Mài	Yīn Linking Vessel		陰維脈
Yīn Xū			陰虛
Yíng Spring point			榮穴
Yuán Qì	Original energy		原氣
Yuán Source point			原穴
Zàng Fǔ organs		Zàng Fǔ	臟腑
Zàng Fǔ patterns		Zàng Fǔ Biàn Zhèng	臟腑不和辨証分型
Zhēn Qì	True energy		貞氣

Term used in text	English term/name (if different)	Pīn Yīn 拼音 (if different)	Traditional Chinese characters
Zhèng Qì	Upright energy		宗氣
Zhì	Stagnation		滯
Zhì	Willpower		志
Zhōu dynasty			周朝

Notes

1   'Energy' is a very poor English translation of Qì. Ellis *et al.* (1989, p.385) translate it as gas, smell, breath, weather, manner, air and the active aspect of matter in the body. I have translated it as energy because I find that most people understand energy, which, by default, means they understand Qì.

2   Tiān Dì Rén is typically translated as Heaven, Earth, Human. However, they are also referred to as the Three Powers and the Three Regions – just to make it confusing.

Appendix 2

Acupuncture Point Terms – English, Pīn Yīn and Traditional Chinese Characters

Term used in text	English term/name	Pīn Yīn 拼音	Traditional Chinese characters
BL 1	Urinary Bladder 1	Jīng Míng	睛明
BL 2	Urinary Bladder 2	Cuàn Zhú	攢竹
BL 7	Urinary Bladder 7	Tōng Tiān	通天
BL 8	Urinary Bladder 8	Luò Què	絡卻
BL 9	Urinary Bladder 9	Yù Zhěn	玉枕
BL 10	Urinary Bladder 10	Tiān Zhù	天柱
BL 11	Urinary Bladder 11	Dà Zhù	大杼
BL 12	Urinary Bladder 12	Fēng Mén	風門
BL 13	Urinary Bladder 13	Fèi Shū	肺俞
BL 14	Urinary Bladder 14	Jué Yīn Shū	厥陰俞
BL 15	Urinary Bladder 15	Xīn Shū	心俞
BL 16	Urinary Bladder 16	Dū Shū	督俞
BL 17	Urinary Bladder 17	Gé Shū	隔俞
BL 18	Urinary Bladder 18	Gān Shū	肝俞
BL 19	Urinary Bladder 19	Dǎn Shū	膽俞
BL 20	Urinary Bladder 20	Pí Shū	脾俞
BL 21	Urinary Bladder 21	Wèi Shū	胃俞
BL 22	Urinary Bladder 22	Sān Jiāo Shū	三焦俞
BL 23	Urinary Bladder 23	Shèn Shū	腎俞
BL 24	Urinary Bladder 24	Qì Hǎi Shū	氣海俞
BL 25	Urinary Bladder 25	Dà Cháng Shū	大腸俞
BL 26	Urinary Bladder 26	Guān Yuán Shū	關元俞
BL 27	Urinary Bladder 27	Xiǎo Cháng Shū	小腸俞
BL 28	Urinary Bladder 28	Páng Guāng Shū	膀胱俞

cont.

Term used in text	English term/name	Pīn Yīn 拼音	Traditional Chinese characters
BL 29	Urinary Bladder 29	Zhōng Lǔ Shū	中膂俞
BL 30	Urinary Bladder 30	Bái Huán Shū	白環俞
BL 32	Urinary Bladder 32	Cì Liáo	次髎
BL 36	Urinary Bladder 36	Chéng Fú	承扶
BL 37	Urinary Bladder 37	Yīn Mén	殷門
BL 39	Urinary Bladder 39	Wěi Yáng	委陽
BL 40	Urinary Bladder 40	Wěi Zhōng	委中
BL 41	Urinary Bladder 41	Fù Fēn	附分
BL 42	Urinary Bladder 42	Pò Hù	魄戶
BL 43	Urinary Bladder 43	Gāo Huāng Shū	膏肓俞
BL 44	Urinary Bladder 44	Shén Táng	神堂
BL 46	Urinary Bladder 46	Gé Guān	膈關
BL 47	Urinary Bladder 47	Hún Mén	魄門
BL 49	Urinary Bladder 49	Yì Shè	意舍
BL 50	Urinary Bladder 50	Wèi Cāng	胃倉
BL 52	Urinary Bladder 52	Zhì Shì	志室
BL 53	Urinary Bladder 53	Bāo Huāng	胞肓
BL 54	Urinary Bladder 54	Zhì Biān	秩邊
BL 55	Urinary Bladder 55	Hé Yáng	合陽
BL 56	Urinary Bladder 56	Chéng Jīn	承筋
BL 57	Urinary Bladder 57	Chéng Shān	承山
BL 58	Urinary Bladder 58	Fēi Yáng	飛陽
BL 59	Urinary Bladder 59	Fū Yáng	跗陽
BL 60	Urinary Bladder 60	Kūn Lún	昆侖
BL 61	Urinary Bladder 61	Pú Cān	僕參
BL 62	Urinary Bladder 62	Shēn Mài	申脈
BL 63	Urinary Bladder 63	Jīn Mén	金門
BL 64	Urinary Bladder 64	Jīng Gǔ	京骨
BL 65	Urinary Bladder 65	Shù Gǔ	束骨
BL 66	Urinary Bladder 66	Zú Tōng Gǔ	足通谷
BL 67	Urinary Bladder 67	Zhì Yīn	至陰
CV 1	Conception Vessel 1	Huì Yīn	會陰
CV 2	Conception Vessel 2	Qū Gǔ	曲骨
CV 3	Conception Vessel 3	Zhōng Jí	中極
CV 4	Conception Vessel 4	Guān Yuán	關元
CV 5	Conception Vessel 5	Shí Mén	石門
CV 6	Conception Vessel 6	Qì Hǎi	氣海

Term used in text	English term/name	Pīn Yīn 拼音	Traditional Chinese characters
CV 8	Conception Vessel 8	Shén Què	神闕
CV 9	Conception Vessel 9	Shuī Fēn	水分
CV 12	Conception Vessel 12	Zhōng Wǎn	中脘
CV 14	Conception Vessel 14	Jù Què	巨闕
CV 15	Conception Vessel 15	Jiū Wěi	鳩尾
CV 17	Conception Vessel 17	Dàn Zhōng[1]	膻中
CV 18	Conception Vessel 18	Yù Táng	玉堂
CV 19	Conception Vessel 19	Zǐ Gōng	紫宮
CV 21	Conception Vessel 21	Xuán Jī	璇機
CV 22	Conception Vessel 22	Tiān Tú	天突
CV 23	Conception Vessel 23	Lián Quán	廉泉
CV 24	Conception Vessel 24	Chéng Jiāng	承漿
GB 1	Gall Bladder 1	Tóng Zǐ Liáo	瞳子髎
GB 2	Gall Bladder 2	Tīng Huì	聽會
GB 8	Gall Bladder 8	Shuài Gǔ	率谷
GB 9	Gall Bladder 9	Tiān Chōng	天沖
GB 12	Gall Bladder 12	Wán Gǔ	完骨
GB 13	Gall Bladder 13	Běn Shén	本神
GB 14	Gall Bladder 14	Yáng Bái	陽白
GB 15	Gall Bladder 15	Tóu Lín Qì	頭臨泣
GB 18	Gall Bladder 18	Chéng Líng	承靈
GB 20	Gall Bladder 20	Fēng Chí	風池
GB 21	Gall Bladder 21	Jiān Jǐng	肩井
GB 24	Gall Bladder 24	Rì Yuè	日月
GB 25	Gall Bladder 25	Jīng Mén	京門
GB 26	Gall Bladder 26	Dài Mài	帶脈
GB 27	Gall Bladder 27	Wǔ Shū	五樞
GB 28	Gall Bladder 28	Wéi Dào	維道
GB 29	Gall Bladder 29	Jū Liáo	居髎
GB 30	Gall Bladder 30	Huán Tiào	環跳
GB 31	Gall Bladder 31	Fēng Shì	風市
GB 33	Gall Bladder 33	Xī Yáng Guān	膝陽關
GB 34	Gall Bladder 34	Yáng Líng Quán	陽陵泉
GB 35	Gall Bladder 35	Yáng Jiāo	陽交
GB 36	Gall Bladder 36	Wài Qiū	外丘
GB 37	Gall Bladder 37	Guāng Míng	光明
GB 38	Gall Bladder 38	Yáng Fǔ	陽輔
GB 39	Gall Bladder 39	Xuán Zhōng	懸鐘

cont.

Term used in text	English term/name	Pīn Yīn 拼音	Traditional Chinese characters
GB 40	Gall Bladder 40	Qiū Xū	丘墟
GB 41	Gall Bladder 41	Zú Lín Qì	足臨泣
GB 42	Gall Bladder 42	Dì Wǔ Huì	地五會
GB 43	Gall Bladder 43	Xiá Xī	俠谿
GB 44	Gall Bladder 44	Zú Qiào Yīn	足竅陰
GV 1	Governing Vessel 1	Cháng Qiáng	長強
GV 3	Governing Vessel 3	Yāo Yáng Guān	腰陽關
GV 4	Governing Vessel 4	Mìng Mén	命門
GV 7	Governing Vessel 7	Zhōng Shū	中樞
GV 8	Governing Vessel 8	Jīn Suō	筋縮
GV 9	Governing Vessel 9	Zhì Yáng	至陽
GV 10	Governing Vessel 10	Líng Tái	靈台
GV 11	Governing Vessel 11	Shén Dào	神道
GV 12	Governing Vessel 12	Shēn Zhù	身柱
GV 13	Governing Vessel 13	Táo Dào	陶道
GV 14	Governing Vessel 14	Dà Zhuī	大椎
GV 15	Governing Vessel 15	Yǎ Mén	啞門
GV 16	Governing Vessel 16	Fēng Fǔ	風府
GV 20	Governing Vessel 20	Bǎi Huì	百會
GV 23	Governing Vessel 23	Shàng Xīng	上星
GV 24	Governing Vessel 24	Shén Tíng	神庭
GV 26	Governing Vessel 26	Shuǐ Gōu	水溝
HT 1	Heart 1	Jí Quán	極泉
HT 2	Heart 2	Qīng Líng	青靈
HT 3	Heart 3	Shào Hǎi	少海
HT 4	Heart 4	Líng Dào	靈道
HT 5	Heart 5	Tōng Lǐ	通里
HT 6	Heart 6	Yīn Xī	陰郄
HT 7	Heart 7	Shén Mén	神門
HT 8	Heart 8	Shào Fǔ	少府
HT 9	Heart 9	Shào Chōng	少沖
KI 1	Kidney 1	Yǒng Quán	湧泉
KI 2	Kidney 2	Rán Gǔ	然谷
KI 3	Kidney 3	Tài Xī	太谿
KI 4	Kidney 4	Dà Zhōng	大鐘
KI 5	Kidney 5	Shuǐ Quán	水泉
KI 6	Kidney 6	Zhào Hǎi	照海
KI 7	Kidney 7	Fù Liū	復溜

Term used in text	English term/name	Pīn Yīn 拼音	Traditional Chinese characters
KI 8	Kidney 8	Jiāo Xìn	交信
KI 9	Kidney 9	Zhú Bīn	築賓
KI 10	Kidney 10	Yīn Gǔ	陰谷
KI 11	Kidney 11	Héng Gǔ	橫骨
KI 12	Kidney 12	Dà Hè	大赫
KI 13	Kidney 13	Qì Xuè	氣穴
KI 14	Kidney 14	Sì Mǎn	四滿
KI 16	Kidney 16	Huāng Shū	肓俞
KI 18	Kidney 18	Shí Guān	石關
KI 19	Kidney 19	Yīn Dū	陰都
KI 21	Kidney 21	Yōu Mén	幽門
KI 22	Kidney 22	Bù Láng	步廊
KI 23	Kidney 23	Shén Fēng	神封
KI 24	Kidney 24	Líng Xū	靈墟
KI 25	Kidney 25	Shén Cáng	神藏
KI 26	Kidney 26	Yù Zhōng	彧中
KI 27	Kidney 27	Shū Fǔ	俞府
LI 1	Large Intestine 1	Shāng Yáng	商陽
LI 2	Large Intestine 2	Èr Jiān	二間
LI 3	Large Intestine 3	Sān Jiān	三間
LI 4	Large Intestine 4	Hé Gǔ	合谷
LI 5	Large Intestine 5	Yáng Xī	陽谿
LI 6	Large Intestine 6	Piān Lì	偏歷
LI 7	Large Intestine 7	Wēn Liù	溫溜
LI 8	Large Intestine 8	Xià Lián	下廉
LI 9	Large Intestine 9	Shàng Lián	上廉
LI 10	Large Intestine 10	Shǒu Sān Lǐ	手三里
LI 11	Large Intestine 11	Qū Chí	曲池
LI 12	Large Intestine 12	Zhǒu Liáo	肘髎
LI 14	Large Intestine 14	Bì Nào	臂臑
LI 15	Large Intestine 15	Jiān Yú	肩髃
LI 17	Large Intestine 17	Tiān Dǐng	天鼎
LI 18	Large Intestine 18	Fú Tú	扶突
LI 20	Large Intestine 20	Yíng Xiāng	迎香
LR 1	Liver 1	Dà Dūn	大敦
LR 2	Liver 2	Xíng Jiān	行間
LR 3	Liver 3	Tài Chōng	太沖
LR 4	Liver 4	Zhōng Fēng	中封

cont.

Term used in text	English term/name	Pīn Yīn 拼音	Traditional Chinese characters
LR 5	Liver 5	Lǐ Gōu	蠡溝
LR 6	Liver 6	Zhōng Dū	中都
LR 8	Liver 8	Qū Quán	曲泉
LR 9	Liver 9	Yīn Bāo	陰包
LR 11	Liver 11	Yīn Lián	陰廉
LR 13	Liver 13	Zhāng Mén	章門
LR 14	Liver 14	Qí Mén	期門
LU 1	Lung 1	Zhōng Fǔ	中府
LU 2	Lung 2	Yún Mén	雲門
LU 3	Lung 3	Tiān Fǔ	天府
LU 4	Lung 4	Xiá Bái	俠白
LU 5	Lung 5	Chǐ Zé	尺澤
LU 6	Lung 6	Kǒng Zuì	孔最
LU 7	Lung 7	Liè Quē	列缺
LU 8	Lung 8	Jīng Qú	經渠
LU 9	Lung 9	Tài Yuān	太淵
LU 10	Lung 10	Yú Jì	魚際
LU 11	Lung 11	Shào Shāng	少商
M-BW-1 (Dìng Chuǎn)	Miscellaneous-Back and Waist-1	Dìng Chuǎn	定喘
M-BW-35 (Huá Tuó Jiā Jǐ)	Miscellaneous-Back and Waist-35	Huá Tuó Jiā Jǐ	華佗夾脊
M-CA-18 (Zǐ Gōng)	Miscellaneous-Chest and Abdomen-18	Zǐ Gōng	子宮
M-HN-1 (Sì Shén Cōng)	Miscellaneous-Head and Neck-1	Sì Shén Cōng	四神聰
M-HN-3 (Yìn Táng)	Miscellaneous-Head and Neck-3	Yìn Táng	印堂
M-HN-8 (Qiú Hòu)	Miscellaneous-Head and Neck-8	Qiú Hòu	球后
M-HN-9 (Tài Yáng)	Miscellaneous-Head and Neck-9	Tài Yáng	太陽
M-HN-14 (Bí Tōng)	Miscellaneous-Head and Neck-14	Bí Tōng	鼻通
M-HN-30 (Bǎi Láo)	Miscellaneous-Head and Neck-30	Bǎi Láo	百勞
M-HN-37 (Hǎi Quán)	Miscellaneous-Head and Neck-37	Hǎi Quán	海泉

Term used in text	English term/name	Pīn Yīn 拼音	Traditional Chinese characters
MN-LE-16 (Xī Yǎn)	Miscellaneous/New-Lower Extremity-16	Xī Yǎn	膝眼
M-LE-27 (Hè Dǐng)	Miscellaneous-Lower Extremity-27	Hè Dǐng	鶴頂
M-LE-34 (Bǎi Chóng Wō)	Miscellaneous-Lower Extremity-34	Bǎi Chóng Wō	百蟲窩
M-UE-1 (Shí Xuān)	Miscellaneous-Upper Extremity-1	Shí Xuān	十宣
M-UE-24 (Luò Zhěn)	Miscellaneous-Upper Extremity-24	Luò Zhěn	落枕
M-UE-29 (Èr Bái)	Miscellaneous-Upper Extremity-29	Èr Bái	二白
M-UE-48 (Jiān Qián)	Miscellaneous-Upper Extremity-48	Jiān Qián	肩前
N-HN-54 (Ān Mián)	New-Head and Neck-54	Ān Mián	安眠
N-UE-14 (Nào Shàng)	New-Upper Extremity-14	Nào Shàng	臑上
N-UE-19 (Yāo Tòng Xué)	New-Upper Extremity-19	Yāo Tòng Xué	腰痛穴
PC 1	Pericardium 1	Tiān Chí	天池
PC 2	Pericardium 2	Tiān Quán	天泉
PC 3	Pericardium 3	Qū Zé	曲澤
PC 4	Pericardium 4	Xī Mén	郄門
PC 5	Pericardium 5	Jiān Shǐ	間使
PC 6	Pericardium 6	Nèi Guān	內關
PC 7	Pericardium 7	Dà Líng	大陵
PC 8	Pericardium 8	Láo Gōng	勞宮
PC 9	Pericardium 9	Zhōng Chōng	中沖
SI 1	Small Intestine 1	Shào Zé	少澤
SI 2	Small Intestine 2	Qián Gǔ	前谷
SI 3	Small Intestine 3	Hòu Xī	後谿
SI 4	Small Intestine 4	Wàn Gǔ	腕骨
SI 5	Small Intestine 5	Yáng Gǔ	陽谷
SI 6	Small Intestine 6	Yǎng Lǎo	養老
SI 7	Small Intestine 7	Zhī Zhèng	支正
SI 8	Small Intestine 8	Xiǎo Hǎi	小海

cont.

Term used in text	English term/name	Pīn Yīn 拼音	Traditional Chinese characters
SI 9	Small Intestine 9	Jiān Zhēn	肩貞
SI 10	Small Intestine 10	Nào Shū	臑俞
SI 11	Small Intestine 11	Tiān Zōng	天宗
SI 14	Small Intestine 14	Jiān Wài Shū	肩外俞
SI 15	Small Intestine 15	Jiān Zhōng Shū	肩中俞
SI 16	Small Intestine 16	Tiān Chuāng	天窗
SI 17	Small Intestine 17	Tiān Róng	天容
SI 19	Small Intestine 19	Tīng Gōng	聽宮
SP 1	Spleen 1	Yǐn Bái	隱白
SP 2	Spleen 2	Dà Dū	大都
SP 3	Spleen 3	Tài Bái	太白
SP 4	Spleen 4	Gōng Sūn	公孫
SP 5	Spleen 5	Shāng Qiū	商丘
SP 6	Spleen 6	Sān Yīn Jiāo	三陰交
SP 8	Spleen 8	Dì Jī	地機
SP 9	Spleen 9	Yīn Líng Quán	陰陵泉
SP 10	Spleen 10	Xuè Hǎi	血海
SP 11	Spleen 11	Jī Mén	箕門
SP 13	Spleen 13	Fǔ Shè	府舍
SP 15	Spleen 15	Dà Héng	大橫
SP 18	Spleen 18	Tiān Xī	天谿
SP 20	Spleen 20	Zhōu Róng	周榮
SP 21	Spleen 21	Dà Bāo	大包
ST 1	Stomach 1	Chéng Qì	承泣
ST 2	Stomach 2	Sì Bái	四百
ST 3	Stomach 3	Jù Liáo	巨髎
ST 4	Stomach 4	Dì Cāng	地倉
ST 6	Stomach 6	Jiá Chē	頰車
ST 8	Stomach 8	Tóu Wéi	頭維
ST 9	Stomach 9	Rén Yíng	人迎
ST 11	Stomach 11	Qì Shè	氣舍
ST 12	Stomach 12	Quē Pén	缺盆
ST 18	Stomach 18	Rǔ Gēn	乳根
ST 21	Stomach 21	Liáng Mén	梁門
ST 25	Stomach 25	Tiān Shū	天樞
ST 28	Stomach 28	Shuǐ Dào	水道
ST 30	Stomach 30	Qì Chōng	氣沖
ST 31	Stomach 31	Bì Guān	髀關

Term used in text	English term/name	Pīn Yīn 拼音	Traditional Chinese characters
ST 32	Stomach 32	Fú Tù	伏兔
ST 34	Stomach 34	Liáng Qiū	梁丘
ST 35	Stomach 35	Dú Bí	犢鼻
ST 36	Stomach 36	Zú Sān Lǐ	足三里
ST 37	Stomach 37	Shàng Jù Xū	上巨虛
ST 38	Stomach 38	Tiáo Kǒu	條口
ST 39	Stomach 39	Xià Jù Xū	下巨虛
ST 40	Stomach 40	Fēng Lóng	豐隆
ST 41	Stomach 41	Jiě Xī	解溪
ST 42	Stomach 42	Chōng Yáng	沖陽
ST 43	Stomach 43	Xiàn Gǔ	陷谷
ST 44	Stomach 44	Nèi Tíng	內庭
ST 45	Stomach 45	Lì Duì	厲兌
TE 1	Sān Jiāo 1	Guān Chōng	關沖
TE 2	Sān Jiāo 2	Yè Mén	液門
TE 3	Sān Jiāo 3	Zhōng Zhǔ	中渚
TE 4	Sān Jiāo 4	Yáng Chí	陽池
TE 5	Sān Jiāo 5	Wài Guān	外關
TE 6	Sān Jiāo 6	Zhī Gōu	支溝
TE 7	Sān Jiāo 7	Huì Zōng	會宗
TE 8	Sān Jiāo 8	Sān Yáng Luò	三陽絡
TE 9	Sān Jiāo 9	Sì Dú	四瀆
TE 10	Sān Jiāo 10	Tiān Jǐng	天井
TE 13	Sān Jiāo 13	Nào Huì	臑會
TE 14	Sān Jiāo 14	Jiān Liáo	肩髎
TE 15	Sān Jiāo 15	Tiān Liáo	天髎
TE 16	Sān Jiāo 16	Tiān Yǒu	天牖
TE 17	Sān Jiāo 17	Yì Fēng	翳風
TE 21	Sān Jiāo 21	Ěr Mén	耳門
TE 23	Sān Jiāo 23	Sī Zhú Kōng	絲竹空

Note

1   CV 17 has at least three different Pīn Yīn names in the current literature. Dàn Zhōng is the name designated for use by WHO in the Western Pacific region, which includes Australia. The other two commonly used Pīn Yīn names are Tán Zhōng (pretty much obsolete now) and Shān Zhōng.

Appendix 3

Acupuncture Point Terms – Pīn Yīn, English and Traditional Chinese Characters

Pīn Yīn 拼音	Term used in the text	English term/name	Traditional Chinese characters
Ān Mián	N-HN-54 (Ān Mián)	New-Head and Neck-54	安眠
Bǎi Chóng Wō	M-LE-34 (Bǎi Chóng Wō)	Miscellaneous-Lower Extremity-34	百蟲窩
Bái Huán Shū	BL 30	Urinary Bladder 30	白環俞
Bǎi Huì	GV 20	Governing Vessel 20	百會
Bǎi Láo	M-HN-30 (Bǎi Láo)	Miscellaneous-Head and Neck-30	百勞
Bāo Huāng	BL 53	Urinary Bladder 53	胞肓
Běn Shén	GB 13	Gall Bladder 13	本神
Bì Guān	ST 31	Stomach 31	髀關
Bì Nào	LI 14	Large Intestine 14	臂臑
Bí Tōng	M-HN-14 (Bí Tōng)	Miscellaneous-Head and Neck-14	鼻通
Bù Láng	KI 22	Kidney 22	步廊
Cháng Qiáng	GV 1	Governing Vessel 1	長強
Chéng Fú	BL 36	Urinary Bladder 36	承扶
Chéng Jiāng	CV 24	Conception Vessel 24	承漿
Chéng Jīn	BL 56	Urinary Bladder 56	承筋
Chéng Líng	GB 18	Gall Bladder 18	承靈
Chéng Qì	ST 1	Stomach 1	承泣
Chéng Shān	BL 57	Urinary Bladder 57	承山
Chǐ Zé	LU 5	Lung 5	尺澤
Chōng Yáng	ST 42	Stomach 42	沖陽
Cì Liáo	BL 32	Urinary Bladder 32	次髎
Cuàn Zhú	BL 2	Urinary Bladder 2	攢竹

Pīn Yīn 拼音	Term used in the text	English term/name	Traditional Chinese characters
Dà Bāo	SP 21	Spleen 21	大包
Dà Cháng Shū	BL 25	Urinary Bladder 25	大腸俞
Dà Dū	SP 2	Spleen 2	大都
Dà Dūn	LR 1	Liver 1	大敦
Dà Hè	KI 12	Kidney 12	大赫
Dà Héng	SP 15	Spleen 15	大橫
Dà Líng	PC 7	Pericardium 7	大陵
Dà Zhōng	KI 4	Kidney 4	大鐘
Dà Zhù	BL 11	Urinary Bladder 11	大杼
Dà Zhuī	GV 14	Governing Vessel 14	大椎
Dài Mài	GB 26	Gall Bladder 26	帶脈
Dǎn Shū	BL 19	Urinary Bladder 19	膽俞
Dàn Zhōng[1]	CV 17	Conception Vessel 17	膻中
Dì Cāng	ST 4	Stomach 4	地倉
Dì Jī	SP 8	Spleen 8	地機
Dì Wǔ Huì	GB 42	Gall Bladder 42	地五會
Dìng Chuǎn	M-BW-1 (Dìng Chuǎn)	Miscellaneous-Back and Waist-1	定喘
Dú Bí	ST 35	Stomach 35	犢鼻
Dū Shū	BL 16	Urinary Bladder 16	督俞
Èr Bái	M-UE-29 (Èr Bái)	Miscellaneous-Upper Extremity-29	二白
Èr Jiān	LI 2	Large Intestine 2	二間
Ěr Mén	TE 21	Sān Jiāo 21	耳門
Fèi Shū	BL 13	Urinary Bladder 13	肺俞
Fēi Yáng	BL 58	Urinary Bladder 58	飛陽
Fēng Chí	GB 20	Gall Bladder 20	風池
Fēng Fǔ	GV 16	Governing Vessel 16	風府
Fēng Lóng	ST 40	Stomach 40	豐隆
Fēng Mén	BL 12	Urinary Bladder 12	風門
Fēng Shì	GB 31	Gall Bladder 31	風市
Fù Fēn	BL 41	Urinary Bladder 41	附分
Fù Liū	KI 7	Kidney 7	復溜
Fǔ Shè	SP 13	Spleen 13	府舍
Fú Tú	LI 18	Large Intestine 18	扶突
Fú Tù	ST 32	Stomach 32	伏兔
Fū Yáng	BL 59	Urinary Bladder 59	跗陽
Gān Shū	BL 18	Urinary Bladder 18	肝俞

cont.

Pīn Yīn 拼音	Term used in the text	English term/name	Traditional Chinese characters
Gāo Huāng Shū	BL 43	Urinary Bladder 43	膏肓俞
Gé Guān	BL 46	Urinary Bladder 46	膈關
Gé Shū	BL 17	Urinary Bladder 17	隔俞
Gōng Sūn	SP 4	Spleen 4	公孫
Guān Chōng	TE 1	Sān Jiāo 1	關沖
Guān Yuán	CV 4	Conception Vessel 4	關元
Guān Yuán Shū	BL 26	Urinary Bladder 26	關元俞
Guāng Míng	GB 37	Gall Bladder 37	光明
Hǎi Quán	M-HN-37 (Hǎi Quán)	Miscellaneous-Head and Neck-37	海泉
Hè Dǐng	M-LE-27 (Hè Dǐng)	Miscellaneous-Lower Extremity-27	鶴頂
Hé Gǔ	LI 4	Large Intestine 4	合谷
Hé Yáng	BL 55	Urinary Bladder 55	合陽
Héng Gǔ	KI 11	Kidney 11	橫骨
Hòu Xī	SI 3	Small Intestine 3	後谿
Huá Tuó Jiā Jǐ	M-BW-35 (Huá Tuó Jiā Jǐ)	Miscellaneous-Back and Waist-35	華佗夾脊
Huán Tiào	GB 30	Gall Bladder 30	環跳
Huāng Shū	KI 16	Kidney 16	肓俞
Huì Yīn	CV 1	Conception Vessel 1	會陰
Huì Zōng	TE 7	Sān Jiāo 7	會宗
Hún Mén	BL 47	Urinary Bladder 47	魄門
Jī Mén	SP 11	Spleen 11	其門
Jí Quán	HT 1	Heart 1	極泉
Jiá Chē	ST 6	Stomach 6	頰車
Jiān Jǐng	GB 21	Gall Bladder 21	肩井
Jiān Liáo	TE 14	Sān Jiāo 14	肩髎
Jiān Qián	M-UE-48 (Jiān Qián)	Miscellaneous-Upper Extremity-48	肩前
Jiān Shǐ	PC 5	Pericardium 5	間使
Jiān Wài Shū	SI 14	Small Intestine 14	肩外俞
Jiān Yú	LI 15	Large Intestine 15	肩髃
Jiān Zhēn	SI 9	Small Intestine 9	肩貞
Jiān Zhōng Shū	SI 15	Small Intestine 15	肩中俞
Jiāo Xìn	KI 8	Kidney 8	交信
Jiě Xī	ST 41	Stomach 41	解溪
Jīn Mén	BL 63	Urinary Bladder 63	金門
Jīn Suō	GV 8	Governing Vessel 8	筋縮

Pīn Yīn 拼音	Term used in the text	English term/name	Traditional Chinese characters
Jīng Gǔ	BL 64	Urinary Bladder 64	京骨
Jīng Mén	GB 25	Gall Bladder 25	京門
Jīng Míng	BL 1	Urinary Bladder 1	睛明
Jīng Qú	LU 8	Lung 8	經渠
Jiū Wěi	CV 15	Conception Vessel 15	鳩尾
Jù Liáo	ST 3	Stomach 3	巨髎
Jū Liáo	GB 29	Gall Bladder 29	居髎
Jù Què	CV 14	Conception Vessel 14	巨闕
Jué Yīn Shū	BL 14	Urinary Bladder 14	厥陰俞
Kǒng Zuì	LU 6	Lung 6	孔最
Kūn Lún	BL 60	Urinary Bladder 60	昆侖
Láo Gōng	PC 8	Pericardium 8	勞宮
Lì Duì	ST 45	Stomach 45	厲兌
Lǐ Gōu	LR 5	Liver 5	蠡溝
Lián Quán	CV 23	Conception Vessel 23	廉泉
Liáng Mén	ST 21	Stomach 21	梁門
Liáng Qiū	ST 34	Stomach 34	梁丘
Liè Quē	LU 7	Lung 7	列缺
Líng Dào	HT 4	Heart 4	靈道
Líng Tái	GV 10	Governing Vessel 10	靈台
Líng Xū	KI 24	Kidney 24	靈墟
Luò Què	BL 8	Urinary Bladder 8	絡卻
Luò Zhěn	M-UE-24 (Luò Zhěn)	Miscellaneous-Upper Extremity-24	落枕
Mìng Mén	GV 4	Governing Vessel 4	命門
Nào Huì	TE 13	Sān Jiāo 13	臑會
Nào Shàng	N-UE-14 (Nào Shàng)	New-Upper Extremity-14	臑上
Nào Shū	SI 10	Small Intestine 10	臑俞
Nèi Guān	PC 6	Pericardium 6	內關
Nèi Tíng	ST 44	Stomach 44	內庭
Páng Guāng Shū	BL 28	Urinary Bladder 28	膀胱俞
Pí Shū	BL 20	Urinary Bladder 20	脾俞
Piān Lì	LI 6	Large Intestine 6	偏歷
Pò Hù	BL 42	Urinary Bladder 42	魄戶
Pú Cān	BL 61	Urinary Bladder 61	僕參
Qì Chōng	ST 30	Stomach 30	氣沖
Qì Hǎi	CV 6	Conception Vessel 6	氣海
Qì Hǎi Shū	BL 24	Urinary Bladder 24	氣海俞

cont.

Pīn Yīn 拼音	Term used in the text	English term/name	Traditional Chinese characters
Qí Mén	LR 14	Liver 14	期門
Qì Shè	ST 11	Stomach 11	氣舍
Qì Xuè	KI 13	Kidney 13	氣穴
Qián Gǔ	SI 2	Small Intestine 2	前谷
Qīng Líng	HT 2	Heart 2	青靈
Qiú Hòu	M-HN-8 (Qiú Hòu)	Miscellaneous-Head and Neck-8	球后
Qiū Xū	GB 40	Gall Bladder 40	丘墟
Qū Chí	LI 11	Large Intestine 11	曲池
Qū Gǔ	CV 2	Conception Vessel 2	曲骨
Qū Quán	LR 8	Liver 8	曲泉
Qū Zé	PC 3	Pericardium 3	曲澤
Quē Pén	ST 12	Stomach 12	缺盆
Rán Gǔ	KI 2	Kidney 2	然谷
Rén Yíng	ST 9	Stomach 9	人迎
Rì Yuè	GB 24	Gall Bladder 24	日月
Rǔ Gēn	ST 18	Stomach 18	乳根
Sān Jiān	LI 3	Large Intestine 3	三間
Sān Jiāo Shū	BL 22	Urinary Bladder 22	三焦俞
Sān Yáng Luò	TE 8	Sān Jiāo 8	三陽絡
Sān Yīn Jiāo	SP 6	Spleen 6	三陰交
Shàng Jù Xū	ST 37	Stomach 37	上巨虛
Shàng Lián	LI 9	Large Intestine 9	上廉
Shāng Qiū	SP 5	Spleen 5	商丘
Shàng Xīng	GV 23	Governing Vessel 23	上星
Shāng Yáng	LI 1	Large Intestine 1	商陽
Shào Chōng	HT 9	Heart 9	少沖
Shào Fǔ	HT 8	Heart 8	少府
Shào Hǎi	HT 3	Heart 3	少海
Shào Shāng	LU 11	Lung 11	少商
Shào Zé	SI 1	Small Intestine 1	少澤
Shén Cáng	KI 25	Kidney 25	神藏
Shén Dào	GV 11	Governing Vessel 11	神道
Shén Fēng	KI 23	Kidney 23	神封
Shēn Mài	BL 62	Urinary Bladder 62	申脈
Shén Mén	HT 7	Heart 7	神門
Shén Què	CV 8	Conception Vessel 8	神闕
Shèn Shū	BL 23	Urinary Bladder 23	腎俞

Pīn Yīn 拼音	Term used in the text	English term/name	Traditional Chinese characters
Shén Táng	BL 44	Urinary Bladder 44	神堂
Shén Tíng	GV 24	Governing Vessel 24	神庭
Shēn Zhù	GV 12	Governing Vessel 12	身柱
Shí Guān	KI 18	Kidney 18	石關
Shí Mén	CV 5	Conception Vessel 5	石門
Shí Xuān	M-UE-1 (Shí Xuān)	Miscellaneous-Upper Extremity-1	十宣
Shǒu Sān Lǐ	LI 10	Large Intestine 10	手三里
Shū Fǔ	KI 27	Kidney 27	俞府
Shù Gǔ	BL 65	Urinary Bladder 65	束骨
Shuài Gǔ	GB 8	Gall Bladder 8	率谷
Shuǐ Dào	ST 28	Stomach 28	水道
Shuǐ Fēn	CV 9	Conception Vessel 9	水分
Shuǐ Gōu	GV 26	Governing Vessel 26	水溝
Shuǐ Quán	KI 5	Kidney 5	水泉
Sì Bái	ST 2	Stomach 2	四白
Sì Dú	TE 9	Sān Jiāo 9	四瀆
Sì Mǎn	KI 14	Kidney 14	四滿
Sì Shén Cōng	M-HN-1 (Sì Shén Cōng)	Miscellaneous-Head and Neck-1	四神聰
Sī Zhú Kōng	TE 23	Sān Jiāo 23	絲竹空
Tài Bái	SP 3	Spleen 3	太白
Tài Chōng	LR 3	Liver 3	太沖
Tài Xī	KI 3	Kidney 3	太谿
Tài Yáng	M-HN-9 (Tài Yáng)	Miscellaneous-Head and Neck-9	太陽
Tài Yuān	LU 9	Lung 9	太淵
Táo Dào	GV 13	Governing Vessel 13	陶道
Tiān Chí	PC 1	Pericardium 1	天池
Tiān Chōng	GB 9	Gall Bladder 9	天沖
Tiān Chuāng	SI 16	Small Intestine 16	天窗
Tiān Dǐng	LI 17	Large Intestine 17	天鼎
Tiān Fǔ	LU 3	Lung 3	天府
Tiān Jǐng	TE 10	Sān Jiāo 10	天井
Tiān Liáo	TE 15	Sān Jiāo 15	天髎
Tiān Quán	PC 2	Pericardium 2	天泉
Tiān Róng	SI 17	Small Intestine 17	天容
Tiān Shū	ST 25	Stomach 25	天樞
Tiān Tú	CV 22	Conception Vessel 22	天突

cont.

Pīn Yīn 拼音	Term used in the text	English term/name	Traditional Chinese characters
Tiān Xī	SP 18	Spleen 18	天谿
Tiān Yǒu	TE 16	Sān Jiāo 16	天牖
Tiān Zhù	BL 10	Urinary Bladder 10	天柱
Tiān Zōng	SI 11	Small Intestine 11	天宗
Tiáo Kǒu	ST 38	Stomach 38	條口
Tīng Gōng	SI 19	Small Intestine 19	聽宮
Tīng Huì	GB 2	Gall Bladder 2	聽會
Tōng Lǐ	HT 5	Heart 5	通里
Tōng Tiān	BL 7	Urinary Bladder 7	通天
Tóng Zǐ Liáo	GB 1	Gall Bladder 1	瞳子髎
Tóu Lín Qì	GB 15	Gall Bladder 15	頭臨泣
Tóu Wéi	ST 8	Stomach 8	頭維
Wài Guān	TE 5	Sān Jiāo 5	外關
Wài Qiū	GB 36	Gall Bladder 36	外丘
Wán Gǔ	GB 12	Gall Bladder 12	完骨
Wàn Gǔ	SI 4	Small Intestine 4	腕骨
Wèi Cāng	BL 50	Urinary Bladder 50	胃倉
Wéi Dào	GB 28	Gall Bladder 28	維道
Wèi Shū	BL 21	Urinary Bladder 21	胃俞
Wěi Yáng	BL 39	Urinary Bladder 39	委陽
Wěi Zhōng	BL 40	Urinary Bladder 40	委中
Wēn Liù	LI 7	Large Intestine 7	溫溜
Wǔ Shū	GB 27	Gall Bladder 27	五樞
Xī Mén	PC 4	Pericardium 4	郄門
Xī Yǎn	MN-LE-16 (Xī Yǎn)	Miscellaneous/New-Lower Extremity-16	膝眼
Xī Yáng Guān	GB 33	Gall Bladder 33	膝陽關
Xiá Bái	LU 4	Lung 4	俠白
Xià Jù Xū	ST 39	Stomach 39	下巨虛
Xià Lián	LI 8	Large Intestine 8	下廉
Xiá Xī	GB 43	Gall Bladder 43	俠谿
Xiàn Gǔ	ST 43	Stomach 43	陷谷
Xiǎo Cháng Shū	BL 27	Urinary Bladder 27	小腸俞
Xiǎo Hǎi	SI 8	Small Intestine 8	小海
Xīn Shū	BL 15	Urinary Bladder 15	心俞
Xíng Jiān	LR 2	Liver 2	行間
Xuán Jī	CV 21	Conception Vessel 21	璇機
Xuán Zhōng	GB 39	Gall Bladder 39	懸鐘

Pīn Yīn 拼音	Term used in the text	English term/name	Traditional Chinese characters
Xuè Hǎi	SP 10	Spleen 10	血海
Yǎ Mén	GV 15	Governing Vessel 15	啞門
Yáng Bái	GB 14	Gall Bladder 14	陽白
Yáng Chí	TE 4	Sān Jiāo 4	陽池
Yáng Fǔ	GB 38	Gall Bladder 38	陽輔
Yáng Gǔ	SI 5	Small Intestine 5	陽谷
Yáng Jiāo	GB 35	Gall Bladder 35	陽交
Yǎng Lǎo	SI 6	Small Intestine 6	養老
Yáng Líng Quán	GB 34	Gall Bladder 34	陽陵泉
Yáng Xī	LI 5	Large Intestine 5	陽谿
Yāo Tòng Xué	N-UE-19 (Yāo Tòng Xué)	New-Upper Extremity-19	腰痛穴
Yāo Yáng Guān	GV 3	Governing Vessel 3	腰陽關
Yè Mén	TE 2	Sān Jiāo 2	液門
Yì Fēng	TE 17	Sān Jiāo 17	翳風
Yì Shè	BL 49	Urinary Bladder 49	意舍
Yǐn Bái	SP 1	Spleen 1	隱白
Yīn Bāo	LR 9	Liver 9	陰包
Yīn Dū	KI 19	Kidney 19	陰都
Yīn Gǔ	KI 10	Kidney 10	陰谷
Yīn Lián	LR 11	Liver 11	陰廉
Yīn Líng Quán	SP 9	Spleen 9	陰陵泉
Yīn Mén	BL 37	Urinary Bladder 37	殷門
Yìn Táng	M-HN-3 (Yìn Táng)	Miscellaneous-Head and Neck-3	印堂
Yīn Xī	HT 6	Heart 6	陰郄
Yíng Xiāng	LI 20	Large Intestine 20	迎香
Yǒng Quán	KI 1	Kidney 1	湧泉
Yōu Mén	KI 21	Kidney 21	幽門
Yú Jì	LU 10	Lung 10	魚際
Yù Táng	CV 18	Conception Vessel 18	玉堂
Yù Zhěn	BL 9	Urinary Bladder 9	玉枕
Yù Zhōng	KI 26	Kidney 26	彧中
Yún Mén	LU 2	Lung 2	雲門
Zhāng Mén	LR 13	Liver 13	章門
Zhào Hǎi	KI 6	Kidney 6	照海
Zhì Biān	BL 54	Urinary Bladder 54	秩邊
Zhī Gōu	TE 6	Sān Jiāo 6	支溝
Zhì Shì	BL 52	Urinary Bladder 52	志室

cont.

Pīn Yīn 拼音	Term used in the text	English term/name	Traditional Chinese characters
Zhì Yáng	GV 9	Governing Vessel 9	至陽
Zhì Yīn	BL 67	Urinary Bladder 67	至陰
Zhī Zhèng	SI 7	Small Intestine 7	支正
Zhōng Chōng	PC 9	Pericardium 9	中沖
Zhōng Dū	LR 6	Liver 6	中都
Zhōng Fēng	LR 4	Liver 4	中封
Zhōng Fǔ	LU 1	Lung 1	中府
Zhōng Jí	CV 3	Conception Vessel 3	中極
Zhōng Lǚ Shū	BL 29	Urinary Bladder 29	中膂俞
Zhōng Shū	GV 7	Governing Vessel 7	中樞
Zhōng Wǎn	CV 12	Conception Vessel 12	中脘
Zhōng Zhǔ	TE 3	Sān Jiāo 3	中渚
Zhǒu Liáo	LI 12	Large Intestine 12	肘髎
Zhōu Róng	SP 20	Spleen 20	周榮
Zhú Bīn	KI 9	Kidney 9	築賓
Zǐ Gōng	CV 19	Conception Vessel 19	紫宮
Zǐ Gōng	M-CA-18 (Zǐ Gōng)	Miscellaneous-Chest and Abdomen-18	子宮
Zú Lín Qì	GB 41	Gall Bladder 41	足臨泣
Zú Qiào Yīn	GB 44	Gall Bladder 44	足竅陰
Zú Sān Lǐ	ST 36	Stomach 36	足三里
Zú Tōng Gǔ	BL 66	Urinary Bladder 66	足通谷

Note

1   CV 17 has at least three different Pīn Yīn names in the current literature. Dàn Zhōng is the name designated for use by WHO in the Western Pacific region, which includes Australia. The other two commonly used Pīn Yīn names are Tán Zhōng (pretty much obsolete now) and Shān Zhōng.

Appendix 4

Cautions and Contraindications When Using Acupuncture

I need to include a caveat here. Every author who attempts to compile a list of points that are contraindicated or cautionary will run into the same problem that has existed for the history of Chinese medicine. That problem is there isn't just one list!

All experienced (theoretically and/or practically) Chinese medicine practitioners will have their own list of points that they show caution with; they might even have some points that they never needle. Their reasons will be wide-ranging, and if these reasons have come from their experience, then they are valid, even if those points are different to those of another, equally experienced, Chinese medicine practitioner.

If they continue to research and learn, then the list will likely become more refined in some areas, and possibly expand in others.

This is my list as at the time of writing. I say that because it will, in all likelihood, be refined or expand in the coming years. You may notice that I take a fairly cautious approach to my needling, but that's just my style. I'd rather be safe than sorry!

Part 1: Points that are contraindicated

Table A4.1 Pregnancy contraindicated points

Points	Comments
LI 4	This is my current list of seven points that I avoid from the time the woman is ovulating (if she is actively trying to fall pregnant) until she starts her menstrual period or falls pregnant.
GB 21	
SP 1	
SP 6	
BL 60	If she has her menstrual period, then I can use these points again.
BL 67*	If she is pregnant, then I won't use these points again until she reaches 38 weeks. At this stage the points will be helpful to prepare the pregnant woman for labor.
KI 6	* I may consider BL 67 to turn a breeched baby prior to 38 weeks.

cont.

Points	Comments
All points on the low back	I appreciate that this is a safety-first approach, but I avoid every single point on the lower back and the entire abdomen, as well as the sacral foramen. This is from the time the woman is ovulating (if she is actively trying to fall pregnant) until after she gives birth.
All points in the sacral foramen (BL 31–BL 34)	
All points on the abdomen	

It is worth noting that not all insurance providers will cover you if you treat a woman who is pregnant. This is certainly the case in Australia, but I am unsure about other countries around the world. It would be smart to check with your insurance provider prior to treating women who are pregnant.

Table A4.2 My current taboo-to-needle points

Points	Reasoning
ST 1	I was never trained in how to needle these points, so until I find someone who gives me practical training, I will avoid needling them.
ST 9	
ST 10	
ST 18	It is generally considered that needling the nipple is contraindicated.
CV 1	I avoid this point because of its location. In Australia, there are potential legal concerns based on perceived sexual misconduct.
CV 8	It is generally considered that needling the umbilicus is contraindicated.
M-HN-8 (Qiú Hòu)	I was never trained in how to needle this point, so until I find someone who gives me practical training, I will avoid needling it.

Part 2: Points to use caution on

These points are not contraindicated to needle; they are points listed purely to remind you to be cautious when needling. Take a second to remind yourself of what angle and depth you need to consider when needling.

Table A4.3 Points to use caution on – condition/region

Condition/region	Points	Reasoning
Blood vessels	BL 1, BL 40 GB 28 HT 1–HT 7 LI 17, LI 18 LR 10–LR 12 LU 5, LU 8, LU 9 M-CA-18 (Zǐ Gōng), M-HN-8 (Qiú Hòu), M-HN-9 (Tài Yáng) PC 3, PC 5–PC 7 SI 5, SI 16, SI 17 SP 11–SP 13 ST 1, ST 2, ST 9–ST 13, ST 41, ST 42 TE 4, TE 17 Any other points that are located near blood vessels.	To avoid needling into blood vessels, always consider your angle and depth of needle insertion (if you are unsure).

Condition/region	Points	Reasoning
Brain/temples	BL 10 GB 1, GB 3, GB 12, GB 20 GV 15, GV 16 M-HN-9 (Tài Yáng), N-HN-54 (Ān Mián) TE 17, TE 22, TE 23 Any other points that are located near the brain/temples need to be evaluated (however briefly) before needle insertion.	Never needle these points deeply on a superior oblique angle (for the brain) or perpendicular angle (for the temples).
Eyes	BL 1 M-HN-8 (Qiú Hòu) ST 1 Any other points that are located in the eye socket. O'Connor and Bensky (1981, pp.147, 150–151, 367, 370) suggest at least four more extra points in the eye socket.	Never needle these points deeply on an oblique angle towards the eyeball. Never needle these points without having had sufficient clinical observation/training and practice.
Heart	CV 14–CV 16 KI 21, KI 22 ST 19, ST 20 Any other points that are located near the heart.	To avoid needling into the heart, never needle these points deeply on a perpendicular/oblique or oblique angle in the direction of the heart.
Kidneys	BL 22, BL 23, BL 51, BL 52 GB 25 Any other points that are located near the kidneys.	To avoid needling into the kidneys, never needle these points deeply on a perpendicular or perpendicular/oblique angle in the direction of the kidneys.
Liver	GB 25 LR 13 SP 16 ST 19–ST 21 Any other points that are located near the liver.	To avoid needling into the liver, never needle these points deeply on a perpendicular/oblique or oblique angle in the direction of the liver.
Lungs/ pneumothorax	BL 11–BL 21, BL 41–BL 50 GB 21–GB 24 HT 1 KI 22–KI 27 LI 16 LR 14 LU 1, LU 2 PC 1 SI 9, SI 10, SI 12–SI 15 SP 17–SP 21 ST 11–ST 18 TE 15 Ā Shì points on the chest, flanks, shoulders, upper back, mid-back. Any other points that are located near the lungs.	To avoid puncturing the lungs (pneumothorax), never needle these points deeply on a perpendicular or perpendicular/oblique angle in the direction of the lungs.

cont.

Condition/region	Points	Reasoning
Nerves	BL 1, BL 40 GB 28, GB 30 GV 3–GV 16 HT 4–HT 7 LR 10–LR 12 M-CA-18 (Zǐ Gōng) PC 3, PC 5–PC 7 SI 5, SI 8 SP 12, SP 13 ST 2, ST 41 TE 17 Any other points that are located near nerves.	To avoid needling into nerves, always consider your angle and depth of needle insertion (if you are unsure).
Peritoneal cavity	CV 2–CV 15 GB 25–GB 28 KI 11–KI 21 LR 13 SP 13–SP 16 ST 19–ST 30 Any other points that are located over the peritoneal cavity.	To avoid needling into the peritoneal cavity, never needle these points deeply on a perpendicular or perpendicular/oblique angle. Obviously, the depth will be different depending on the patient's frame/size. This should be factored in before needling.
Sex organs	BL 35 CV 1 GV 1 Any other points that are located near the sex organs.	To avoid needling into the sex organs, never needle these points deeply on a perpendicular/oblique or oblique angle in the direction of the sex organs.
Spinal cord	GV 3–GV 16 M-BW-35 (Huá Tuó Jiā Jǐ), M-HN-30 (Bǎi Láo) Any other points that are located on, or near, the spine.	To avoid needling into the spinal cord, never needle these points deeply perpendicularly, or perpendicular/oblique in a medial direction.
Spleen	GB 25 LR 13 SP 16 ST 19–ST 21 Any other points that are located near the spleen.	To avoid needling into the spleen, never needle these points deeply on a perpendicular/oblique or oblique angle in the direction of the spleen.
Tendons	BL 38, BL 39, BL 59, BL 60, BL 62 GB 33, GB 34, GB 39, GB 41 HT 4–HT 7 KI 3–KI 7, KI 10 LI 5 LR 4, LR 8 LU 5, LU 7, LU 9 M-LE-27 (Hè Dǐng), M-UE-29 (Èr Bái) PC 3–PC 7 SI 5 SP 5 ST 41 TE 4–TE 6, TE 10 Any other points that are located near tendons.	To avoid needling into tendons, always consider your angle and depth of needle insertion (if you are unsure).

Condition/region	Points	Reasoning
Urinary bladder	CV 2–CV 4 KI 11–KI 13 ST 28–ST 30 Any other points that are located near the urinary bladder.	To avoid needling into the urinary bladder, never needle these points deeply on a perpendicular/oblique or oblique angle in the direction of the urinary bladder.

Appendix 5

Special Point Category Tables

Table A5.1 Yīn Yáng organ special point categories

Zàng Fǔ channels	Front Mù Collecting point	Back Shù Transporting point	Yuán Source point	Luò Connecting point	Xì Cleft point	Horary point	Lower Hé (Uniting) Sea point	Alternative Front Mù Collecting[i] point
Gall Bladder	GB 24	BL 19	GB 40	GB 37	GB 36	GB 41	GB 34	LR 14
Heart	CV 14	BL 15	HT 7	HT 5	HT 6	HT 8	-	CV 15
Kidneys	GB 25	BL 23	KI 3	KI 4	KI 5	KI 10	-	CV 4 & CV 6
Liver	LR 14	BL 18	LR 3	LR 5	LR 6	LR 1	-	GB 24
Lungs	LU 1	BL 13	LU 9	LU 7	LU 6	LU 8	-	CV 17
Large Intestine	ST 25	BL 25	LI 4	LI 6	LI 7	LI 1	ST 37	CV 4 & CV 12
Pericardium	CV 17	BL 14	PC 7	PC 6	PC 4	PC 8	-	CV 14
Sān Jiāo	CV 5	BL 22	TE 4	TE 5	TE 7	TE 6	BL 39	CV 21
Small Intestine	CV 4	BL 27	SI 4	SI 7	SI 6	SI 5	ST 39	ST 25
Spleen	LR 13	BL 20	SP 3	SP 4	SP 8	SP 3	-	SP 15
Stomach	CV 12	BL 21	ST 42	ST 40	ST 34	ST 36	ST 36	ST 21
Urinary Bladder	CV 3	BL 28	BL 64	BL 58	BL 63	BL 66	BL 40	CV 5

Table A5.2 Five Shū/Transporting points

Zàng Fǔ channels	Jǐng Well point	Yíng Spring point	Shù (Transport) Stream point	Jīng (Flow) River point	Hé (Unite) Sea point
Gall Bladder	GB 44	GB 43	GB 41	GB 38	GB 34
Heart	HT 9	HT 8	HT 7	HT 4	HT 3
Kidneys	KI 1	KI 2	KI 3	KI 7	KI 10
Liver	LR 1	LR 2	LR 3	LR 4	LR 8
Lungs	LU 11	LU 10	LU 9	LU 8	LU 5
Large Intestine	LI 1	LI 2	LI 3	LI 5	LI 11
Pericardium	PC 9	PC 8	PC 7	PC 5	PC 3
Sān Jiāo	TE 1	TE 2	TE 3	TE 6	TE 10
Small Intestine	SI 1	SI 2	SI 3	SI 5	SI 8
Spleen	SP 1	SP 2	SP 3	SP 5	SP 9
Stomach	ST 45	ST 44	ST 43	ST 41	ST 36
Urinary Bladder	BL 67	BL 66	BL 65	BL 60	BL 40

Table A5.3 Yīn Yáng channel Five Element points

Zàng Fǔ channels	Wood point	Fire point	Earth point	Metal point	Water point
Gall Bladder	GB 41	GB 38	GB 34	GB 44	GB 43
Heart	HT 9	HT 8	HT 7	HT 4	HT 3
Kidneys	KI 1	KI 2	KI 3	KI 7	KI 10
Liver	LR 1	LR 2	LR 3	LR 4	LR 8
Lungs	LU 11	LU 10	LU 9	LU 8	LU 5
Large Intestine	LI 3	LI 5	LI 11	LI 1	LI 2
Pericardium	PC 9	PC 8	PC 7	PC 5	PC 3
Sān Jiāo	TE 3	TE 6	TE 10	TE 1	TE 2
Small Intestine	SI 3	SI 5	SI 8	SI 1	SI 2
Spleen	SP 1	SP 2	SP 3	SP 5	SP 9
Stomach	ST 43	ST 41	ST 36	ST 45	ST 44
Urinary Bladder	BL 65	BL 60	BL 40	BL 67	BL 66

Table A5.4 Wǔ Xíng Mother and Child points

Zàng Fǔ channels	Shēng/Generating cycle		Kè/Controlling cycle	
	Wǔ Xíng Mother point	Wǔ Xíng Child point	Wǔ Xíng Mother point	Wǔ Xíng Child point
Gall Bladder	GB 43	GB 38	GB 44	GB 34
Heart	HT 9	HT 7	HT 3	HT 4
Kidneys	KI 7	KI 1	KI 3	KI 2
Liver	LR 8	LR 2	LR 4	LR 3
Lungs	LU 9	LU 5	LU 10	LU 11
Large Intestine	LI 11	LI 2	LI 5	LI 3
Pericardium	PC 9	PC 7	PC 3	PC 5
Sān Jiāo	TE 3	TE 10	TE 2	TE 1
Small Intestine	SI 3	SI 8	SI 2	SI 1
Spleen	SP 2	SP 5	SP 1	SP 9
Stomach	ST 41	ST 45	ST 43	ST 44
Urinary Bladder	BL 67	BL 65	BL 40	BL 60

Table A5.5 Huì Meeting points

Treats	Point
Blood vessels	LU 9
Bone	BL 11
Fǔ	CV 12
Marrow	GB 39
Qì	CV 17
Tendons/sinews	GB 34
Xuè	BL 17
Zàng	LR 13

Table A5.6 Eight Extraordinary Vessels (Qí Jīng Bā Mài) confluent (opening and coupled) points

Eight Extraordinary Vessels (Qí Jīng Bā Mài)	Confluent (opening and coupled) points
Chōng Mài	SP 4
Dài Mài	GB 41
Dū Mài	SI 3
Rèn Mài	LU 7
Yáng Qiāo Mài	BL 62
Yáng Wéi Mài	TE 5
Yīn Qiāo Mài	KI 6
Yīn Wéi Mài	PC 6

Table A5.7 Window of Heaven/Windows of the Sky points

BL 10	PC 1
CV 22	SI 16
GV 16	SI 17
LI 18	ST 9
LU 3	TE 16

Table A5.8 Ma Dan-Yang Heavenly Star points

BL 40	LI 4
BL 57	LI 11
BL 60	LR 3
GB 30	LU 7
GB 34	ST 36
HT 5	ST 44

Table A5.9 Spirit Gate/Shén Mén points

Points	Treats
KI 22 (Bù Láng) – Veranda/Corridor Walk	Water and Fire elements
KI 23 (Shén Fēng) – Spirit Seal	Earth element
KI 24 (Líng Xū) – Spirit Burial Ground	Metal element
KI 25 (Shén Cáng) – Spirit Storehouse	Fire element
KI 26 (Yù Zhōng) – Lively Center	Wood element
KI 27 (Shū Fǔ) – Palace Treasury Transporter	Water and Metal elements

Table A5.10 Urinary Bladder Wǔ Shén/Five Spirits points

Wǔ Shén/Five Spirits	Urinary Bladder channel points
Pò	BL 42 (Pò Hù) – Corporeal/Grounded Soul Door
Shén	BL 44 (Shén Táng) – Spirit Hall
Hún	BL 47 (Hún Mén) – Ethereal/Heavenly Soul Gate
Yì	BL 49 (Yì Shè) – Thought Abode
Zhì	BL 52 (Zhì Shì) – Willpower Residence

Table A5.11 Four Seas points

Four Seas	Points
Sea of Blood/Xuè	BL 11 ST 37 ST 39
Sea of Food	ST 30 ST 36
Sea of Marrow	GV 16 GV 20
Sea of Qì	CV 17 GV 14 GV 15 ST 9

Table A5.12 Six Command points

Six Command	Points
Abdomen	ST 36
Chest	PC 6
Face (head and mouth)	LI 4
Neck (head)	LU 7
Low back	BL 40
Resuscitation	GV 26

Table A5.13 Sūn Sī Miǎo Ghost points

BL 62	LU 11
CV 1	M-HN-37 (Hǎi Quán)
CV 24	PC 7
GV 16	PC 8
GV 23	SP 1
GV 26	ST 6
LI 11	

Note

1   The alternative Front Mù Collecting points are a selection of points that I consider to be superior or on an equal (or even slightly lesser) footing to the standard Front Mù Collecting points. These are my own selection based in a large part on clinical experience. I tend to use them as replacements for the original Front Mù Collecting points, in conjunction with them or ignored in favor of the original proven set of Front Mù Collecting points. I include them here to give you something else to think about/trial.

References

Aurelius, M. (2004) *Meditations: Living, Dying and the Good Life*, trans. Gregory Hays. London: Phoenix. Originally written c. 170 CE.

Beinfield, H. and Korngold, E. (1991) *Between Heaven and Earth: A Guide to Chinese Medicine*. New York, NY: Ballantine Books.

Bertschinger, R. (2013) *The Great Intent: Acupuncture Odes, Songs and Rhymes*. London: Singing Dragon.

Bisio, T. (2004) *A Tooth from the Tiger's Mouth*. New York, NY: Fireside.

Boethius, A. (1999) *The Consolation of Philosophy*, trans. Victor Watts. London: Penguin Books. Originally written 524 CE.

Carey, D. and De Muynck, M. (2007) *Acutonics: There's No Place Like Ohm* (2nd edn). Llano, NM: Devachan Press.

Chang, C.S. (1977) *The Development of Neo-Confucian Thought*. Westport, CT: Greenwood Press. First English edition published 1957.

Chen, P. (2004) *Diagnosis in Traditional Chinese Medicine*. Taos, NM: Complementary Medicine Press.

Cheng, X.N. (ed.) (2010) *Chinese Acupuncture and Moxibustion* (3rd edn). Beijing: Foreign Languages Press.

Collinson, D., Plant, K. and Wilkinson, R. (2000) *Fifty Eastern Thinkers*. London: Routledge.

Cotterell, A. (1995) *China: A History*. London: Pimlico.

De Botton, A. (2000) *The Consolations of Philosophy*. London: Penguin Books.

Deadman, P., Al-Khafaji, M. and Baker, K. (2007) *A Manual of Acupuncture*. Hove: Journal of Chinese Medicine Publications.

Dechar, L.E. (2006) *Five Spirits: Alchemical Acupuncture for Psychological and Spiritual Healing*. New York, NY: Chiron Publications/Lantern Books.

Descartes, R. (1954) *The Geometry of Rene Descartes*, trans. David Eugene Smith and Marcia L. Latham. New York, NY: Dover Publications, Inc. Originally published 1637 CE.

Ellis, A., Wiseman, N. and Boss, K. (1989) *Grasping the Wind*. Brookline, MA: Paradigm Publications.

Ellis, A., Wiseman, N. and Boss, K. (1991) *Fundamentals of Chinese Acupuncture*. Brookline, MA: Paradigm Publications.

Feng, G.F. and English, J. (trans.) (2008) *Chuang Tsu Inner Chapters* (4th edn). Portland, OR: Amber Lotus Publishing. Originally written c. 300–200 BCE.

Flaws, B. (trans.) (2004) *The Classic of Difficulties: A Translation of the Nan Jing* (3rd edn). Boulder, CO: Blue Poppy Press. Originally written c. 0–200 CE.

Flaws, B. and Wolfe, H.L. (2008) *Sticking to the Point: A Step-by-Step Approach to TCM Acupuncture Therapy*. Boulder, CO: Blue Poppy Press.

Franglen, N. (2014) *The Handbook of Five Element Practice*. London: Singing Dragon.

Fung, Y.L. (1952) *A History of Chinese Philosophy: Volume I*, trans. Derk Bodde. Princeton, NY: Princeton University Press. Originally published 1931.

Fung, Y.L. (1953) *A History of Chinese Philosophy: Volume II*, trans. Derk Bodde. Princeton, NJ: Princeton University Press. Originally published 1934.

Furley, D. (ed.) (1999) *From Aristotle to Augustine: Routledge History of Philosophy Volume 2.* London: Routledge.

Hartmann, D. (2009) *Acupoint Dictionary* (2nd edn). Sydney: Churchill Livingstone Elsevier.

Hecker, H.U., Steveling, A., Peuker, E.T. and Kastner, J. (2005) *Practice of Acupuncture*, trans. Ursula Vielkind. Stuttgart: Thieme.

Hicks, A., Hicks, J. and Mole, P. (2010) *Five Element Constitutional Acupuncture* (2nd edn). Edinburgh: Elsevier Churchill Livingstone.

Hinrichs, T.J. and Barnes, L.L. (eds) (2013) *Chinese Medicine and Healing: An Illustrated History.* Cambridge, MA: Belknap Press of Harvard University Press.

Jarmey, C. and Tindall, J. (2005) *Acupressure for Common Ailments.* London: Gaia Books.

Kaatz, D. (2005) *Characters of Wisdom: Taoist Tales of the Acupuncture Points.* Soudorgues: Petite Bergerie Press.

Kaatz, D. (2009) *Receiving Spirit: The Practice of Five Element Acupuncture.* Soudorgues: Petite Bergerie Press.

Kaptchuk, T. (2000) *Chinese Medicine: The Web That Has No Weaver.* London: Rider Books.

Lade, A. (1989) *Acupuncture Points: Images and Functions.* Seattle, WA: Eastland Press.

Larre, C. and Rochat De La Vallee, E. (1997) *The Eight Extraordinary Meridians.* Cambridge: Monkey Press.

Lau, D.C. (trans.) (1979) *Confucius: The Analects.* London: Penguin Books. Originally written c. 400–300 BCE.

Lau, D.C. (trans.) (2001) *Tao Te Ching: A Bilingual Edition.* Hong Kong: Chinese University Press. Originally written c. 550–250 BCE.

Lau, D.C. (trans.) (2003) *Mencius: A Bilingual Edition.* Hong Kong: Chinese University Press. Originally written c. 300 BCE.

Legge, D. (2011) *Close to the Bone* (3rd edn). Woy Woy: Sydney College Press.

Li, S.Z. (2007) *Clinical Application of Commonly Used Acupuncture Points.* Potters Bar: Donica Publishing.

Li, S.Z. (2010) *An Exposition on the Eight Extraordinary Vessels: Acupuncture, Alchemy and Herbal Medicine*, trans. Charles Chase and Miki Shima. Seattle, WA: Eastland Press. Originally published 1578 CE.

Lian, Y.L., Chen, C.Y., Hammes, M. and Kolster, B.C. (2000) *The Seirin Pictorial Atlas of Acupuncture: An Illustrated Manual of Acupuncture Points*, trans. Colin Grant. Cologne: Konemann.

Liang, C.J. (1996) *The Great Thoughts of China: 3000 Years of Wisdom That Shaped a Civilization.* New York, NY: John Wiley & Sons.

McDonald, J. (1986) *Acupuncture Point Dynamics, Volume 1.* Self-published.

McDonald, J. (1989) *Acupuncture Point Dynamics, Volume 2.* Self-published.

McDonald, J. and Penner, J. (1994) *Zang Fu Syndromes: Differential Diagnosis and Treatment.* Toluca Lake, CA: Lone Wolf Press.

Maciocia, G. (2004) *Diagnosis in Chinese Medicine: A Comprehensive Guide.* Edinburgh: Churchill Livingstone.

Maciocia, G. (2006) *The Channels of Acupuncture.* Edinburgh: Elsevier Churchill Livingstone.

Maciocia, G. (2009) *The Psyche in Chinese Medicine.* Edinburgh: Elsevier Churchill Livingstone.

Maciocia, G. (2015) *The Foundations of Chinese Medicine* (3rd edn). Edinburgh: Elsevier Churchill Livingstone.

Maclean, W. and Lyttleton, J. (1998) *Clinical Handbook of Internal Medicine: Volume 1.* Macarthur: University of Western Sydney.

Maclean, W. and Lyttleton, J. (2002) *Clinical Handbook of Internal Medicine: Volume 2.* Macarthur: University of Western Sydney.

Maclean, W. and Lyttleton, J. (2010) *Clinical Handbook of Internal Medicine: Volume 3.* Hong Kong: Pangolin Press.

Marchment, R. (2004) *Chinese for TCM Practitioners.* Melbourne: Ji Sheng.

Martin, E.A. (1994) *Concise Medical Dictionary.* Oxford: Oxford University Press.

Matsumoto, K. and Birch, S. (1983) *Five Elements and Ten Stems: Nan Ching Theory, Diagnostics and Practice*. Brookline, MA: Paradigm Publications.

Matsumoto, K. and Birch, S. (1986) *Extraordinary Vessels*. Brookline, MA: Paradigm Publications.

Mi, H.F. (2004) *The Systematic Classic of Acupuncture and Moxibustion*, trans. Yang Shou-zhong and Charles Chase. Boulder, CO: Blue Poppy Press. Originally published 282 CE.

Mou, B. (ed.) (2009) *History of Chinese Philosophy: Routledge History of World Philosophies Volume 3*. London: Routledge.

Ni, M.S. (trans.) (1995) *The Yellow Emperor's Classic of Medicine*. Boston, MA: Shambhala. Originally written c. 200–0 BCE.

O'Connor, J. and Bensky, D. (trans. and eds) (1981) *Acupuncture: A Comprehensive Text*. Seattle, WA: Eastland Press. Originally published 1974.

Phillips, J. (2017) *The Living Needle: Modern Acupuncture Techniques*. London: Singing Dragon.

Quirico, P.E. and Pedrali, T. (2007) *Teaching Atlas of Acupuncture Volume 1: Channels and Points*, trans. Ornella Vecchio Bottino. Stuttgart: Thieme.

Ross, J. (1995) *Acupuncture Point Combinations: The Key to Clinical Success*. Edinburgh: Churchill Livingstone.

Ross, J. (1985) *Zang Fu: The Organ Systems of Traditional Chinese Medicine* (2nd edn). Edinburgh: Churchill Livingstone.

Rossi, E. (2007) *Shen: Psycho-Emotional Aspects of Chinese Medicine*. Edinburgh: Churchill Livingstone Elsevier.

Schnyer, R.N. and Allen, J.J.B. (2001) *Acupuncture in the Treatment of Depression*. Edinburgh: Elsevier Churchill Livingstone.

Seneca (1997) *On the Shortness of Life*, trans. C.D.N. Costa. London: Penguin Books. Originally written c. 49 CE.

Shi, X.M. (2007) *Shi Xue-min's Comprehensive Textbook of Acupuncture and Moxibustion: Volume One*, trans. Liang Hui *et al.* Beijing: People's Medical Publishing House.

Sionneau, P. and Gang, L. (1996) *The Treatment of Disease in TCM. Volume 1: Diseases of the Head and Face Including Mental/Emotional Disorders*. Boulder, CO: Blue Poppy Press.

Soulie de Morant, G. (1994) *Chinese Acupuncture*, trans. Lawrence Grinnell, Claudy Jeanmougin and Maurice Leveque. Brookline, MA: Paradigm Publications. Originally published 1972.

Spinoza, B. (2006) *The Essential Spinoza: Ethics and Related Writings*, trans. Samuel Shirley. Cambridge: Hackett Publishing Company. *Ethics* originally published 1677 CE.

Sūn, T. (2011) *The Art of War: The New Illustrated Edition*, trans. Samuel B. Griffith. Baulkham Hills: Lifetime Distributors 'The Book People' Pty Ltd. Originally written c. 450–350 BCE.

Sun, P.L. (ed.) (2011) *The Treatment of Pain with Chinese Herbs and Acupuncture* (2nd edn). Edinburgh: Churchill Livingstone Elsevier.

Thompson, G.M. (2012) *The Guide to Chinese Horoscopes*. London: Watkins Publishing.

Twicken, D. (2013) *Eight Extraordinary Channels: Qi Jing Ba Mai*. London: Singing Dragon.

Unschuld, P.U. (1985) *Medicine in China: A History of Ideas*. Berkeley, CA: University of California Press.

Unschuld, P.U. (trans.) (1986) *Medicine in China: Nan Ching – The Classic of Difficult Issues*. Berkeley, CA: University of California Press. Originally written c. 0–200 CE.

Unschuld, P.U. (2009) *What is Medicine? Western and Eastern Approaches to Healing*, trans. Karen Reimers. Berkeley, CA: University of California Press.

Wang, B. (1997) *Yellow Emperor's Canon Internal Medicine*, trans. Nelson Liansheng Wu and Andrew Qi Wu. Beijing: China Science and Technology Press. Originally published c. 762 CE.

Wang, J.Y. and Robertson, J.D. (2008) *Applied Channel Theory in Chinese Medicine: Wang Ju-Yi's Lectures on Channel Therapeutics*. Seattle, WA: Eastland Press.

Wang, Z.Z. (2014) *The Classic of Supporting Life with Acupuncture and Moxibustion: Zhēn Jiǔ Zī Shēng Jīng Volumes I–III*, trans. Yue Lu. Portland, OR: Chinese Medicine Database. Originally published 1180–1195 CE.

WHO (2007) *WHO International Standard Terminologies on Traditional Medicine in the Western Pacific Region*. Manila: World Health Organization.

Wu, J.N. (trans.) (1993) *Ling Shu or The Spiritual Pivot*. Washington, DC: University of Hawaii Press. Originally written c. 200–0 BCE.

Yang, J.Z. (2010) *The Great Compendium of Acupuncture and Moxibustion: Zhen Jiu Da Cheng Volume V*, trans. Lorraine Wilcox. Portland, OR: Chinese Medicine Database. Originally published 1601 CE.

Yang, J.Z. (2011) *The Great Compendium of Acupuncture and Moxibustion: Zhen Jiu Da Cheng Volume VIII*, trans. Yue Lu. Portland, OR: Chinese Medicine Database. Originally published 1601 CE.

Further Reading

Baldry, P.E. (2005) *Acupuncture, Trigger Points and Musculoskeletal Pain* (3rd edn). Edinburgh: Elsevier Churchill Livingstone.

Beijing College of Traditional Chinese Medicine (1980) *Essentials of Chinese Acupuncture*. Beijing: Foreign Languages Press.

Bertschinger, R. (2015) *Essential Texts in Chinese Medicine: The Single Idea in the Mind of the Yellow Emperor*. London: Singing Dragon.

Bynum, W. (2008) *The History of Medicine: A Very Short Introduction*. Oxford: Oxford University Press.

Chaitow, L. (1990) *The Acupuncture Treatment of Pain* (3rd edn). Rochester, VT: Healing Arts Press.

Chen, E. (1995) *Cross-Sectional Anatomy of Acupoints*. Edinburgh: Churchill Livingstone.

Chen, H.F., Li, D.F. and Han, C.P. (2011) *Chinese External Medicine*. Beijing: People's Medical Publishing House.

Ching, N. (2017) *The Art and Practice of Diagnosis in Chinese Medicine*. London: Singing Dragon.

Dolowich, G. (2003) *Archetype Acupuncture: Healing with the Five Elements*. Aptos, CA: Jade Mountain Publishing.

Flaws, B. and Finney, D. (1996) *A Compendium of TCM Patterns and Treatments*. Boulder, CO: Blue Poppy Press.

Hammer, L. (2005) *Dragon Rises, Red Bird Flies: Psychology and Chinese Medicine*. Seattle, WA: Eastland Press.

Lin, A. and Flaws, B. (1991) *The Dao of Increasing Longevity and Conserving One's Life*. Boulder, CO: Blue Poppy Press.

Lindberg, D.C. (2007) *The Beginnings of Western Science* (2nd edn). Chicago, IL: University of Chicago Press.

Lu, S.J. (2009) *Acupuncture in the Treatment of Musculoskeletal and Nervous System Disorders* (2nd edn), trans. Rodger Watts and Shuzhang Mao. Potters Bar: Donica Publishing.

Maciocia, G. (2008) *The Practice of Chinese Medicine: The Treatment of Diseases with Acupuncture and Chinese Herbs* (2nd edn). Edinburgh: Churchill Livingstone Elsevier.

Manning, C.A. and Vanrenen, L.J. (1988) *Bioenergetic Medicines East and West: Acupuncture and Homeopathy*. Berkeley, CA: North Atlantic Books.

Ni, Y.T. (1996) *Navigating the Channels of Traditional Chinese Medicine*. San Diego, CA: Complementary Medicine Press.

Reichert, B. (2011) *Palpation Techniques: Surface Anatomy for Physical Therapists*, trans. Michelle Hertrich. Stuttgart: Thieme.

Robinson, B.H. (2007) *Biomedicine: A Textbook for Practitioners of Acupuncture and Oriental Medicine*. Boulder, CO: Blue Poppy Press.

Scheid, V. (2007) *Currents of Tradition in Chinese Medicine 1626 to 2006*. Seattle, WA: Eastland Press.

Sionneau, P. and Gang, L. (1996) *The Treatment of Disease in TCM. Volume 2: Diseases of the Eyes, Ears, Nose, and Throat.* Boulder, CO: Blue Poppy Press.

Sionneau, P. and Gang, L. (1997) *The Treatment of Disease in TCM. Volume 3: Diseases of the Mouth, Lips, Tongue, Teeth, and Gums.* Boulder, CO: Blue Poppy Press.

Sionneau, P. and Gang, L. (1998) *The Treatment of Disease in TCM. Volume 4: Diseases of the Neck, Shoulders, Back, and Limbs.* Boulder, CO: Blue Poppy Press.

Sionneau, P. and Gang, L. (1998) *The Treatment of Disease in TCM. Volume 5: Diseases of the Chest, Abdomen, and Rib-side.* Boulder, CO: Blue Poppy Press.

Sionneau, P. and Gang, L. (1999) *The Treatment of Disease in TCM. Volume 6: Diseases of the Urogenital System and Proctology.* Boulder, CO: Blue Poppy Press.

Sionneau, P. and Gang, L. (2000) *The Treatment of Disease in TCM. Volume 7: General Symptoms.* Boulder, CO: Blue Poppy Press.

Sun, P.L. (2007) *The Management of Post-operative Pain with Acupuncture.* Edinburgh: Churchill Livingstone Elsevier.

Unschuld, P.U. (trans.) (2003) *Huang Di Nei Jing Su Wen: Nature, Knowledge, Imagery in an Ancient Chinese Medical Text.* Berkeley, CA: University of California Press. Originally written c. 200–0 BCE.

WHO (2009) *WHO Standard Acupuncture Point Locations in the Western Pacific Region.* Manila: World Health Organization.

Wiseman, N. and Ellis, A. (1996) *Fundamentals of Chinese Medicine.* Brookline, MA: Paradigm Publications.

Wiseman, N. and Ye, F. (1998) *A Practical Dictionary of Chinese Medicine* (2nd edn). Brookline, MA: Paradigm Publications.

Yang, J.Z. (2010) *The Great Compendium of Acupuncture and Moxibustion: Zhen Jiu Da Cheng Volume I*, trans. Sabine Wilms. Portland, OR: Chinese Medicine Database. Originally published 1601 CE.

About the Author

David Hartmann has been an acupuncturist for over 20 years, having graduated from the Australian College of Natural Medicine (now Endeavour) in 1996. David also completed a Master of Acupuncture in 2009 (Southern Cross University) and is interested in pursuing a PhD in coming years.

He has been a Chinese medicine (TCM) lecturer for the past 15 years in Australia, and was Head of the TCM Department for over a decade during that time; David has also developed a Bachelor of Acupuncture degree.

David has presented at conferences and done stand-alone workshops/seminars throughout Australia, New Zealand, the USA, Germany, the Netherlands and Denmark. He has also written a previous textbook titled *Acupoint Dictionary 2e* (2009). His love for Chinese medicine comes from always wanting to know more, and with more than 2000 years of knowledge to draw on, he won't go hungry for learning.

During his 20-year career David has treated most disorders and has a particular love for balancing his clients' Shén. This translates roughly into 'Spirit', which includes, but is not limited to, emotional disorders, stress, anxiety, sleep disorders and memory problems. It also includes a person's self-esteem, focus, concentration, drive, determination, willpower, courage, decision making and even how you balance yourself between your 'dreaming' state and your 'doing/being' state.

David doesn't always limit himself to just Chinese medicine. Where necessary, he will also consider looking into a patient's numerology, view different Eastern/Western archetype systems and interpret drawings, just to name a few. Sometimes a patient with very complex or chronic disorders needs to be more holistically treated.

David also loves history and philosophy. It doesn't matter from what era; he just wants to learn from the world's ancestors. A lot of ancients had fascinating things to say, that are as relevant today as they were hundreds or thousands of years ago. This is what David is inspired by and what drives him to be the best person he can be, for himself, his family and for everyone around him.

Aside from Chinese medicine, David spends his leisure time in Brisbane, Australia, with his three amazing daughters and his incredible wife. They are his inspiration and his absolute love.

Index